Praise for Other Books by Nicholas J. Gonzalez, MD

The Trophoblast and the Origins of Cancer
"Everyone interested in cancer, of how medical research should work, should read this book."

—J.P. Jones, PhD, retired vice president of research and
development, the Procter & Gamble Company

What Went Wrong: The Truth behind the Clinical Trial of the Enzyme Treatment of Cancer
"This tragic tale tends to support a growing suspicion that the cancer cartel of organizations, government agencies, and vested interests is devoted more to preserving their enormous profits and reputations than to the prevention and cure of cancer."

—Paul J. Rosch, MD, president, the American Institute of Stress; clinical
professor of medicine and psychiatry, New York Medical College

**Conquering Cancer: Volume One—50 Pancreatic and Breast
Cancer Patients on The Gonzalez Nutritional Protocol**
"Conventional cancer treatment overpromises and under delivers—science, clinicians, and patients are confirming this grave reality. For twenty-seven years, Dr. Nicholas Gonzalez rigorously applied a nutrition-based protocol in the care of terminal cancers and degenerative diseases. Within these pages are the astounding, unparalleled, and paradigm-shifting records of patients whose lives were not only prolonged, but vitalized by this elegant work."

—Kelly Brogan, MD, author of the *New York
Times* bestseller *A Mind of Your Own*

For more information,
visit The Nicholas Gonzalez Foundation website at
www.dr-gonzalez.com.

NUTRITION AND THE AUTONOMIC NERVOUS SYSTEM

NUTRITION AND THE AUTONOMIC NERVOUS SYSTEM:

The Scientific Foundations of The Gonzalez Protocol

Nicholas J. Gonzalez, MD

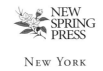

NEW SPRING PRESS

NEW YORK

NOTICE

This book is intended for general informational purposes only, not as a medical manual. The materials presented in no way are meant to be a substitute for professional medical care or attention by a qualified practitioner, nor should they be construed as such. Always check with your doctor if you have any questions or concerns about your condition or before starting or modifying a program of treatment. New Spring Press LLC and the author(s) are not responsible or liable, directly or indirectly, for any form of damages whatsoever resulting from the use (or misuse) of information contained in or implied by this book.

Cover photograph © roxxephotography.com. Used with permission.
Book design by Debra Tremper, Six Penny Graphics

Publisher's Cataloging-in-Publication
(Provided by Quality Books, Inc.)

Gonzalez, Nicholas J., 1947-2015, author.
    Nutrition and the autonomic nervous system : the scientific foundations of the Gonzalez protocol / Nicholas J. Gonzalez.
        pages cm
        Includes bibliographical references.
        ISBN 978-0-9985460-0-1
        ISBN 978-0-9985460-1-8

    1. Autonomic nervous system--Diseases--Nutritional aspects. 2. Autonomic nervous system--Diseases--Diet therapy. 3. Autonomic nervous system--Physiology. I. Title.

RC407.G66 2017   616.85'690654
                                    QBI17-900009

Contents

Foreword

The author of this book, Dr. Nicholas Gonzalez, and I were professional colleagues for more than 25 years. During our long working relationship, I was always one of the first to read Nick's drafts, after he had done numerous rewrites himself. Reading this manuscript brought back memories of the first time I reviewed it, many years ago. Nick had not completed this work; he started it in the early 2000s, but put it aside as other issues took priority.

Nick and I met when I was in medical school; he was the intern and I was the third-year medical student on an internal medicine team at Vanderbilt University Medical Center. He was already engaged in his study of the work of William Donald Kelley, DDS, the brilliant and eccentric orthodontist who had developed a nutritional method for treating cancer and other illnesses, using individualized protocols involving diet, nutritional supplements and detoxification routines. Dr. Kelley believed that regulation of the autonomic nervous system explained how his methods worked.

The autonomic nervous system is in charge of the functions of our bodies that we do not consciously direct, such as digestion or heart rate. The autonomic system has two parts, the sympathetic and parasympathetic nervous systems, with different and frequently opposing actions. The sympathetic nervous system, the "fight-flight-freeze" system, is in charge of the stress response; among other activities, it raises heart rate and blood pressure, and slows digestion so that the body's resources can go towards dealing with immediate threats. The parasympathetic system is in charge of the "rest-digest" functions; it stimulates the digestive tract and all its accessory organs such as the pancreas, but slows the heart and drops the blood pressure. In normal physiology, these two systems take turns depending on the need of the hour, the sympathetic system being active in times of stress and the parasympathetic system being dominant when repair is needed.

All this is well known to any first or second year medical student, but by the time most of us graduate and move on to our clinical work, the functions of the autonomic nervous system are not considered on a day-to-day basis. But in Dr. Kelley's work, and subsequently in Nick's practice and my own, the autonomic nervous system is the core of the recommendations we make. As described in this book, Dr. Kelley empirically found that some patients did well on an alkalinizing, plant-based diet, with supplementation of magnesium and potassium, while other patients prospered on an acid-forming diet, high in protein and fat, with calcium supplementation. He then found in the work of Francis Pottenger, Sr, MD, the theoretical explanation for why this could be so.

Dr. Pottenger, in his book *Symptoms of Visceral Disease*, described how disease could be caused by autonomic imbalance.[1] Dr. Pottenger theorized that in some individuals, either the sympathetic or parasympathetic system was overly active, bringing about disease states that could be ameliorated if the overactive system was toned down. He found that the administration of magnesium would suppress the sympathetic system, potassium stimulated the parasympathetic system, and calcium stimulated the sympathetic system. Dr. Kelley, recognizing the same pattern that he himself had noted, realized that Dr. Pottenger's findings about autonomic physiology explained his own clinical observations. Dr. Kelley then synthesized all of this into the treatment program he utilized, stipulating that based on the balance between the activity of the two halves of the autonomic nervous system, different types of people might have different dietary needs, respond differently to nutritional supplements, and even have different "normal" parameters for various blood tests.

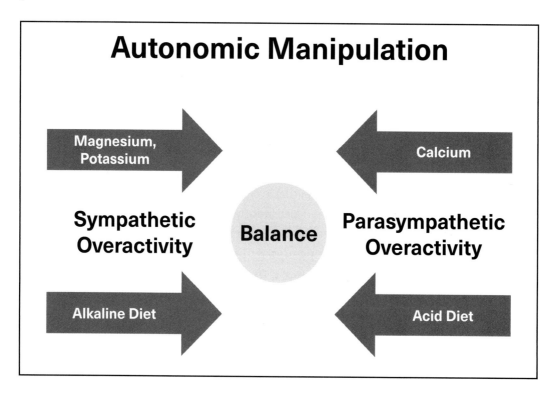

1   Pottenger, F.M., *Symptoms of Visceral Disease*. 1944, St. Louis, MO: C.V. Mosby Company.

At the time Nick met Dr. Kelley, in 1981, Kelley had already put these premises together. During the next six years, as Nick reviewed Dr. Kelley's charts for the research project that would eventually be published as the book One Man Alone,[2] Nick was filled with questions for Dr. Kelley about how this theoretical model of autonomic balance worked in practice. Not only did he have questions about Kelley's patient files, he also asked about patients he was seeing in his orthodox medical training—for during this same time period, Nick completed his third and fourth year of medical school, his medical internship, and an immunology fellowship.

Early in our relationship, Nick told me that one of the best things about these principles of autonomic imbalance was that it helped make sense out of many of the bits and pieces that would float past in the medical and nutritional literature. As an example, researchers have found that breast cancer patients who were prescribed beta-blockers (for reasons other than breast cancer, such as hypertension or heart disease) do better than patients who were not prescribed this medication.[3] In Kelley's model, breast cancer patients have an overactive sympathetic nervous system, and beta-blockers specifically block the beta-adrenergic receptor of the sympathetic nervous system, helping bring these patients' metabolisms closer to balance.

In another study, administration of calcium supplements slightly raised the risk of heart attacks.[4] Later analyses, pooling the results of many studies, suggested that there was no such increased risk.[5] Calcium, as a stimulator of the sympathetic nervous system, could well be an instigator of heart attacks if given in large doses to patients whose sympathetic nervous systems are already too active. In the Kelley model, patients with overactive parasympathetic nervous systems need and thrive on high doses of calcium supplements, while patients with overactive sympathetic systems need very little. The patients in the study showing increased risk might well have been made up mostly of those with overactive sympathetic systems. Larger analyses, pooling data from many studies with patients of a variety of metabolic types, would show no risk.

In contrast to Kelley, Nick and myself, others in the integrative nutritional world state that everyone should be on the same diet, which might be anywhere from vegan to low-carb—usually the diet that the prescribing practitioners feel best eating for themselves. With our methods, I will find myself recommending for some patients a diet with less animal protein than works for me, and for others a diet with much much more. Two of my patients, who were included in our article in *Alternative Therapies in*

---

2   Gonzalez, N.J., *One Man Alone; An Investigation of Nutrition, Cancer, and William Donald Kelley.* 2010, New York, NY: New Spring Press.

3   Barron, T.I., L. Sharp, and K. Visvanathan, *Beta-adrenergic blocking drugs in breast cancer: a perspective review.* Ther Adv Med Oncol 2012. **4**(3): p. 113–125.

4   Xiao, Q., et al., *Dietary and supplemental calcium intake and cardiovascular disease mortality: the National Institutes of Health-AARP diet and health study.* JAMA Intern Med, 2013. **173**(8): p. 639–46.

5   Waldman, T., et al., *Calcium Supplements and Cardiovascular Disease: A Review.* Am J Lifestyle Med, 2015. **9**(4): p. 298–307.

Health and Medicine,[6] illustrate this point; one, with pancreatic cancer, was told to eat a near-vegetarian diet, the other, with lymphoma, was told to eat large amounts of animal protein. Both patients are alive and well today, nearly ten years since the publication of this article. Each continues to eat the prescribed diet with relish. The vast majority of the time, patients feel well with the recommendations we give.

However, in some cases, patients will modify things not because they feel unwell, but because they have read something that contradicts our advice. As an example, a few months after Nick's death, I saw one of his patients, a parasympathetic dominant patient with a low-grade lymphoma of the skin. His disease had improved at first, but then stabilized with a small patch of disease remaining. As most clinicians know, with a change of physicians sometimes new information comes forward. I routinely ask whether patients are having any trouble tolerating their supplements. He said no, rather tentatively, and paused; then he said, "Well, I'm not actually taking the calcium supplements that Dr. Gonzalez told me to take. I read that calcium needs to be balanced with magnesium, so I've been taking a product with extra magnesium." The extra magnesium was making his system too alkaline and suppressing his weak sympathetic system, keeping his parasympathetic system relatively overactive and preventing the protocol from bringing his system into balance. The advice he found about balancing calcium with magnesium is valid for people with other metabolic types, but not for him. From my point of view, his modification of his protocol was preventing progress against his disease.

Another example involves a patient whose sympathetic system was overactive; such patients are accustomed to having the quick responses of a metabolism that is on red alert all day long, ready to react and react quickly. Sympathetic dominants are usually very busy people, rushing through their day checking things off their to-do list. Their nervous system is accustomed to this frenetic activity, and when they begin a treatment protocol that is designed to tone down the sympathetic system, they may feel somewhat lethargic, contemplative for the first time in years, possibly depressed as they sense some unpleasant realities in their lives that were previously ignored in a sea of busyness. If they relax and allow their nervous systems to readjust, they can learn to appreciate this state and even find that they become more effective—they listen to others more carefully, they plan more thoughtfully, and they spend less energy pointlessly.

But some patients resist this process. A long-time patient of Nick's illustrates this principle. She would call periodically, reporting mild lack of energy. He would remind her of the goal of toning down her sympathetic nervous system. She would then start reading the nutritional literature or going to other practitioners, looking for a solution for her low energy, and start some herb or supplement that would make her feel better by stimulating her sympathetic system. A few months later, she would call Nick because

6   Gonzalez, N.J. and L.L. Isaacs, *The Gonzalez therapy and cancer: a collection of case reports.* Altern Ther Health Med 2007. **13**(1): p. 46–55.

of a worsening in her medical condition. He would then find out what she had started this time, explain why it was counterproductive, and tell her to stop it; her condition would then improve, until the next time she decided it was time to find out why she did not have the energy to complete her extensive to-do list. This cycle repeated for years.

Another, sadder story involves a patient of mine, who also had an overactive sympathetic system along with a metastatic carcinoma in his abdomen that he and I could feel on exam. After receiving his protocol from me, he had not followed it completely and his disease was dramatically worse when he returned for his six-month checkup, with a mass in his abdomen the size of a cantaloupe. I pointed out that he would never know if it would work for him if he did not follow through 100%; he then called a few months later to report that he had taken my words to heart and that his tumor had markedly reduced in size. When I spoke with him a few months later, he had continued to improve, but he did report some low grade fatigue and depression. I explained that the diet and supplements were designed to tone down the sympathetic system and that this could create these symptoms. I counseled him to be patient.

About six months later, he called and asked, "Do the enzymes ever stop working?" His cancer had resurged with a vengeance; the mass had regrown and he had developed fluid in his abdomen, putting pressure on his stomach and making adherence to his protocol challenging. On further questioning, I learned that a few months earlier he had visited his family physician and reported his symptoms of fatigue and mild depression. His physician then prescribed Adderall, a potent sympathetic stimulant, and the patient opted to proceed without checking with me. On this medication, not surprisingly his fatigue and depression resolved—and his disease exploded.

Balanced patients, those whose sympathetic and parasympathetic systems are equally or nearly equally active, need only to have this balance maintained with their nutritional supplements. The diets for balanced patients have a great deal of flexibility; such patients will at times crave red meat and other acid-forming foods, and at other times desire only salads, citrus and other more alkalinizing foods. I saw one such patient recently, a long-term patient of Nick's who is a health professional; she reported that she did indeed have shifts in her food preferences, with days of eating meat followed by days of eating leafy greens.

She then told me enthusiastically about a meditation program that she had begun. I started to feel a little nervous as she spoke. Some forms of meditation have been shown to stimulate the parasympathetic nervous system,[7] which could cause a balanced patient to shift into parasympathetic dominance. Dr. Kelley once told me that meditation was bad for people with an overactive parasympathetic system, and that such patients

---

7   Amihai, I. and M. Kozhevnikov, *Arousal vs. relaxation: a comparison of the neurophysiological and cognitive correlates of Vajrayana and Theravada meditative practices.* PLoS One, 2014. **9**(7): p. e102990.

should instead consider watching action movies or playing video games to stimulate the underactive sympathetic system.

As I started to express my reservations, she said, "Oh, I don't meditate every day. There are some days that it just doesn't seem like the right thing to do." I then told her that it would be interesting to see if her preferences about meditation correlated with her food choices, and asked her to keep track of that going forward. She said, "I can already answer that. The days I want to meditate, I don't want red meat. The days that meditation doesn't feel right, I want to eat a steak." After many years on her protocol, she was able to recognize how her metabolism was functioning on any given day, and adjust both her diet and her activities to bring her system into balance, almost instinctively. On days when her sympathetic system was a trifle overactive, she would meditate and eat more lightly; on days when her parasympathetic system was overactive, she would eat more animal protein and skip the meditation.

The principles detailed in this book, when used correctly, can be a powerful tool to improve health and well-being. As with any kind of medical knowledge, these principles are best learned in an apprenticeship or internship setting, such as Nick had with Dr. Kelley, and as I had with Nick. The prevailing mindset of the medical world, whether using pharmaceuticals, diet or nutritional supplements, is biased towards a "one size fits all" model that takes some time and training to unlearn.

Drs. Pottenger, Gellhorn and Kelley used their observational skills and clinical acumen to create medical theories that deserve wider recognition than they have received. I hope that the publication of this book will help speed the day when their work becomes part of standard medical treatment.

Linda L. Isaacs, MD

Acknowledgments

While several people were involved in the actual development and publication of this book, the person who deserves the highest acknowledgment is Dr. Nick Gonzalez himself. Despite his long days treating patients in his private practice, Nick was driven to write about his scientific theories and spent nights and weekends documenting his conclusions. Thankfully, we now have the benefit of his teachings to share and help heal the world.

I'd also like to thank the following people for their contributions to this book and their continued support of Nick's legacy:

- Colin A. Ross, MD, our medical editor and advisor
- Linda L. Isaacs, MD, for contributing our foreword and providing her expertise and guidance
- The board members of The Nicholas Gonzalez Foundation, for their devotion to our mission of preserving and promoting Dr. Gonzalez's legacy. To learn more, visit www.thegonzalezprotocol.com.
- Author Bridge Media, for the expert editing and publishing guidance
- Six Penny Graphics, for our formatting and cover art
- Nick's patients, who continue to inspire us with their dedication to continuing their treatment and preserving Nick's legacy

Mary Beth Gonzalez

Introduction

When I first read the manuscript of this book, it was an inspiring and revolutionary experience for me as a psychiatrist. Dr. Gonzalez has opened the door to a whole new way of thinking about mental disorders. He did so by his usual method, evident in his series of books about John Beard, Donald Kelley, the trophoblast model of cancer, and the treatment of cancer with pancreatic enzymes. In this book, Dr. Gonzalez provides a thorough, scholarly, evidence-based review of the autonomic nervous system, including how it functions and how it is regulated. His understanding of the autonomic nervous system is a core component of his model for the treatment of cancer.

All doctors have been taught about the autonomic nervous system and its two major divisions, the sympathetic nervous system and the parasympathetic nervous system. This book provides a great deal of historical information I had never been taught and likewise a great deal of detail about how the system works, all based on hundreds of scientific experiments, peer-reviewed papers, and textbooks.

Before reading this book, I knew that mammals under threat can respond with fight, flight, or freeze. I knew that fight-flight involves activation of the sympathetic nervous system, increased adrenaline, hyperalertness, the shunting of blood away from digestion and sexual activity toward the muscles, pupil dilation (to scan for danger more effectively), and increased aggression. I knew that freeze and submission involve the opposite: activation of the parasympathetic nervous system, reduction in pulse and blood pressure, the shunting of blood away from the muscles, and so on. This is a thoroughly proven picture of the autonomic nervous system.

Reading the manuscript, I learned a lot more, much of it directly relevant to my work as a psychiatrist specializing in the effects of psychological trauma. When I wrote a paper about Dr. Gonzalez's trophoblast model of cancer, I went to a lot of trouble to formulate every component of the model in a fashion that can be scientifically tested, and I outlined how that could be done.[1] In this book, Dr. Gonzalez offers the same thing: a model of the autonomic nervous system and its relevance to cancer, psychiatry,

---

1   Colin A. Ross, "The Trophoblast Model of Cancer," *Nutrition and Cancer* 67: 61–67.

and many branches of medicine that is highly specified and scientifically testable. This is not "alternative" or "complementary" medicine. It is mainstream scientific medicine with animal models, basic science neurophysiology, human data, and novel testable scientific predictions.

To summarize briefly:

The story begins with Pavlov's dog experiments. Pavlov received a Nobel Prize in Medicine and Physiology in 1904. He is best known for his experiments in which he conditioned dogs to salivate at the sound of a bell, by ringing a bell at the same time that he offered them food. He induced a conditioned reflex: the bell was the conditioned stimulus, and salivation was the conditioned response. But Pavlov did much more than this.

One of Pavlov's experiments was to condition dogs by ringing a bell at the same time that they jumped up on a table to get food. After enough conditioning trials, they would jump up on the table when a bell was rung, even when there was no food on the table. In the next experimental step, Pavlov began to give the dogs an electric shock when they jumped up on the table. There were many variations on this experiment, and there have been many since, conducted by others.

Basically, an animal is trained to respond to a conditioned stimulus with a conditioned response. Then, in a second step, the conditioned stimulus is paired with a noxious stimulus such as an electric shock. In some experiments, the shock is inescapable or inconsistent and can't be controlled. Pavlov observed that not all dogs responded in the same way when the ringing of the bell was followed by an electric shock. He divided the animals into four groups; groups II and III can be collapsed together.

The Group I dogs responded by becoming agitated, angry, and aggressive. When the handlers came to get them from their kennels to take them to the experimental room, they would attack, bite, and go into fight mode. Their behavior would escalate further in the experimental room, and they would not settle down back in their kennels. These dogs went into sympathetic overdrive.

The Group IV dogs responded very differently. They became passive, frightened, and withdrawn in their kennels, and more so when taken to the experimental room. Pushed to the extreme, Group IV animals might go to sleep, freeze, salivate excessively, or urinate or defecate on themselves. They did not return to normal baseline back in their kennels.

Group II dogs, in contrast, remained well adjusted in their kennels, before and after the experiments. They did not like the shock experiments, but they could shake off the effects once the experiments were over. Pavlov described these groups of dogs in detail and at length.

The next step in the story is Dr. Funkenstein, a Harvard doctor whom Dr. Gonzalez met in 1969. Dr. Funkenstein published dozens of papers in professional journals describing his experiments at Harvard. He repeated and extended Pavlov's observations.

He divided his experimental animals into three genetically determined groups. Most animals, he said, had a balanced autonomic nervous system (Group II), while a smaller percentage was either sympathetic dominant (Group I) or parasympathetic dominant (Group III). These three groups responded to conditioning trials in the same way that Pavlov's dogs did.

Funkenstein went on to develop an array of different experimental challenges. One was the mecholyl test. Mecholyl is still available on the market and is an antihypertensive that can be used to treat high blood pressure. Funkenstein observed that when he gave mecholyl to Group I dogs, their blood pressure went down a bit, returned to baseline in three to five minutes, and then became slightly elevated. With Group II dogs, the blood pressure went down more, and then returned to baseline in five to eight minutes and did not go above baseline. With the Group III dogs, the blood pressure dropped drastically and did not return to baseline after fifteen or more minutes.

The mecholyl causes the peripheral arterioles to dilate, which then stimulates, via baroreceptors, a sympathetic counterresponse to bring blood pressure back to normal. The Group I dogs overresponded due to their sympathetic dominance, the Group II dogs had a balanced response, and the Group III dogs could not mount a sufficient sympathetic counterresponse to get back to baseline. After conducting mecholyl challenges on hundreds of normal volunteers, Funkenstein found that 80 to 90 percent of human beings are autonomic balanced, while 10 to 20 percent are either sympathetic or parasympathetic dominant.

Now the psychiatry part:

Based on mecholyl challenges with psychiatric patients, Funkenstein found that only 30 to 50 percent are autonomic balanced. The rest are either sympathetic or parasympathetic dominant. There are measurement and methodological details about all of this, all discussed at length in the peer-reviewed literature; here, I am giving a summary.

Funkenstein found, not surprisingly, that Group I people tend to be hostile, angry, and aggressive, and these qualities increase under experimental stress. He called this "anger out." Group III people tend to be passive and melancholic, and these qualities increase under experimental stress. He called this "anger in." These categories correspond to what are currently called externalizing disorders and internalizing disorders in psychiatry.

Funkenstein then went on to study responses to treatment in Group I and III psychiatric patients. He observed that when given electroconvulsive therapy (ECT), Group I patients got worse while Group III patients improved. He reasoned that this was because ECT activates an already overactivated sympathetic nervous system in Group I patients but counteracts an overactivated parasympathetic nervous system in Group III patients.

Conversely, Funkenstein found that when given the tranquilizer chlorpromazine, Group I patients improved while Group III got worse. The chlorpromazine oversedated the already endogenously "sedated" parasympathetic-dominant group but helpfully down-regulated the sympathetic-dominant group. Here we have the foundation of a system for predicting medication response based not on genetic analysis, as in pharmacogenetics, but on autonomic nervous system balance, which is a genetically determined trait with a bell-shaped distribution in the general population. This distribution of autonomic types is a prediction of the Pavlov-Funkenstein-Gellhorn-Gonzalez model: it is a scientifically testable hypothesis that can be validated, modified, or refuted by experiment.

In addition, Funkenstein stated that Group I individuals respond better to psychotherapy than Group III individuals do. Again, this prediction needs to be empirically investigated, but it is consistent with a truly biopsychosocial psychiatry. What we have here is a simple, inexpensive, nontoxic biological challenge that can be administered in an office and can potentially predict responses to both medication and psychotherapy. If valid, and adopted, the model could place psychiatry squarely within mainstream, scientific, biological medicine.

The next person in the story is Ernst Gellhorn, who was born in Breslau, Germany, in 1893. Gellhorn obtained his MD from the University of Heidelberg and immigrated to the United States in 1929. He was a professor of physiology at the University of Minnesota from 1943 to 1960. There, he studied the hypothalamus and published hundreds of papers, plus a series of books, about his work.

Gellhorn made original contributions to our understanding of the autonomic nervous system. He showed that the control center for the sympathetic nervous system is in the posterior hypothalamus, while the control system for the parasympathetic nervous system is in the anterior hypothalamus, and he demonstrated that these two centers feed back to each other via nerve tracts in the hypothalamus. He described "the law of reciprocity," according to which anything that up-regulates the sympathetic nervous system down-regulates the parasympathetic nervous system, and vice versa.

Gellhorn made a number of technical innovations, including using tiny cannulae to study the hypothalamus in experimental animals. He demonstrated a whole series of facts about how the autonomic nervous system is regulated in his elegant, replicated experiments. For example, he showed that introducing Pentothal to the anterior hypothalamus turned off the parasympathetic arm of the system, resulting in sympathetic dominance and increased heart rate and blood pressure. This was accompanied by hostile, aggressive behavior. Conversely, turning off the posterior hypothalamus resulted in the opposite effect: parasympathetic dominance, slowed heart rate, reduced blood pressure, and docile behavior or even sleep. Gellhorn also demonstrated that if he stimulated or activated either the posterior or the anterior hypothalamus, he got the opposite effects of those observed with Pentothal.

This is interesting, but his subsequent experiments were even more remarkable. Gellhorn introduced strychnine to the cerebral cortex, which increased activity in the cortex and subsequently increased activity in the posterior hypothalamus. In other words, he demonstrated that the cortex regulates the hypothalamus and the balance of the autonomic nervous system. When he infused Pentothal into the cortex, he observed the opposite effect, with the animals becoming somnolent rather than activated. I'm leaving out some of the experimental details discussed by Dr. Gonzalez in the later pages of this book.

Gellhorn also challenged animals with either norepinephrine or mecholyl and found that they belonged to the same three groups described by Funkenstein. If he tranquilized the posterior hypothalamus beforehand, he found that mecholyl had no effect (because the counterresponse of sympathetic activation was blocked). If he tranquilized the anterior hypothalamus, he found that norepinephrine had no effect (because the counterresponse of parasympathetic activation was blocked). All of this fits exactly with what he knew about the regulation of the autonomic nervous system.

In addition, Gellhorn did a series of experiments demonstrating that the musculature and peripheral nervous system feed back on and regulate the hypothalamus and thereby the balance in the autonomic nervous system. These experiments are described by Dr. Gonzalez.

Overall, Gellhorn demonstrated that the hypothalamus is regulated bottom up from the periphery, top down from the cortex, and internally by the law of reciprocity. All of this regulatory traffic, he showed, is bidirectional: the hypothalamus also regulates the cortex and the periphery. Gellhorn also replicated Funkenstein's work on the three autonomic groups in normal controls and psychiatric patients. He showed that chlorpromazine down-regulates the posterior hypothalamus while amphetamines up-regulate it.

Building on this, Dr. Gonzalez proposed that, because serotonin is involved in regulation of the anterior hypothalamus, selective serotonin reuptake inhibitors (SSRIs) will up-regulate the parasympathetic nervous system and therefore have a good effect in individuals who are sympathetic dominant. Inversely, SSRIs will cause symptom exacerbation in parasympathetic-dominant individuals because they will drive them further into parasympathetic dominance.

Alternatively, however, noradrenergic antidepressants, such as some of the tricyclics, will activate the posterior hypothalamus and therefore have a desirable effect for individuals who are parasympathetic dominant, but will be toxic for individuals who are sympathetic dominant. All of these predictions may or may not be accurate, but they are testable scientific hypotheses of potential clinical importance. They are grounded in neurophysiology, animal models, human experimentation, and what we know about how the autonomic nervous system is regulated.

This model of balanced, sympathetic-dominant, and parasympathetic-dominant individuals is a core element of Dr. Gonzalez's treatment for cancer. He predicted, and observed in his practice, that sympathetic-dominant individuals are more prone to solid tumors, while parasympathetic-dominant individuals are more prone to leukemia and lymphomas. Dr. Gonzalez's prediction about tumor type and autonomic dominance, although not supported by any research data at present, is also a scientifically testable hypothesis. His nutritional support for his patients is based in great detail on his analysis of autonomic balance. Dr. Gonzalez described some of this in a posthumously published paper[2] and went into it in detail in the present volume.

The dietary protocol developed by Dr. Kelley was empirically derived. It was based on trial and error in Dr. Kelley's clinical practice. Once the ten Kelley diets were established, one could infer the supplements and minerals that needed to be added to the diets from the known minerals and vitamins in the types of food prescribed. The diets, supplements, and autonomic types then became part of an integrated nutritional model that also predicts tumor type (solid versus immune cancers) and the risk for developing cancer. Of course, no single model can account for everything, or predict everything, nor does any cancer treatment model have a 100 percent success rate.

The purpose of this book is twofold: 1) to demonstrate that Dr. Gonzalez read widely and thought carefully about the autonomic nervous system and 2) to demonstrate that his theory of nutritional types is grounded in science. His writing about both topics is scholarly, medical, and scientific, at a level well beyond that of the average clinician. The present volume provides the foundation for a training manual for The Gonzalez Protocol. In editing this volume for publication, I corrected minor typos and added the tables in chapter 6; otherwise, everything is as Dr. Gonzalez wrote it. As stated in the notice for this book, however, the present volume is not a treatment manual and does not include enough information for readers to use The Gonzalez Protocol in clinical practice. An adequate training course is in development, and this book will be part of the required reading for it.

With publication of this book, no critic can now claim that there is "no scientific evidence" for Dr. Gonzalez's model of sympathetic-parasympathetic balance or his model of nutritional types. His model is based on a body of replicated scientific data derived from many different types of experiments, conducted in multiple species, and published by authors with appointments at leading universities.

Colin A. Ross, MD

---

2   Nicholas J. Gonzalez, "A Case of Insulin-Dependent Diabetes," *Alternative Therapies in Health and Medicine* 20, no. 4 (2016): 63–85.

NUTRITION AND THE AUTONOMIC NERVOUS SYSTEM

Part I:
A History Lesson

by Nicholas J. Gonzalez, MD

CHAPTER I:

Dr. Beard and the Placenta

The roots of my work with cancer and other degenerative diseases go back to the early years of the twentieth century and the brilliant Scottish biologist John Beard. Beard, who taught at the University of Edinburgh until his death in 1923, was not a physician but a research biologist who spent much of his life studying embryonic development in mammals, including humans. Beard made numerous important discoveries regarding fetal growth, many that are still quoted in the mainstream scientific literature.

Beard's main area of interest, which occupied the better part of his professional life, was the placenta. The development of the mammalian fetus differs from that of reptiles, birds, amphibians, and all other complex life forms because its growth occurs inside the mother's uterus, not outside in an egg. It is the placenta, the anchor attaching the developing fetus to the mother's uterus, that allows for such internal survival. Here, the blood supply of the mother, carrying nutrients and oxygen, connects with the blood supply of the embryo, saturated with the end products of metabolism such as carbon dioxide. Here, the fetal blood can absorb needed nutrition in a perfectly predigested form and transfer its wastes to the mother for disposal. Without the placenta, in utero development of mammals would be impossible.

The placenta is complex in structure, shaped at full term like a disk, perhaps two inches thick and ten inches in diameter and weighing about five hundred grams (about a pound). Its formation begins within days of conception, after the primitive fetus—called at this point a blastocyst—makes its way into the uterine cavity. At that point, the growing blastocyst consists of several dozen indistinct ameboid-like cells shaped into a microscopic ball. As the blastocyst grows, a single and distinctive layer of cells called the trophoblast forms on its surface, reacting to signals from the lining of the uterine cavity. These trophoblastic cells ultimately grow into the life-sustaining placenta. I like to think of the trophoblast layer as a microscopic capsule, or cellular shell, surrounding the central blastocyst. As these trophoblasts take form, they begin secreting a collection of powerful enzymes that enable the embryo to invade the uterus and quickly establish a firm foothold.

Beard was especially fascinated by the microscopic appearance of early placental cells, this trophoblastic layer of tissue that so effectively attaches to the uterine wall. Early in his studies, Beard made a simple but extraordinary observation, noting that these trophoblast cells resembled, in their microscopic appearance, cancer cells. Although by today's standards we may look back at the nineteenth and early twentieth century as primitive times in terms of modern molecular biology, the development of microscopy during the nineteenth century had already opened the way for a generation of pathologists to catalogue the differences between normal and cancer cells. Scientists such as Beard knew what cancer cells looked like.

In their form and structure, malignant cells differ from those of normal tissues primarily by a lessening of what scientists call differentiation. All cells of all tissues in all organisms have a distinctive appearance that is unmistakable, unique for the tissue of origin, reflecting the particular function of that cell. It is this quality of uniqueness, of specificity, that defines differentiation. The cells lining the small intestine look like, and only like, cells lining the small intestine; nerve cells look like nerve cells; pancreas cells look like pancreas cells; muscle cells look like muscle cells. Even cell types within an organ can vary greatly, depending on their specific function. For example, the pancreatic cells that secrete insulin appear far different from their neighbors in the pancreas that secrete the digestive enzymes such as trypsin.

Cancer cells lose this specificity, this differentiation. They may resemble cells from the tissue in which they develop, but as the cancer cells become more aggressive, the similarity becomes less pronounced. In fact, pathologists define certain aggressive tumor cells as "poorly differentiated," meaning they appear so primitive and indistinct that an experienced microscopist, unless aware of the patient's history, often cannot identify the tissue of origin.

Placental cells not only look like cancer cells under the microscope, Beard realized, but even more significantly, the trophoblastic cells behave like cancer cells. Even during Beard's time, cancer biologists had identified the behavioral characteristics of cancer cells that distinguished them from those of normal tissues. First, cancer cells can invade; they produce a host of enzymes enabling them to break down tissue barriers efficiently and spread through normal tissue with deadly efficacy. Second, cancer cells and malignant tissues develop their own blood supply, through the process known as angiogenesis, allowing the tumor to grow effectively wherever it chooses to grow. And third, cancer cells and tumors, unlike normal tissues and organs, grow without restraint or inhibition; normal tissues grow as needed and when needed but only as appropriate.

For example, the lining of the large intestine is sloughed off every five days or so and is completely replaced from precursor cells in the intestinal lining. If a surgeon removes a kidney, the remaining kidney can double in size and actually increase its function to compensate for the loss. If a portion of the liver, in fact up to 80 percent, is surgically excised, the remaining liver cells start reproducing until the missing liver completely regenerates. But the growth stops, usually on signal, just at the right time. Cancer cells, however, grow without restriction and without regard for boundaries, until the tumor jeopardizes the life of the host organism.

Indeed, as Beard discovered, trophoblastic cells do effectively invade the uterus, just as a tumor might. The placenta, just like a tumor, early on begins generating its own complex blood supply, allowing for its rapid growth and continued invasion of the maternal uterus. However, while early on the placenta aggressively invades the uterus and proliferates wildly, in most cases at some point the invasion slows, and the growth comes to a halt. I say in most cases because even a hundred years ago physicians knew that occasionally the placenta, just like a tumor, does not stop growing as it should and instead becomes a very aggressive cancer called choriocarcinoma. Choriocarcinoma is a cancer of uncontrolled placental growth that in Beard's day would kill usually within months. Today, this particular malignancy can be controlled quite effectively with chemotherapy and represents one of the few successes in the drug war against cancer.

Beard knew that during its development, at some critical point, the placenta changed in character from an aggressive, invading, angiogenic, proliferating tissue to a docile, tame, and stable organ. In his research, Beard uncovered a fundamental truth about the nature of trophoblastic growth: in every species of mammal that he studied, he learned that the placenta stops growing at a very specific point in embryological development that is quite unique for each species. In the human, he proposed, the placenta changes from its aggressive to noninvasive form on day fifty-six after conception. Today, a hundred years later, this milestone in fetal-placental development first identified by Beard has been confirmed.

Beard correctly, as it turned out, realized that something important happened on day fifty-six that turned the tumor-like trophoblastic tissue into the mature placenta. And he then made a leap of faith: he assumed that if he could understand the switch that guided this remarkable transformation, he would have the answer to cancer.

Beard devoted years of his life struggling to unravel the process that turned the cancer-like and potentially deadly trophoblast into a life-sustaining organ. He realized the signal could be coming from the mother or from the fetus, and he systematically analyzed, at least with the scientific tools available to him at that time, the various possibilities. He investigated the development of the fetal nervous system and the endocrine system of both the embryo and the mother (at least the endocrine system as understood at that time). He thought about blood supply and immune function. The pathologist Virchow had already uncovered the underlying concepts of modern immunology, and Beard probably had some knowledge of Virchow's pioneering work.

But nothing made sense in Beard's mind until he considered the embryonic pancreas. The pancreas sits in the back of the upper abdominal cavity, behind the stomach in what anatomists call the retroperitoneal space. It is a complex piece of metabolic machinery, actually two organs in one, consisting of both endocrine and exocrine tissues. Endocrine cells secrete hormones into the blood system that act on distant tissues; in this case, the islet cells of the pancreas secrete glucagon and insulin, used to regulate blood sugar levels.

The exocrine pancreas, the bulk of the pancreas, manufactures the various digestive enzymes, which it releases into the small intestine during and after a meal. Scientists identify three main classes of pancreatic enzymes: the proteolytic class, consisting of trypsin and chymotrypsin among others, which digest proteins; the lipases, which break down fats; and the amylases, which cleave starches into simple sugars. Even in Beard's day, the major classes of pancreatic enzymes, and their respective functions, were well known.

After his years of research and his many false starts, Beard came to a very pivotal conclusion. He believed that the very day the placenta stopped invading, stopped growing, and metamorphosed from an aggressive tumor-like tissue to the essential placenta was the very day the fetal pancreas became active. This is an astonishing phenomenon to have uncovered, when one considers the somewhat primitive tools that were available to Beard at that time. But the more he studied the problem of placental growth in animal models, the more convinced he was that some product from the fetal pancreas ultimately signaled the placenta to slow and eventually stop its growth. Based on his animal studies, Beard concluded that the primary signaling factor must be the proteolytic, protein-digesting enzymes—particularly trypsin.

Recent embryological research confirms that the fetal pancreas does begin manufacturing and secreting digestive enzymes very early in development. This is an interesting finding in itself, because the fetus receives all the nutrients required for growth in a perfectly predigested form from the blood supply of the mother and has no need for an activated pancreas or for pancreatic enzymes until it takes its first meal the day of its birth—nine months after conception. Yet the fetal pancreas does produce enzymes, and in a not insignificant amount, early in development, beginning approximately two months into a nine-month gestation.

Beard was the first to suspect, and document, that the fetal pancreas produced enzymes early in development. And he hypothesized that the fetus produced enzymes for one primary, essential reason: to slow placental growth, to keep the organ under control. And if the proteolytic pancreatic enzymes did this, Beard assumed that these same enzymes should be able to control cancer—because he increasingly believed that cancer was nothing more than placenta-like cells growing without the influence of adequate pancreatic enzymes.

Early in his research, Beard used analogies: trophoblastic cells behaved like cancer cells; the placenta was like a tumor. But as he came to master the intricacies of embryonic development, he began to believe that the connection between cancer and trophoblastic cells was even more direct, going to the very origin of cancer itself.

After a hundred years of study, scientists still debate the origin of cancer cells. Although in recent years the field has been changing rapidly, most researchers today believe that cancer cells arise because of mutations in the genetic material, which in turn cause mature differentiated cells performing their normal functions in an organ to become less differentiated, capable of invasion, able to stimulate angiogenesis (blood vessel formation), and distinguished by uncontrolled cell division and the ability to migrate to distant sites. Such a process requires that mature cells become less mature, less specialized, and less restrained.

When I studied pathology in medical school in 1980, my textbook of pathology, written by the famous Dr. Stanley L. Robbins, suggested that cancer cells might arise through quite a different mechanism, involving uncontrolled growth of stem cells. In recent years, stem cells have been the subject of intensive research around the world, with media reports on a regular basis extolling stem cells as the hope against all manner of serious illness, from cancer to Parkinson's disease. These small cells are also the cause of enormous controversy, with politicians dueling over the ethics of embryonic stem cell research.

In essence, stem cells are primitive, undifferentiated cells that form nests in every organ of the body. Upon proper signaling, they can start dividing and ultimately form the mature, functional tissues of an organ. They are absolutely necessary for life, serving as an essential source of new cells to replace those lost due to normal turnover and the usual wear and tear, as well as injury, aging, or disease. For example, as mentioned, every five days the lining of the large intestine sloughs off and needs to be replaced. Throughout the lining of the large intestine, microscopic indentations, known as crypts, harbor nests of these primitive stem cells, which continually migrate to the surface of the intestine.

As they move upward, these cells transform from their ameboid-like state with no distinctive appearance or functional ability, into the very specialized microscopic lining of the gut. Without these active cells, intestinal action—both digestion and absorption of nutrients—would quickly come to a halt. Fortunately, most of the time the replication and differentiation of these crypt stem cells proceeds smoothly and appropriately, with stem cell division, movement, and differentiation precisely regulated.

Stem cells are also needed for repair of damaged tissue, such as a liver that has been reduced by surgery or skin that must heal after a wound. Eighty percent of the human liver can be removed, and yet the stem cells ensconced within the remaining vital liver can rather quickly, within a period of several months, regenerate the missing tissue, down to the particular anatomic landmarks of the organ; a liver so regenerated seems normal to a T. If, say due to kidney cancer, one of our two must be surgically extracted, within a period of months the remaining kidney will most commonly double in size and take on the added job of its missing twin.

Wound healing cannot occur without epidermal stem cells. Though we take this process for granted, it is an obvious indication of the power of these cells. Even a small razor cut could never heal were it not for stem cells.

Over the past decade, we have learned a lot about these rather remarkable cells. For example, we know that a variety of signals—hormonal, neurological, and peptide, among others—stimulate stem cells into action. We know further that, whatever the organ, during the process of differentiation, as the primitive stem cells transform into mature, highly specialized adult cells as replacements for those lost due to whatever reason, they lose their power to migrate, to divide, to grow uncontrollably. Maturity brings, in some respects, quiescence, an inability to move or replicate.

Usually, the whole process of stem cell activation, replication, or maturation works wonderfully, such as along the gut lining, minute to minute, throughout the years of our lives. However, should stem cells be activated but the signals for differentiation go awry, they can remain primitive, retaining the ability to migrate, even to invade, to grow without restriction and spread to distant organs. So such cells, unless tightly regulated, can, many now believe, form deadly cancers.

More and more evidence indicates that cancer may actually arise in just this way, as the result of stem cells behaving badly, and not due to some process by which mature, highly differentiated normal cells turn ugly.

Beard may have been the first to recognize what we today call stem cells, though he didn't use that term. In one of his great achievements, he recognized that each tissue in every species he studied contained nests of primitive undifferentiated cells. In his writings, Beard argued convincingly that such cells exist in every tissue of every organ of every animal species. He further proposed that these primitive undifferentiated cells, which under the microscope resembled to him nothing other than the primitive trophoblastic cells, represented residual placental cells left over from early fetal development. Beard claimed these cells migrated from the primitive yolk sac of the developing mammalian fetus and ended up dispersed throughout the body. He wasn't sure why these placental cells were present, but he found them wherever he looked.

Beard claimed further that contrary to what researchers believed at that time—and what many still believe today—cancer tumors do not arise through some process of de-differentiation, whereby mature, specialized cells turn primitive, aggressive, and invasive, all the while replicating wildly. No, instead, he maintained, all tumors, whether originating in the brain or the skin of the foot, arose from these misplaced placental cells that had lost their normal restraints. In the final summation of his life's work, he said that this ultimate controlling signal, this factor that determined the behavior of these misplaced placental cells, was none other than the proteolytic enzymes such as trypsin. All cancer, he believed, not just the well-documented choriocarcinoma, developed from placental cells left over from our embryonic stage of being that normally would be kept under control by the circulating pancreatic enzymes. Should the pancreas, for whatever reason, fail to synthesize or release adequate amounts of the these "ferments," as Beard called enzymes, some of these residual trophoblastic cells hidden away in the nooks and crannies of our tissues could quickly grow out of control.

When Beard presented his theories in a series of lectures and papers during the period 1902–1915, his colleagues greeted his ideas largely with scorn, ridicule, and hostility. However, a number of physicians, both in Europe and in America, took Beard very seriously and, working with him, treated advanced cancer patients with injectable pancreatic enzyme preparations. A series of articles from the mainstream academic literature of the time documented tumor regression and even "cure" among patients treated according to Beard's precepts. Dr. Margaret Cleaves, a New York physician with an office on Madison Avenue, described one of the first cases of response to enzyme therapy in a letter published in the December 8, 1906 issue of *Medical Record* (70: 918). Dr. Cleaves wrote the following:

> Two illustrative cases will be briefly mentioned: one a postoperative (two operations), and now inoperable cancer of the tongue; only a stump left. . . . Treatment instituted in February, 1906. . . . The patient is now living in good physical condition and keeping appointments with her dentist to have teeth lost by ravages of the disease, replaced.
>
> The second illustrative case is one of postoperative and inoperable cancer of the rectum. . . . There were three operations, the last nine months since. At that time the mesenteric glands were found enlarged and indurated. Pain, which had persisted for two years necessitating the use of opiates, increased, and when the patient was first seen, six months since, the characteristics of progressive malignant disease were present. There were obstinate constipation, loss of appetite, strength and flesh, pain, discharge, odor, sense of weight, bearing down, and a sinking feeling in the pelvis, with inability to stand or walk save for a few moments only, and very short distances. . . .
>
> Treatment [with pancreatic enzymes] has been thorough and vigorous. . . . Masses have been absorbed and eliminated; the rectal tissues are soft and flexible; the cauliflower condition has undergone tumefaction, degeneration, and elimination—in part, by its being thrown off per rectum, and indirectly by absorption. The patient walks, drives, does some professional work, eats most heartily, functions well. (Cleaves 1906, 918)

In a second report, published in the March 23, 1907 issue of the *Journal of the American Medical Association* (48: 1030), Dr. Richard A. Goeth of San Antonio, Texas, reported on a series of advanced cancer patients treated with injectable pancreatic enzymes according to Beard's hypothesis. Dr. Goeth described a particularly extraordinary case of a woman with advanced, metastatic breast cancer who enjoyed a complete regression of her disease with the pancreatic enzyme extract:

> Case 4.—This woman, whom I am treating at present, has a cancer in one breast with secondary nodules in both axillae [armpits] and around the diseased breast. I began the treatment in this case about the beginning of January, 1907, and have had the same experience as in the previous case, i.e., there has been considerable sloughing of the canecrous [sic] tissue, producing a wound a little larger than a hen's egg. Every gland that was infected with the cancer has become intensely inflamed and painful and the entire tumor mass is sloughing away rapidly. . . .

> This patient is recovering from all the bad symptoms, and I feel sure that it will be my second cure in a short time. Even now I consider her cured, as her general health is improving daily. The patient told me to-day that she felt much better all the time. However, up to this time she has had no faith in the treatment, and only came to me because the Roentgen-ray [X-ray] treatment had failed completely and her case had progressed until it was entirely inoperable. (Goeth 1907, 1030)

Such cases are the first I know of in the medical literature documenting destruction of tumors without surgical intervention. Yet despite the extraordinary successes, Beard's work was largely despised and ultimately forgotten, and when he died in 1923, he died in obscurity, his work relegated to no more than a footnote in medical history. Few scientists at the time could accept his theories about placental growth, the similarity of the placenta to cancer, and its regulation by fetal pancreatic enzymes. No one at the time but Beard could find the primitive undifferentiated "placental cells" he claimed to see in every mammalian tissue.

Unfortunately, Beard was one hundred years ahead of his time; eighty years would pass before other scientists would prove the fetal pancreas became active early in embryonic life. World War I, its terrible destruction, the influenza epidemic of 1918, and the fascination with radiation therapy as a cancer "cure" seemed to push Beard aside. Decades would pass before histologists and molecular biologists would identify primitive stem cells—Beard's misplaced placental cells—in every tissue in every organ. Nearly one hundred years would pass before these primitive cells, which Beard saw so clearly, would be seen increasingly as the cell line that, if not properly controlled, could develop into malignancy.

When I read Beard's crowning achievement, his 1911 book *The Enzyme Treatment of Cancer* summarizing his thesis, I realized how frustrated he was by the disregard given his work by the orthodox research establishment. To Beard, cancer presented no mystery at all; it was a question of misplaced placental cells, growing without restraint because of inadequate pancreatic enzyme production.

After Beard's death, periodically other physicians and scientists rediscovered his work. During the 1920s and 1930s, a St. Louis physician, Dr. F. L. Morse, reported a number of cancer patients successfully treated with pancreatic enzymes. When he presented his well-documented findings to the St. Louis Medical Society in 1934—a proceeding documented in the *Weekly Bulletin of the St. Louis Medical Society* (28: 599–603)—his colleagues attacked him viciously and relentlessly. One physician at the session, a Dr. M. G. Seelig, remarked, "While I heartily agree with Dr. Allen when he strikes the note of encouragement, I recoil at the idea of witlessly spreading the hope of a cancer cure which is implicit in the remarks of Dr. Morse this evening."

Had it not been for the strange hand of fate, the ongoing hostility to Beard's work would have caused it to be lost forever.

CHAPTER II

Dr. Pottenger's Cats

There is another line of thought that underlies my current approach to cancer and other illnesses. This is the work of the American physicians Francis Pottenger Sr. and his son, Francis Pottenger Jr. Although he doesn't appear to have been aware of Beard's work, Dr. Pottenger Sr. began his research career during the 1910s, when Beard's career was winding down. Pottenger, like Beard, was a man of many talents; a lung specialist by training, he was highly regarded in orthodox medical circles for his work with tuberculosis. Additionally, his son's studies of cat nutrition have made him a hero of the alternative medical world.

For a ten-year period, beginning in the early 1930s, Pottenger Jr. completed a series of very simple but elegant studies with cats. He isolated two populations of cats in roomy, comfortable outdoor chambers. All cats received the same exact diet, but with one difference: one group received uncooked, completely raw meat and milk, while the second group received only cooked meat and milk. In experiments repeated year after year, Pottenger carefully documented the health and well-being of the different populations of cats, and the results were always the same.

The raw foods cats, in generation after generation, were extremely healthy, happy cats. X-rays documented ideal bone structure, a perfectly formed dental arch, and perfect teeth. The cats exhibited healthy skin, protection against infectious diseases, and an absence of degenerative disease such as arthritis and cancer. Interestingly, the cats lived harmoniously together, in a well-organized, stable social structure, as benevolent as a cat society could be.

However, for the cooked food cats, life was quite different. In these animals, by the third generation, Pottenger reported a variety of abnormalities in bone structure and teeth. The cats suffered rampant allergies, infectious and skin diseases, and degenerative diseases such as arthritis, heart disease, and colitis. The social structure broke down in the cooked food group, with uncontrolled violence, cannibalism, and destructive behavior epidemic. After the fourth generation, the cooked food cats could no longer reproduce, and the line would die out.

In a series of extraordinary papers, Pottenger documented the results of a simple change in diet, the use of cooked foods, in the health of his cats. And of course, he made connections to the epidemic of degenerative diseases in civilized society, which relied then—and relies now—so heavily on cooked foods.

Pottenger Jr.'s achievements in pulmonary medicine and experimental nutrition were, in my opinion at least, outstanding. But his father's work, in the far different field of neurophysiology, remains one of the least read—and perhaps one of the most important—books in medicine: *Symptoms of Visceral Disease*, whose editions span the period 1919 to 1944.

Pottenger was one of the pioneers describing the function of the autonomic nervous system, the elaborate network of nerves that connects to, and controls the metabolism of, all the tissues, organs, and glands of the body. The word *autonomic* was first used by J. N. Langley, the English scientist, during the early years of the twentieth century as a take on the word *automatic*, to describe the nerves that can function automatically, without the direct intervention of our conscious brain. The autonomic system directs processes such as blood pressure and heart rate, immune function, and the activity of all the endocrine glands in the body, including the thyroid and adrenal glands. Autonomic nerves directly control all digestion, including the secretion of hydrochloric acid in the stomach, the production and release of digestive enzymes from the pancreas, the secretion of bile from the liver, the movement of food along the intestines, and the absorption and utilization of nutrients.

The autonomic system can itself be divided into two components: the sympathetic and parasympathetic branches, which are very distinct anatomically and functionally. Each branch connects to every tissue, organ, and gland in the body but produces opposing effects. For example, the sympathetic system when active increases heart rate, blood pressure, and cardiac output and stimulates the endocrine glands, such as the thyroid and adrenals. Adrenaline production increases.

However, when sympathetic nerves fire, the entire digestive system turns off: the pancreas stops secreting enzymes, the liver stops producing and releasing bile, and peristalsis (the rhythmic contraction of the intestines that moves food along) slows down. Blood shunts away from the intestinal organs to the muscles and the brain. In addition, the sympathetic neurons inhibit immune function. Overall, the sympathetic system tends to stimulate metabolism and in effect cause the breakdown of tissues, such as fats and muscle, to produce energy.

Traditionally, scientists describe the sympathetic nervous system as the "flight or fight system," the nerves that activate during any physical or emotional stress. An active sympathetic system shifts metabolism to aid the body in dealing with a stressful event. Heart output increases, to provide a quick flow of oxygen, energy, and nutrients where it is needed most: to the brain for quick thinking, and to the muscles for rapid physical response. Activities not crucial in a moment of stress, such as digestion, shut down so that energy can be conserved for more essential needs.

In contrast, the parasympathetic system, when it fires, slows the heart rate, reduces blood pressure, and turns on the entire digestive tract. The production and secretion of all digestive juices increases, including acid in the stomach, pancreatic enzymes, and bile from the liver. Peristalsis, the movement of digestion products through the intestines, becomes strong and blood shunts away from the muscles to the intestines, so that the digestion, absorption, and utilization of nutrients proceed efficiently. In addition, parasympathetic nerves enhance immune function and slow down the secretion of thyroid and adrenal hormones. Overall, metabolism slows down.

The parasympathetic system is the regeneration system of the body, directing the digestion of food and the absorption and utilization of nutrients to allow for the repair and rebuilding of tissues and organs. This system is especially active at night, during rest, when the body recovers from the damage of the day's activity.

Though scientists think of the sympathetic system as the "stress" system and the parasympathetic nerves as being more involved with routine metabolism, in fact the two systems operate together, in every moment of our lives, adjusting metabolism to suit each situation we face. This system allows us to adapt, constructively, to the physical and emotional world around us.

Pottenger did much to outline the intricate function of the two branches of the autonomic nervous system. In that work, he was truly brilliant. But he also made a series of observations that directly relate to our treatment approach some fifty years later. Pottenger was an excellent observer, involved not only in research but also in patient care. During his early clinical work in the 1920s, Pottenger noticed that some of his patients were born with a very strong, perhaps overly developed, sympathetic nervous system and a correspondingly weak parasympathetic system.

In these patients, all the tissues, organs, and glands normally stimulated by the sympathetic system, such as the heart, the muscles, the left hemisphere of the brain, and the endocrine glands, were very highly developed, very efficient, perhaps too active. In contrast, the tissues, organs, and glands normally stimulated by the weak parasympathetic system—such as the right brain hemisphere and the entire digestive system, including the pancreas and the liver—were very weak and inefficient.

In these "sympathetic dominants," Pottenger identified a series of ailments related to their autonomic imbalance. Emotionally, these patients were very anxious, irritable, reactive, and easily upset, in keeping with their overly developed stress response system and high levels of circulating adrenaline from sympathetic nerve firing. Such patients tended to be disciplined and good at routines. Structurally, they were usually thin, because of their strong thyroid and adrenal function. They needed little sleep and often slept lightly and fitfully. In these patients, Pottenger reported strong muscles but terrible digestion: such patients were subject to a wide range of digestive problems such as food intolerances, ulcers, colitis, irritable bowel, chronic ingestion, and hiatal hernias.

In other patients, Pottenger identified a strong parasympathetic system and a correspondingly weak sympathetic system. In this group, Pottenger claimed, all the tissues, organs, and glands normally stimulated by the strong parasympathetic system—such as the right hemisphere of the brain; the entire digestive tract, with the pancreas and liver; and the immune system—were overly developed and overly active. However, in these patients, the organs controlled by the weak sympathetic system, such as the heart, the muscular system, and the endocrine glands such as the thyroid, were very sluggish and inefficient.

Pottenger described these patients as calm, emotionally stable, and even keeled, very slow to anger but at times prone to depression. They were, Pottenger said, undisciplined but very creative. This group suffered degenerative musculoskeletal illnesses, as well as low adrenal and low thyroid function, correlating with their weak sympathetic tone. Such patients had a diminished capacity to deal with acute stress, and as a result of their low endocrine output, such patients could easily become overweight. Even minor stresses could be exhausting.

Pottenger described a third group, with a more balanced autonomic nervous system and equally strong and equally efficient sympathetic and parasympathetic nerves. In addition, all the tissues, organs, and glands stimulated by these nerves in this group were equally developed, equally efficient, and equally active. These balanced people had a personality profile between the two extremes. They dealt with stress efficiently but were not overly reactive; disciplined when needed, they could also be creative. Their digestive and endocrine systems were very efficient, neither overly strong nor weak. Of the three groups, balanced patients were the most resilient and generally healthiest. If stressed enough, they could suffer illnesses of either the sympathetic or the parasympathetic group but usually in a less severe form.

By the 1930s, Pottenger realized not only that did these different groups—the sympathetic dominants, the parasympathetic dominants, and the balanced patients—differ remarkably in their basic metabolism, personalities, and health profiles, but also that each group responded quite differently to specific nutrients. Pottenger spent many years studying the effect of individual nutrients, particularly the minerals calcium, magnesium, and potassium, on autonomic function. He found that magnesium tended to block sympathetic activity, while calcium stimulated sympathetic firing. He discovered, in 1936, that potassium activated parasympathetic nerves. Much of his innovative work has, seventy years later, been confirmed. Scientists now know that magnesium does block—and calcium does stimulate—sympathetic nerve firing, while potassium stimulates parasympathetic activity, just as Pottenger claimed.

After years of trial and error, Pottenger learned that he could use these three nutrients to bring an out-of-balance autonomic system into balance. And, as the sympathetic and parasympathetic systems came into equilibrium, his patients felt better and did better, whatever their underlying disease might have been. For example, he learned that sympathetic-dominant patients did very well with the minerals magnesium and potassium, which respectively blocked their strong sympathetic nerves while stimulating the weak parasympathetic outflow. But these sympathetic patients did very poorly with calcium, which stimulated their already too strong sympathetic system.

Parasympathetic-dominant patients, on the other hand, did very well with large doses of calcium, which stimulated their weak sympathetic system. But such patients did very poorly with supplemental magnesium and potassium. With the careful use of these basic nutrients, Pottenger claimed, he could bring his patients to health.

Increasingly, Pottenger believed that disease, whatever its form, from allergies to cancer to eczema, had as a major cause autonomic system imbalance. Health, he came to believe, resulted when the two branches of the autonomic system, and in turn, all the tissues and organs they control, were equally strong, efficient, and in physiological balance.

CHAPTER III:

Dr. Kelley's Mother

After the last edition of Pottenger's book in 1944, his work—like that of John Beard decades earlier—was largely forgotten. Periodically, as with Beard, Pottenger's research would be rediscovered. But it would take the eccentric and controversial dentist William Kelley, who during the 1960s developed an elaborate nutritional therapy, to bring both Beard and Pottenger together into a revolutionary and very controversial approach to cancer and other illnesses.

Kelley grew up in a small farming community in rural Kansas during the hardest years of the Depression. Though his father worked for the railroad, Kelley's parents owned some acreage and grew much of their food, particularly necessary during the Depression years. Kelley's mother was very knowledgeable about nutrition, folk medicine, and herbal medicine and firmly believed the basis of good health was healthy soil and wholesome, natural food. During her childhood, her family was too poor to afford doctors and relied on natural medicines and local healers almost exclusively. She was a resourceful woman; after her husband died of a heart attack at age fifty-six, she raised her three boys by herself during the toughest years of the Depression in an area particularly hard hit. All three became quite successful: Dr. Kelley's older brother was a famed dental surgeon; his younger brother, a literary scholar, was an expert in Elizabeth and Robert Browning, the nineteenth-century English poets.

Kelley graduated in 1954 from the Dental College of Baylor University in Dallas and then completed postgraduate training in orthodontics. By the early 1960s, he maintained a very successful orthodontic practice in Grapevine, Texas, in those days a small suburb outside of Dallas. It was through his dental work that Kelley first developed a serious interest in nutrition, which even by 1960 was his true passion—though, he later admitted, a largely theoretical one, as he lived in those days largely on "junk" food. His two particular weaknesses were pizza and chocolate, but any junk food would do.

However, in 1961, when he was thirty-five years old, his junk food lifestyle caught up with him. In that year, he became very ill with what was clinically diagnosed as pancreatic cancer, though he never had a biopsy. He had been very sick for a number of months, with a variety of debilitating symptoms, and by the time he was tentatively diagnosed, he had lost some fifty pounds on his 6'3" frame and was bedridden, weak, and exhausted. His doctors thought the disease was far advanced, with evidence of spread to the liver, lungs, and bones. Kelley reported his liver was so enlarged he could actually feel the tumors protruding through his abdominal skin. Of course, this was before the advent of sophisticated radiographic studies such as CT scans and MRI, but his doctors thought he had only six weeks to live.

But Kelley, when he looked at his life, realized he couldn't afford to die. He and his wife had adopted four children, and at the time he became ill, all his children were still quite young. When Kelley's doctors told him he had only six weeks to live, he began checking through his life insurance policies and savings accounts, which he had entrusted to the care of his accountants. Unfortunately, he learned his life insurance policies had lapsed, and his other accounts were empty; all had been squandered on expenses and poor investments. Kelley feared that if he died, his four young children would end up back in the orphanage.

Kelley knew that orthodox medicine could do nothing for him. In desperation, he tried to manipulate his diet, in the hopes that perhaps food might control his cancer. Because of the large tumors protruding from his liver, he could tell immediately the effect of individual foods. Certain foods, particularly cooked animal foods such as red meat and poultry, made him feel immediately worse and caused his tumors to enlarge. Other foods, particularly raw fruits, leafy greens, and freshly made vegetable juice, made him feel somewhat stronger and seemed to at least stabilize his liver tumors. Gradually, through trial and error, he began to design a diet for himself, consisting almost entirely of fresh raw vegetables, fruits, nuts, seeds, and whole grains, with limited animal protein including an egg daily and freshly made yogurt—but absolutely no fish, no poultry, and no red meat.

Kelley had help in his battle against his illness. When his doctors first diagnosed him, Kelley called his elderly mother, who still lived in the house in Kansas where Kelley had been raised. She told her son that he simply couldn't die and that she would help nurse him back to health. She left her home in Kansas and moved in with Dr. Kelley in Grapevine.

Mrs. Kelley told her son that if he was to get well—and there was no choice but that he had to get well—he would have to follow her instructions. She mixed up for him a special fourteen-grain breakfast cereal that he ate raw, ground up, and soaked in juice and yogurt. Mrs. Kelley claimed the cereal would help "kill the cancer." She made up mixtures of fresh vegetable juice that she made him drink every several hours. She poured fresh organic fruits and vegetables and nuts into him, even though his appetite had long gone.

She insisted that nearly all his foods be raw; raw foods, she said, contained large amounts of "enzymes" and other nutrients that would also help kill his cancer but that cooking would destroy. In retrospect, Mrs. Kelley's treatment was quite remarkable. This was 1961, when health food stores were small and hard to find and the word "organic" was largely unknown.

In addition to his rigorous diet, Kelley, with his mother's help, began experimenting with supplemental vitamins, minerals, and trace elements. Certain nutrients seemed to have a positive effect on the way he felt, while others made him weaker and seemed to stimulate tumor growth. Specifically, he seemed to do better with beta-carotene and the B vitamins thiamine, riboflavin, niacin, pyridoxine, and folic acid. Moderately large doses of vitamin C, in the three- to four-gram range, improved his energy almost at once, as did the fat-soluble vitamins A, D, and E.

He particularly noticed an improvement with the minerals magnesium and potassium and the trace elements chromium and manganese, but he felt worse when he took calcium supplements and the B vitamins pantothenic acid, inositol, and choline, as well as B12. Nutrient by nutrient, he worked out his supplement protocol. He wasn't sure why these nutrients helped him; he knew only that they did.

In addition to the diet and supplements, Kelley's mother also strongly suggested that he begin daily coffee enemas, which she insisted would help the liver get rid of "toxins" produced as the body fought the tumors. But on this point, Kelley became stubborn; he was feeling better, he said, and didn't need the enemas. His mother only reported, "You will need them."

Kelley was lucky in the most unlucky way. He was unlucky of course that he had pancreatic cancer, but he had an unusual advantage because his tumors were so extensive and so big he had a very obvious and accessible marker to gauge the progress of his treatment. He was also lucky because his pancreatic cancer caused him to think about enzymes.

In Beard's model, all patients with cancer suffer a deficiency in pancreatic enzymes. With pancreatic cancer, the enzyme deficiency is particularly pronounced because the tumor itself will destroy normal enzyme manufacturing cells in the pancreas. Because of this severe enzyme deficiency, patients such as Dr. Kelley invariably develop severe chronic digestive problems such as bloating, pain with meals, indigestion, and reflux. Kelley, despite his therapeutic diet, did suffer all these symptoms, to the point that he began to wonder if he could continue eating.

In desperation, he went to his local pharmacy, run by a friend of his from the town country club who already knew about Kelley's illness. Kelley described his symptoms to the pharmacist, who immediately recommended Kelley start taking with each meal large doses of a prescription form of pancreatic enzyme capsules. Kelley bought a caseload of the enzymes and that day began taking the tablets with each meal.

To Kelley's relief, the enzyme capsules helped immediately, though not completely, with his digestive problems. He started taking large doses, six, then eight tablets with each meal. Because he still noticed belching, bloating, and pain between meals, he began taking doses away from meals. To his astonishment, he noticed that when he took the enzymes on an empty stomach away from food, within half an hour he could feel pain in his liver tumors.

He tried increasing the dose, and the pain worsened. The tumors—which he could palpate through his skin—felt tender to the touch, softer, and inflamed. He discussed this with his mother, who told him without surprise that the enzymes were attacking the cancer. "That's what enzymes are supposed to do," she said, from her years of folk wisdom.

Kelley began taking the enzymes around the clock, both with meals and on an empty stomach, and within days he began to feel stronger. His appetite revived, he gained weight for the first time in months, and his energy and stamina improved. He was convinced the enzymes, as his mother said, were attacking his tumor. For the first time, Kelley began to feel that there was a chance he might survive.

But his optimism quickly came to a crashing halt. After he had been on the enzymes for only a week, he began to deteriorate rapidly. His appetite and sleep worsened, and his abdominal pain increased. His liver felt enlarged, and he felt himself growing weaker by the hour. He thought he was dying. He confided in his mother that the brief period of improvement was the calm before the storm: he thought it was all over.

She yelled at him and told him he wasn't dying, but that he was too toxic. She explained that his body was overloaded with waste materials from the dying tumor, and that if he didn't start doing the coffee enemas as she had suggested earlier, the tumor wastes would poison him to death. In desperation, he agreed to her suggestion and did his first coffee enema with an enema bag his mother had purchased from the local pharmacy and with coffee she brewed in his percolator. To his astonishment, his energy came back, at least for several hours. When he felt his symptoms returning, his mother brewed more coffee, he did another enema, and his symptoms again resolved—at least for several hours. In the days that followed, she introduced him to juice fasting and other routines that she claimed would help his liver and kidneys work better.

Even though he was still largely bedridden, his mother would not let him close down his practice. Frankly, he needed the money. His mother set up a very rigorous schedule of rest, juices, enemas, enzymes, patient care, more rest, more enzymes, more juices, food . . . etc. The first months were very difficult, but he made it to three months, six months, one year. He described feeling quite ill even into his second year, but eventually, three years later, he was cured. He would always suffer residual damage: a tumor had eaten through his right hip, and he would never walk normally again. And during his ordeal his hair turned completely white and never regained its original color. In addition, he suffered persistent heart rhythm disturbances, affecting the timing mechanism in the right atrium. But he was alive.

CHAPTER IV:

Dr. Kelley in Theory and in Practice

As Kelley improved, he began analyzing the various aspects of his own treatment and why it worked. He read extensively in the medical literature and learned of Max Gerson, the American physician who for thirty years had treated patients with a largely vegetarian diet and, to Kelley's surprise, coffee enemas. Gerson believed, as did Mrs. Kelley, that coffee enemas helped the liver detoxify the body more efficiently of tumor and other metabolic wastes. He was also surprised to learn that coffee enemas had been a recommended therapy in many nursing texts and in the Merck Manual, a compendium of orthodox treatments. The texts indicated that patients invariably reported feeling better with the enemas, though no one was quite sure why.

He particularly reviewed the literature on pancreatic enzymes and learned of the work of John Beard. He also studied the nutritional literature, trying to understand why certain vitamins and minerals had helped him and others seemed to feed the tumor. However, thirty years ago the research on specific vitamins and minerals and their effect on cancer was often contradictory, just as it is today.

Nonetheless, Kelley's recovery became legendary in the small, close-knit community of Grapevine. Gradually, as he reestablished his full-time dental practice, he found himself besieged not by dental patients, but by an endless stream of terminal cancer patients wanting his "therapy." Even his doctors, whom he had known for years as friends, began referring cancer patients to him for his odd nutritional treatment. Kelley's days as an orthodontist were in effect over, and by the late 1960s, Kelley was well known—perhaps notorious is a better word—in the alternative medicine underground. He was arrested for practicing medicine without a license but released, apparently because so many officials in the area had been grateful patients. He continued offering his nutritional approach to patients, though never completely free from government harassment.

Kelley initially treated all his patients as he had treated himself, with a primarily vegetarian, raw foods diet emphasizing fresh organic fruits and vegetables, nuts, seeds, whole grains, the powerful fourteen-grain raw cereal, and very limited animal protein— an egg a day, some freshly made yogurt, but absolutely no red meat, poultry, or fish. He prescribed the supplementary nutrients he had found useful in his own situation, as well as large doses of orally ingested pancreatic enzymes, taken around the clock, the exact dose depending on the extent of the cancer. He prescribed for all patients daily coffee enemas and the other detoxification routines he had learned from his mother.

In 1969, Kelley published the first edition of his thirty-two-page pamphlet, "One Answer to Cancer." In this small book, he outlined his own personal battle with presumed cancer, his ultimate victory over the disease, and the treatment program he used in his practice. The self-published book became an immediate underground classic, quickly selling several hundred thousand copies through a strictly word-of-mouth network. The book in fact became successful enough that the attorney general of Texas instituted proceedings against Kelley, claiming his publication of the book constituted the practice of medicine.

After years of litigation with the state, and enormous legal expenses, Kelley ultimately lost and was forbidden to publish any book related to medicine again. When I have discussed this case with lawyers, none believes that such an outcome could occur in the United States of America, with all its protections for freedom of speech. But apparently, such freedom did not apply to Dr. Kelley.

Despite his legal travails, Kelley continued his practice and was widely rumored in the cancer underground to have many remarkable successes with his therapy. He also had failures, of course, but Kelley admitted years later that he had had enough successes that he might have kept doing what he had been doing, treating each patient that same way, except for another life-changing event.

In 1970, Kelley treated a young woman who came to him not for cancer, but for allergies. Her allergies were so severe that on several occasions she had nearly died from anaphylactic shock. She reacted so strongly to iodine, I have been told, that she could not be within ten miles of the ocean, because the miniscule amounts of iodine in the wind blown in from the sea could send her to the emergency room. By the time Kelley met her, she had been to dozens of doctors, both orthodox and unconventional, with no success: she had tried allergy desensitization injections, which ended up giving her hepatitis through a contaminated needle. She had tried elimination diets, rotation diets, fasts, single-food diets, organic food, bland food, homeopathy—but she continued to worsen to the point that she could not continue school or hold a job.

Kelley treated the young woman with his usual therapy, the vegetarian "Kelley Diet," with the fourteen-grain cereal, large amounts of freshly made vegetable juices, fruits, nuts, seeds, whole grains, the supplements that had helped him, and the coffee enemas. And on this regimen, initially the young woman improved, but after several months, she began to deteriorate very rapidly. She lost all strength, lapsed into a severe and relentless depression, and ended up in bed, too weak to leave her room. Kelley, who had developed a particular fondness for this patient, first tried to manipulate her diet: he made the diet stricter, eliminating eggs and yogurt; he increased the amount of raw food and the daily intake of vegetable juices. He increased the number of coffee enemas as well, but the young woman only worsened.

Kelley then began experimenting with different doses of nutrients. During his own period of experimentation with supplements, Kelley had seemed to respond particularly well when he increased the doses of the minerals magnesium and potassium in his program. He suggested that this patient do the same, and she upped her intake of both nutrients. Within half an hour, she lapsed into a cataclysmic depression that lasted for three days. The patient insisted the magnesium and potassium made her sick, but Kelley could not accept that these essential nutrients could have this effect on anyone. After she stabilized somewhat, he suggested she try another single capsule of each; again, she lapsed into a three-day depression.

Eventually, the patient's mother called in near desperation; her daughter was semiconscious. Kelley thought about the patient, and thought about her some more, and then did the only thing he hadn't done: he told her mother to stop the raw vegetarian diet and all the supplements and start feeding her daughter large servings of raw blenderized organic red meat. Off the supplements and within hours of her first dose of meat, the patient sat up for the first time in days. She began eating red meat every few hours, and every few hours she felt herself growing stronger.

After several days, Kelley then suggested, though cautiously, she start taking all the nutrients that had made him worse during his own battle with cancer—the B vitamins niacinamide, pantothenic acid, choline, inositol, and B12. He prescribed large doses of calcium and the trace minerals selenium and zinc but told her to avoid all magnesium and potassium. To his relief, the patient responded exceptionally well, particularly to calcium, which had made him feel so much worse.

Within weeks, on the largely fatty red meat diet and the supplements Kelley had always avoided in his treatment, the patient improved substantially. Kelley learned, always through trial and error, that she seemed to tolerate certain vegetables, particularly the root vegetables such as carrots and potatoes, but became immediately worse with leafy greens and citrus fruit. Gradually, he worked out a precise diet and supplement program for the patient. Within months, she was completely well, for the first time in her adult life. Kelley immediately tried the meat diet and the new supplement protocol on a number of his problem patients, who, like this young woman, had only worsened on his Kelley Diet therapy. Kelley reported being astonished that there were patients who would not get well unless they ate large quantities of fatty red meat, sometimes three and four times a day.

Kelley began to experiment with his problem patients, varying the amount of animal protein and the other foods. He began a process of identifying different "metabolic types" based on dietary needs. He referred to himself as a "vegetarian" and his meat-eating allergy patient as a "carnivore."

At that point, Kelley still believed strongly that whether a patient required fruits and nuts or meat for good health, the food needed to be raw for maximum benefit. As his mother had taught him, raw foods contain many nutrients, not only vitamins but also enzymes, that cooking destroys, and these nutrients and enzymes were critical to the success of the therapeutic protocol.

A voracious reader of the scientific literature, Kelley found considerable support in the medical literature for his clinical observation. He learned that for some several thousand years, from the time of the Egyptians, and the later time of Hippocrates in Greece, physicians had recommended raw foods, including raw meat, as therapeutic. More recently, the early twentieth-century American physician Dr. Edward Howell promoted raw foods in his practice and over a sixty-year period treated thousands of very sick patients with raw foods.

A scientist as well as a clinician, Howell studied the biochemical effect of raw foods in the body. He pointed out in his writings that humans are the only species of animal that cooks its food, and he proposed, as did Francis Pottenger, that this simple process we all take for granted has had profound effects on our individual health and the health of our civilization. Raw foods, whether plant-based foods such as fruit and vegetables or raw animal products, contain, in addition to vitamins, minerals, and trace elements, large quantities of enzymes. Howell claimed these enzymes are absorbed like a nutrient and are as important to our metabolism, and our health, as any of the other better-known vitamins, minerals, and trace elements.

Enzymes are a type of protein, complex molecules made up of amino acid chains. Enzymes function as catalysts, which enable complicated reactions that would otherwise require considerable heat and time to occur quickly and efficiently at low temperature. For example, certain chemical reactions involved in energy production in our cells would, without enzymes, require temperatures in the range of a thousand or more degrees. Such temperatures are not compatible with life. With the aid of enzymes, thousands of complicated reactions occur very efficiently each second in every cell in our body within a very narrow and very low temperature range. In fact, without enzymes, there could be no life as we know it.

Each cell of every plant and animal is a reservoir of enzymes. When we eat raw foods of either plant or animal origin, we absorb huge quantities of vital enzymes that can be used, Howell claimed, in our own cells for efficient metabolism. However, enzymes, like most proteins, become clumped and inactive with even moderately high temperatures. Howell proposed that the human predilection for cooked foods left us all severely enzyme deficient and this deficiency could account for the epidemics of degenerative and infectious disease in civilized countries.

Kelley was familiar with the work of Howell, and of Max Gerson, who like Howell had developed an intensive largely raw foods vegetarian approach to treating degenerative disease. So it wasn't surprising, faced with Howell's compelling argument, that Kelley assumed all his patients, whether vegetarian or carnivore, would require raw foods. He assumed raw foods were best for all. He continued to assume this until he met his next problem patient, a young man who today would most likely be classified as suffering from severe chronic fatigue and environmental illness.

The patient arrived in Kelley's office virtually too weak to sit in the chair opposite Kelley's desk. He had a long, sad story: a very brilliant student, he was pursing graduate studies in the sciences when, after a period of severe stress related to his work and a failing romance, his health had suddenly collapsed. Almost overnight, he developed severe, unrelenting exhaustion and depression, which responded to none of the medications available at the time. He could barely concentrate enough to read the newspaper, let alone his scientific journals and texts. His memory was failing, and he had gone from being a motivated, ambitious student to a morose patient who barely left his room.

He had chronic digestive problems, such as bloating and diarrhea alternating with constipation. He had severe headaches after eating any type of fat, yet fruits and vegetables left him spacey and grains left him more tired and more depressed. He had arthritic-type joint pains. He felt his vision was deteriorating. He had been to many doctors and many major medical centers, as was true with so many of Kelley's patients. No diagnostic test had revealed much, and no therapy had helped.

He had tried a number of alternative-type treatments popular in the early 1970s such as megavitamin therapy, but these approaches left him feeling worse. He felt hopeless, convinced he had cancer or some other terrible illness that his doctors had missed. At age twenty-nine, this young man saw his once-promising life coming to an end.

Kelley first tried the patient on the vegetarian raw foods "Kelley Diet," with the associated supplements, but on this the patient quickly worsened. He then switched the young man to the raw meat diet and the "carnivore" complement of supplements. Initially, the young man improved, but not as much or as significantly as the allergy patient who had done so well on raw meat. In fact, over a period of weeks on raw meat and limited raw vegetables, this young man took a turn for the worse.

Kelley tried a mixed diet, of raw meat and animal products along with generous amounts of raw vegetables, raw fruits, sprouted raw grains and seeds, and sprouted beans. He began testing supplements, one by one, to see if he could uncover a combination that might help. Again, the patient initially improved but then began to worsen. Kelley was perplexed, as he had been when his young allergy patient worsened so dramatically on the "perfect" raw foods vegetarian diet.

Kelley tried a variety of combinations of raw foods, to no effect. He tried different combinations of nutritional supplements, again to no effect. Eventually, Kelley suggested to the patient the one thing he would never have thought reasonable: he told the young man to start cooking all his foods. He told him to start eating soups and stews, with meat and vegetables, and to stop the juices, salads, and sprouts. He also suggested large doses of the whole range of vitamins, minerals, and trace elements, far larger than Kelley had ever used with his previous patients, including nutrients he had previously prescribed for both his vegetarian and his carnivore patients.

Within days, the patient began to improve. Although the improvement was less striking, more gradual than the improvement in the case of the young allergy patient, after a period of some eight months, the young man was essentially well and able to resume his schoolwork.

This patient's response completely contradicted Howell, Gerson, and other proponents of raw foods. Kelley accepted that raw foods do contain nutrients such as vitamin C and folic acid that cooking largely inactivates. He accepted Howell's argument that cooking also destroys natural food enzymes present in all raw foods, and that optimal health requires these enzymes. However, he suspected that this patient was so debilitated and deteriorated in so many ways that he lacked the digestive capability to break down raw foods and use the nutrients. Although cooking may destroy certain nutrients and useful enzymes, it has the effect of predigesting the food, breaking down proteins in animal foods and cell walls in plant foods to make many nutrients more available. With cooking, the basic proteins, fats, carbohydrates, and many other heat-stable nutrients are made more easily accessible.

Food scientists have known for years, for example, that in our intestines, more beta-carotene, a vitamin A precursor, will be absorbed from cooked rather than raw carrots. As valuable as raw carrots may be, much of the beta-carotene remains locked behind the tough plant cell walls. And recently, scientists have found that men who consume frequent servings of cooked—but not raw—tomato products have reduced levels of heart disease and prostate cancer. Cooked tomato products release large quantities of lycopene, an antioxidant related to beta-carotene that is thought to provide the beneficial effect. Kelley began to suspect that this particular patient was so debilitated that no system, including digestion, worked with any level of efficiency. On the raw foods diet Kelley had initially prescribed, this particular patient was unable to use the food effectively and was, Kelley believed, essentially starving to death.

With this lesson at hand, Kelley began carefully to monitor each of his patients' responses to particular foods, diets, and nutritional supplements. If a patient didn't respond over time to the initially prescribed diet and supplement regimen, he would try something different. Kelley tried to eliminate all his assumptions. If raw vegetarian didn't work, he might try cooked vegetarian, raw meat, raw balanced, or cooked balanced. He worked as a clinician, through trial and error. If high-dose vitamin C made the patient worse, he would try low dose, and if that didn't work he would try different forms such as the calcium or magnesium salts of vitamin C.

By 1970, Kelley began to classify his patients into three broad categories: vegetarian, carnivore, and balanced metabolizers, with subtypes within each category. Kelley developed his complex therapy out of his clinical experience. He had learned that certain patients did best on a largely vegetarian diet, others with a largely meat diet, and others with a varied diet including both plant and animal products. He learned that certain patients thrived with most of their food eaten raw and others with most of their food cooked. He learned that vegetarian patients did well with very large doses of vitamin C, magnesium, and potassium, but that carnivores did best with low doses of C, minimal if any magnesium and potassium, and large doses of calcium. Experience taught Kelley that these things were true, but on a physiological level, he did not know why.

CHAPTER V:

Dr. Kelley Meets Dr. Pottenger

Kelley, ever the student, continually scoured the medical literature, looking for some explanation for what he had seen in his own practice. It was during the mid-1960s that he first learned of Francis Pottenger's innovative but largely ignored work with nutrition and autonomic function. Kelley was fascinated that Pottenger, in broad strokes, had decades earlier claimed that there were different types of humans—the sympathetic dominants, the parasympathetic dominants, and the balanced metabolizers—that responded very differently to individual nutrients. Pottenger, fifty years earlier, had described what Kelley himself was seeing in his own practice.

Pottenger's claim that these various "types" varied considerably in their biochemistry, neurophysiology, and behavior was a revelation and a confirmation for Kelley. As he worked out his various diets and supplement regimens, Kelley independently recognized that his own patients differed not only in the type of diet and nutrients required for optimal health but also in their fundamental biology, physiology, and psychology. His vegetarian and carnivore patients seemed to Kelley like two entirely different species, and he began to suspect that these variations could result from degrees of sympathetic or parasympathetic nervous system efficiency.

Kelley realized very quickly that the patients he had observed who did best with a vegetarian or largely vegetarian diet were the very same patients Pottenger had described as sympathetic nervous system dominants: patients with a strong sympathetic nervous system and a weak parasympathetic system, who did well with large doses of magnesium and potassium, but who did terribly with supplemental calcium. Kelley's vegetarian patients fit that mold exactly. And Kelley's patients who did best with a largely meat-based diet had to be Pottenger's parasympathetic dominants—those who did best with large doses of calcium but terribly with magnesium and potassium. Kelley's balanced metabolizers, who thrived on a very varied diet and supplement protocol and did best with moderate doses of calcium, magnesium, and potassium must be, Kelley thought,

Pottenger's patients with a balanced autonomic nervous system. What Kelley discovered through trial and error in his small Grapevine, Texas, office, Pottenger had described in elegant biochemical detail in a book that had been out of print for twenty-five years when Kelley was refining his therapy during the early 1970s.

Kelley spent every spare moment studying and relearning autonomic physiology and biochemistry from a more contemporary perspective. He reviewed years of his own patient records, trying to correlate Pottenger's concepts of autonomic function to his own findings. By 1974, Kelley had described in great detail the structural, biochemical, physiological, and psychological qualities of his dietary types, based on Pottenger's concept of autonomic dominance.

In Kelley's vegetarian patients, as with Pottenger's sympathetic dominants, the sympathetic nervous system did seem highly developed, and the tissues normally stimulated by sympathetic function—such as the heart, the muscles, the endocrine system, and the left hemisphere of the brain—tended to be well developed and active, perhaps overly active. Similarly, in these patients the parasympathetic system appeared sluggish, and all the tissues, organs, and glands stimulated by the weak parasympathetic system—such as the stomach, the intestines, the pancreas, and the liver—were inefficient.

Structurally, Kelley's vegetarians, or Pottenger's sympathetic dominants, tended to be very lean, with long and strong bones, narrow faces, and a narrow dental arch. Often, their teeth were crowded and crooked, and as children, they frequently required orthodontia. Their muscles tended to be well developed even with minimal exercise, and sympathetic dominants were often good athletes at sports requiring fine motor skills, such as baseball and tennis. Because of their strong endocrine and thyroid function, they usually were thin, even as they aged—just as Pottenger had claimed.

In terms of their basic biochemistry, Kelley described three functions of particular importance that he believed made sympathetic dominants unique and helped explain their particular dietary needs: inefficient energy metabolism in the cells, an acidic cellular environment, and tight cell membranes.

All our cells produce the energy necessary to maintain life through two related series of chemical reactions: glycolysis, which occurs in the cytoplasm of cells, and the Krebs or tricarboxylic acid cycle, occurring in the mitochondria. Mitochondria are small organelles or "mini organs" scattered throughout the cytoplasm. In glycolysis, the main sugar of the bloodstream, glucose, is broken down through a series of steps to pyruvic acid, a two-carbon acid. In the process, two molecules of adenosine triphosphate (ATP), the basic energy storage molecule in the body, are formed. Pyruvic acid is then converted to acetate, a simple molecule also with two carbons, and acetate moves inside the mitochondria, where it primes the Krebs cycle.

The Krebs cycle, named after the biochemist who first described the system, is a complex series of reactions that produces additional energy as ATP through the movement of electrons. Overall, the coupling of glycolysis and the Krebs cycle produces large amounts of stored energy in the form of ATP. ATP in turn provides the energy needed to fuel every process in the cell. In addition, large amounts of carbon dioxide form as a waste product.

Fruits contain large amounts of simple sugars such as glucose and fructose. The body quickly converts fructose to glucose for use in glycolysis and in turn, through pyruvic acid and acetate, for use in the Krebs cycle. Fats and proteins can be broken down, although more slowly, into acetate and other molecules that also feed directly into the Krebs cycle for energy production. Kelley had long observed that his sympathetic-dominant vegetarian patients invariably craved and did very well with foods such as fruit, which contain simple sugars.

They also thrived with other carbohydrate foods such as grains, but they tended to feel tired and sluggish after eating complex protein foods and fats. He proposed that in these patients, cellular oxidation through the Krebs cycle was a very inefficient process, and simple sugars could more easily and more quickly feed into the Krebs reactions than could complex foods such as proteins and fats. Sugars, he felt, were their ideal fuel.

Furthermore, if efficient, the only waste material from this multistep energy-producing process will be carbon dioxide, which is eventually excreted through the lungs. But Kelley believed that in sympathetic dominants, the oxidation reactions of the tricarboxylic acid cycle occur inefficiently, with a very slow conversion of sugars, proteins, and fats to energy and CO_2. Instead, because of the oxidative inefficiency, these sympathetic cells produce large quantities of acid waste products such as lactic acid and pyruvic acid, which accumulate in the cells, in the fluids between cells, and in the blood. The sympathetic-dominant metabolism tends toward acidosis, which can at times, depending on the level of sympathetic activity, become quite pronounced.

Physiologists have known for a hundred years how critically important the acid-base balance can be in disease and health, and how tightly regulated this balance is in our bodies. Extremes in either direction, acidosis or alkalosis, can be life threatening, and we have complex biochemical mechanisms available in our cells, as well as in the blood and in the fluids of our tissues, to keep acid and base levels under control. We continually produce acid wastes, such as lactic acid, as a product of cellular metabolism, and we produce buffers such as bicarbonate, a powerful antacid, to neutralize excess acidity. Acidic or alkaline molecules can be excreted efficiently through the kidneys, as needed, or released through breathing to maintain the appropriate acid-base levels. For example, carbon dioxide, the waste product of cellular respiration, can be converted to carbonic acid in the body. By increasing the rate of breathing, we can rid ourselves of excessive CO_2 and, in effect, lower the body levels of circulating acid.

Not only did the sympathetic cells produce large amounts of acid wastes, but Kelley believed that the excretion processes of the kidney, which normally removed excess acid into the urine, were also inefficient. The end result, Kelley maintained, is that sympathetic cells, tissues, organs, and fluids such as blood were always loaded with excess acid. This chronic acidosis in turn, through an elaborate feedback mechanism, profoundly affected sympathetic physiology. An acidic environment, Kelley believed, further stimulated sympathetic activity and suppressed parasympathetic firing. In a sense, an active sympathetic nervous system created an environment that encouraged sympathetic dominance.

Kelley came to believe, as Pottenger had earlier, that calcium metabolism was crucial to understanding the differences among the sympathetic, parasympathetic, and balanced types. Although we think of calcium as the main cement and foundation of our bones, calcium is an extremely versatile molecule. On a cellular level, calcium actually functions as a hormone, stimulating a variety of reactions within the cell. In addition, calcium is one of the major molecular components of the membranes of all cells and provides membrane stability. Kelley believed that in his sympathetic-dominant patients, the excess sympathetic tone and the high levels of circulating adrenaline in these patients tended to drive calcium into the cell membranes and into the cell interior.

Contemporary physiologists now know that sympathetic action, and adrenaline, will do just this. In turn, this excessive intracellular calcium tends to produce very strong, very tight cell membranes that impede the passage of nutrients into cells and wastes out of cells. This might explain why Kelley's extreme sympathetic dominants, presumably with the tightest cell membranes, were very resistant to allergies; their membranes served as a barrier, blocking the entry of potentially irritating molecules into the cells, as well as the release from the cells of molecules normally associated with allergic symptoms, such as histamine and serotonin. Kelley's biochemical hypothesis helps explain why, fifty years earlier, Pottenger had noted that his sympathetic patients rarely suffered allergies.

This calcium retention he, and Pottenger earlier, observed in sympathetic-dominant patients had a very important effect above and beyond cell membrane structure. For years, even in Pottenger's time, orthodox physiologists have known that the stimulation of the sympathetic nerves requires the presence of calcium ions, and the more calcium present, the greater the sympathetic output. In effect, a strong sympathetic nervous system causes a cascade of increased calcium retention, and the increased calcium stimulates further sympathetic firing. In a similar way, the acidic environment created by a strong sympathetic nervous system tends to keep that system strong. In essence, the sympathetic-dominant system creates a biochemical environment that perpetuates its own dominance.

Kelley also described, in far greater detail than Pottenger, the psychological makeup of sympathetic-dominant patients. Like Pottenger, Kelley believed that the strong sympathetic and weak parasympathetic systems in these patients could explain the observed behavioral characteristics. Sympathetic nerves, when active, produce two major hormone products, norepinephrine and epinephrine, also known as adrenaline. These two hormones act as neurotransmitters as well as hormones and affect, very predictably, many brain functions. Neurotransmitters are the signaling molecules released by nerves that allow them to communicate to other nerves, or to tissues such as muscle or the pancreatic acinar cells.

Scientists have known for more than fifty years that an injection of the sympathetic neurotransmitter epinephrine into a laboratory animal produces very distinctive reactions associated with an acute stress response. The animal becomes irritable, angry, aggressive, and prone to quick reactions and reflexes, as if the brain is on full alert. These animals have to be handled with care, as they can be unpredictably violent. In a threatening situation, such responses are clearly protective.

In humans, epinephrine enhances alertness, depresses appetite, and reduces sleep needs. During World War II, Japanese authorities fed factory workers in the war industry large doses of amphetamines, a pharmacological sympathetic stimulant, to increase productivity and reduce sleep requirements. On amphetamines, workers could easily go through twenty-four-hour shifts, barely needing breaks for food.

In his human patients, like Pottenger before him, Kelley described his sympathetic patients as irritable, prone to anger and temper outbursts. They slept poorly and lightly, but nonetheless reported excellent energy and concentration. They tended to be very aggressive and controlling, very concerned about position and dominance, all aggressive characteristics, Kelley believed, brought on by high levels of circulating adrenaline. The sympathetic-dominant mind works very fast and responds to situations quickly, oftentimes without evaluating the consequences.

Overall, in sympathetic-dominant patients, thinking tended to be linear and simplistic rather than expansive and three-dimensional. Such patients were good at rote activities requiring discipline and concentration but weren't very creative or imaginative. They made good workers, but not innovators. In the extreme, these patients could suffer agitated depressions, with anger, insomnia, and irritability dominating the clinical picture.

Kelley described the parasympathetic dominants in equal detail. In these patients, all the tissues normally stimulated by the strong parasympathetic nerves—such as the stomach, the intestinal tract, the pancreas, the liver, and the right hemisphere of the brain—tended to be well developed and overly active. In contrast, the tissues normally stimulated by their weak sympathetic nerves, such as the endocrine glands, the muscles, the heart, and the left hemisphere of the brain, were inefficient and sluggish.

In terms of their overall body appearance, Kelley found parasympathetic dominants tended toward a rounded appearance, with large shoulders, a rounded rather than narrow facial structure, and a broad dental arch. Because of their chronic weak sympathetic nervous system tone, parasympathetic dominants usually had flabby, unresponsive muscles—just as Pottenger had described. Even mild exercise could result in severe pain, muscle tears, and hernias. And because of their weak endocrine and thyroid function in particular, these patients gained weight easily.

Biochemically, the cells of parasympathetic-dominant patients efficiently—in fact, too quickly and too efficiently—converted sugars into energy through glycolysis and the complex Krebs cycle. After a meal loaded with carbohydrates, these patients would use the sugar load so rapidly that, ironically, low blood sugar resulted. Because the brain uses blood glucose preferentially as its energy source, without an adequate supply patients can suffer fatigue, sleepiness, and depression. They tended to do far better, in terms of their general energy and well-being, when they ate fatty, high-protein foods. In these patients, proteins and fats only gradually convert into energy, allowing for a slow, steady production of ATP energy on a cellular level.

This efficient energy metabolism produced only minimal amounts of acid wastes. In addition, Kelley believed that the kidneys in these patients proficiently excreted acid molecules and tended instead to reabsorb bicarbonate—the body's main alkaline buffer. As a result, parasympathetic cells, tissues, organs, and body fluids were very alkaline, as opposed to acid. This alkaline environment, Kelley maintained, tended to stimulate the already strong parasympathetic—and suppress the weak sympathetic—nervous systems. In a sense, the alkaline environment of a parasympathetic dominant supported parasympathetic activity and autonomic imbalance.

In contrast to the sympathetic-dominant patients, the parasympathetic cells tended to lose calcium into the bloodstream, and the kidneys rapidly excreted calcium into the urine. As a result, these calcium-deficient parasympathetic cell membranes were loose and leaky, easily allowing the influx of molecules into cells and the efflux of wastes, hormones, neurotransmitters, and other cell products out of cells. Because of these porous membranes, potential allergens easily made their way inside the cells, and the mediators of inflammation, such as histamine, easily left cells to produce the symptoms of allergy—mucus production, asthma, skin rashes, postnasal drip, hives, and irritability. Kelley's biochemical hypothesis neatly explained why Pottenger found his parasympathetic patients to be so prone to allergic reactions.

In Kelley's model, the personality of the parasympathetic dominant contrasted greatly with that of the sympathetic profile and could be explained by the strong parasympathetic and weak sympathetic systems. Such patients produce minimal amounts of the stress hormones norepinephrine and epinephrine that produce protective, aggressive behavior, but large amounts of the parasympathetic neurotransmitters acetylcholine and serotonin. Serotonin, the main parasympathetic neurotransmitter in the brain, has a relaxing, sedating, calming effect. Our bodies manufacture serotonin from the amino acid tryptophan, which physicians used for years as a sleep enhancer. And the Prozac generation of antidepressants work by increasing levels of serotonin in the brain, which tends to produce calm, reduce anger and aggressiveness, and improve sleep.

As a group, parasympathetic-dominant patients tend to be easygoing and friendly, enjoying the company of friends, rarely prone to anger or temper tantrums. Kelley found them usually nonaggressive, at times passive—and as a result, easily taken advantage of by aggressive sympathetic dominants. Predictably, because their levels of the aggressive sympathetic neurotransmitters tend to be low, parasympathetics don't like confrontation. Patients in this group usually sleep very soundly and need long hours of sleep, at times ten to twelve hours. They feel best in the later portions of the day but feel groggy and spacey in the mornings.

In the extreme, these patients can suffer lethargic depressions, characterized by withdrawal and severe melancholy. In the most extreme situation, with serotonin levels far too high, these patients can become paranoid and then defensively violent. When depressed, parasympathetic-dominant patients do better with sympathetic stimulants such as the tricyclic antidepressants, rather than the serotonin reuptake inhibitors.

Parasympathetics do poorly, Kelley claimed, with rote and routine, but are in general very creative and innovative in their perspectives and thinking. These patients have as a group a very well-developed right hemisphere of the brain, where three-dimensional thinking occurs. Many successful artists and creative scientists are parasympathetic dominant, Ernest Hemingway being a classic example. Undisciplined and prone to moodiness and severe depression, Hemingway enjoyed the company of friends, loved sensual pleasures, and of course was very creative in his work. Toward the end of his life, he became paralytically depressed and paranoid: unable to write and enjoy what he loved most, he ended his life in 1962.

The third general type, the balanced metabolizers, fall between the sympathetics and parasympathetics in terms of their structure, biochemistry, physiology, and psychology. Because both branches of the autonomic system tend to be equally developed and equally efficient, Kelley maintained, all the tissues, organs, and glands stimulated by the sympathetic and parasympathetic nerves—the heart, the muscles, the left and right hemispheres of the brain, and the digestive, endocrine, and immune systems—are equally developed, equally efficient, and equally strong. There is no imbalance and no dominance of organ systems.

In terms of their overall structure, Kelley described balanced metabolizers as well proportioned, neither too lean, like the sympathetics, nor overly rounded, like the parasympathetic group. Their facial structure and dental arch are ideally proportional. Their bones and muscles are innately strong and responsive to exercise, though not as responsive as the bones and muscles of the sympathetics. They can be good athletes, with training.

On a cellular level, the balanced cells efficiently produce energy through both glycolysis and the Krebs cycle, which function neither too quickly nor too sluggishly. Their cells can effectively convert sugars as well as proteins and fats into energy and can use a variety of food types equally well, unlike the parasympathetic and sympathetic extremes. Overall, these metabolizers have excellent energy and stamina, unlike the sympathetics, who tend to have excessive energy for short bursts, or the parasympathetics, who tend toward fatigue.

In balanced patients, the cells, tissues, organs, and body fluids are neither too acid nor too alkaline. The kidneys and the bicarbonate buffer systems work efficiently to keep the levels of acid and alkaline molecules under tight control. In turn, the neutral acid-base balance keeps the sympathetic and parasympathetic systems in equilibrium, with neither system overactive because of excessive acidity or alkalinity.

Such metabolizers use calcium efficiently, holding on to the mineral when needed and easily excreting any excess. Calcium enters cell membranes as needed, neither excessively nor too slowly. The membranes of balanced cells allow influx of nutrients as needed and the efflux of wastes as appropriate. If exposed to high levels of allergens in the bloodstream or body fluids, balanced metabolizer cells can respond with the release of histamine and other mediators of allergic reactions—but only if such allergens are present in excessive amounts.

The personality of the balanced types tends to be very resilient and adaptable, not prone to extremes of behavior, in keeping with their balanced autonomic system. These metabolizers produce equivalent amounts of neurotransmitters from both the sympathetic and parasympathetic systems, such as norepinephrine, epinephrine, acetylcholine, and serotonin. Balanced individuals are not prone to anger and irritability on the one hand, or depression on the other, responding with aggressiveness when appropriate yet able to relax when needed for body repair and regeneration. They need six to eight hours of sleep a night in general, though under stress they can function well with less and when relaxed can sleep more at will. The balanced types can adjust to routine as needed but can also be very creative.

In situations of stress, their sympathetic system can turn on fairly strongly—though never as strongly as in a sympathetic dominant. However, under prolonged stress, if the sympathetic system continues to fire, the balanced metabolizer patients can develop sympathetic ailments, such as digestive problems, ulcers, or colitis. If the stress persisted too long, Kelley claimed, the sympathetic system in these patients could actually wear out and shut down, leaving the parasympathetic system to take over by default. In a state of such parasympathetic dominance, the balanced metabolizers could literally change personality and develop the classic parasympathetic illnesses, such as allergies and depression.

CHAPTER VI:

Dr. Kelley and His Ten Metabolic Types

In his writings, Pottenger identified only three basic groups: the sympathetic and parasympathetic dominants, and the balanced autonomic group. By 1974, Kelley had identified ten basic types of patients, based on their dietary and nutritional needs and autonomic dominance: three vegetarian sympathetic-dominant types, three carnivore parasympathetic types, and four balanced autonomic types. In his metabolic scheme, Kelley labeled the different types from 1 to 10, in the order in which he had identified each.

Kelley's three sympathetic-dominant groups were named extreme, moderate, and inefficient sympathetic (vegetarian)—and the three parasympathetic groups extreme, moderate, and inefficient parasympathetic (carnivore)—to correlate with precise gradations of sympathetic and parasympathetic dominance. For example, the patient group Kelley labeled extreme sympathetic-dominant metabolizers, Kelley's Type 1 patients, demonstrated extreme sympathetic dominance, with highly developed—perhaps excessively developed—strength in the organs, such as the heart and thyroid gland, normally stimulated by this system. Conversely, these patients showed very weak parasympathetic function, and the organs normally stimulated by this system, such as the digestive tract including the accessory organs such as the pancreas, were very weak and inefficient. In these patients, the sympathetic traits described by Pottenger and refined by Kelley—such as nervousness, tendency toward anger, good muscle tone, insomnia, and poor digestive function—would be very pronounced.

Kelley's moderate sympathetic-dominant metabolizers, the Type 4 group, were only moderately sympathetic dominant, with moderate parasympathetic inefficiency. In these patients, the sympathetic qualities, such as irritability, good muscle tone, insomnia, and digestive problems, would be less extreme, though still evident. Such patients suffered a tendency toward intermittent digestive problems, rather than chronic debilitating gastrointestinal diseases.

Kelley believed his Type 6 patients, the inefficient sympathetic-dominant metabolizers, like the moderate sympathetics, again showed moderate sympathetic dominance and moderate parasympathetic weakness. But neither system was very efficient, and these patients seemed to be sympathetic dominant by default. For example, an extreme sympathetic-dominant patient might have a sympathetic nervous system operating at 100 percent possible strength and a parasympathetic system at 20 percent of capacity. A moderate sympathetic-dominant patient might have a sympathetic nervous system operating at 70 percent capacity and a parasympathetic system at 30 percent efficiency.

In the case of the inefficient sympathetic dominants, the sympathetic system might be at 30 to 40 percent capacity and the parasympathetic system at 10 to 20 percent. These patients were sympathetic dominant, but neither system worked well, and in turn, none of the tissues, organs, or glands worked effectively. These patients tended to be very sick, requiring intensive dietary and nutritional support during treatment.

Similarly, the extreme parasympathetic-dominant group (Type 2) exhibited very strong, extreme parasympathetic dominance with very strong, in fact overly strong, development of all the organs, such as the digestive system, normally stimulated by this system. Conversely, these patients demonstrated very weak sympathetic function and severe inefficiency in the organs activated by sympathetic nerves. In these patients, the parasympathetic qualities documented by Pottenger, such as a quiet, unassuming nature, would be exaggerated: these were the patients who tended to be passive and unmotivated, often developing severe lethargic depression. They could suffer chronic fatigue and exhaustion even with minimal mental or physical exertion, debilitating environmental allergies, muscle weakness, and muscle diseases. They required excessive sleep, ten to twelve hours a night, and would still wake tired. In these patients, digestion was too vigorous, and they could develop chronic diarrhea.

The moderate parasympathetic-dominant (Type 5) patients showed only moderately strong parasympathetic dominance and moderately weak sympathetic inefficiency. In these patients, the parasympathetic qualities were evident, but not extreme. These patients might still be subdued but were more assertive than the extreme parasympathetics; they might suffer occasional bouts of depression and fatigue, but not chronically. They were prone to moderate allergies, perhaps seasonally, and muscle weakness if they pushed their physical activities. They needed considerable sleep, but not as much as the extreme parasympathetics.

The inefficient parasympathetic-dominant (Type 7) group, like the moderate parasympathetics, showed moderate parasympathetic dominance, but only by default. An extreme parasympathetic patient might have a parasympathetic system firing at 100 percent potential and a sympathetic system at 20 percent capacity. A moderate parasympathetic might have a parasympathetic system at 70 percent efficiency and a sympathetic system at 30 percent. However, the inefficient parasympathetic patients might have a parasympathetic system operating only at 30 to 40 percent of its potential and a sympathetic system at 10 to 20 percent capacity. These were the sickest of the parasympathetic-dominant patients, with severe allergies, debilitating depressions, paranoia, and arthritis.

In all four balanced metabolizer groups identified by Kelley—the Type 10, 8, 9, and 3 patients—both branches of the autonomic system were equally developed and equally strong (or weak). The groups differed not in levels of autonomic dominance, but only in terms of efficiency. For example, the highly efficient balanced metabolizers (Type 10) have both the sympathetic and parasympathetic systems capable of 100 percent activity and efficiency. A moderately efficient balanced metabolizer (Type 8) might exhibit 80 percent sympathetic and 80 percent parasympathetic activity and efficiency.

The moderately inefficient balanced metabolizers (Type 9) might have sympathetic and parasympathetic systems at equal 50 percent potential. The very inefficient balanced metabolizer group (Type 3) might function with each system at only 10 to 20 percent capacity. Of the balanced patients, the last group, the Type 3 patients, would be the sickest, prone to the problems of both inefficient sympathetic and parasympathetic patients such as extreme digestive problems, severe allergies, severe heart and endocrine problems, and severe depressions.

Kelley perceived then two axes of metabolism, a horizontal axis for sympathetic and parasympathetic dominance, and a vertical axis for efficiency. He could plot his patient groups on a graph. They are summarized in Table 6.1.

Table 6.1. Kelley Metabolic Types—Numbered in the Order in Which He Identified Them

Metabolic Type	Sympathetic Efficiency (%)	Parasympathetic Efficiency (%)
1 Extreme Sympathetic Dominant	100	20
4 Moderate Sympathetic Dominant	70	30
6 Inefficient Sympathetic Dominant	30–40	20–30
2 Extreme Parasympathetic Dominant	20	100
5 Moderate Parasympathetic Dominant	30	70
7 Inefficient Parasympathetic Dominant	20–30	30–40
10 Highly Efficient Balanced	100	100
8 Moderately Efficient Balanced	80	80
9 Moderately Inefficient Balanced	50	50
3 Very Inefficient Balanced	10–20	10–20

Kelley outlined the dietary needs for each of the ten types in great detail. These dietary prescriptions developed out of his own clinical experience, long before he learned of Francis Pottenger's system of autonomic dominance.

Type 1 patients were the extreme sympathetic-dominant patients such as Dr. Kelley himself, who did best on a largely raw food, plant-based vegetarian diet. For these patients, Kelley recommended that at least 80 percent of the food be raw or at best very lightly steamed. The diet emphasized unlimited vegetables of all types, and at least a quart of freshly made vegetable juice a day. Though these patients tolerated all vegetables, Kelley learned that this group did especially well with dark leafy green vegetables, such as collards, carrot greens, dark romaine lettuce, and parsley. The diet also allowed unlimited fruit and recommended at least two to three servings a day. These patients did particularly well with citrus fruit.

Grains, because of the protein content, were a mainstay of the diet, and Kelley prescribed for the extreme sympathetic-dominant (vegetarian) patients two to four tablespoons of Mrs. Kelley's fourteen-grain cereal daily, along with unlimited whole-grain breads, brown rice, and raw sprouted grains. The diet included beans as well, either raw as sprouts or cooked. In fact, the diet included several servings of sprouted raw beans and grains daily because Kelley believed that sprouting increases the nutrient and enzyme content of foods such as beans, seeds, and grains. The diet allowed seeds and nuts, particularly almonds, which Kelley felt had an anticancer effect and which also provided a complete protein source.

Though plant foods provided most of the protein needed, Kelley found these extreme sympathetic patients did well with certain limited amounts of animal protein. He allowed a daily egg and a daily serving of freshly made yogurt. But fish, meat, and poultry were excluded from the diet.

Type 2 patients were extreme parasympathetic-dominant metabolizers, the type Kelley first identified in his young allergy patient. For optimal health, these patients required frequent servings of lightly cooked fatty red meat such as beef or lamb up to three times a day. Kelley suggested his extreme carnivore patients eat as much fat as possible and recommended for these patients organ meats such as liver and kidneys, and meaty soups and stews. Kelley did allow three to four daily servings of vegetables on this diet, chosen primarily from root vegetables including carrots, potatoes, sweet potatoes, turnips, and yams.

Kelley found these patients also did well with all types of squash as well as the cruciferous vegetables such as broccoli, Brussels sprouts, cabbage, and cauliflower. However, he learned from experience that carnivore patients did not tolerate leafy greens such as collards, escarole, lettuce, and parsley. The diet forbade all fruit except occasional servings of berries, and fruits such as apples and pears. Kelley allowed only minimal servings of grains, nuts, seeds, and beans as well.

Type 3 patients, the very inefficient balanced metabolizers, such as the young graduate student, did very well with a varied diet that included plant and animal sources of food. However, most if not all of their food needed to be cooked except for freshly made juices, which these patients seemed to tolerate. For these patients, raw salads, raw sprouts, and even raw fruit could not be effectively utilized.

The diet specifically recommended three to four servings of vegetables a day from all classes, including cruciferous vegetables, leafy greens, root vegetables, and squash. All fruits were allowed, but Kelley recommended much of the fruit be cooked such as in compotes, stewed fruit dishes, or baked apples. Freshly made fruit juice was acceptable; juicing, Kelley believed, had the same effect of cooking and enhanced nutrient availability for these very inefficient patients. Instead of whole nuts and seeds, Kelley recommended nut and seed butters, which again provided nutrients in a more easily assimilated form. The diet allowed unlimited amounts of whole-grain breads, cereals, and brown rice. These patients were to eat eggs daily, as much whole natural cheese and yogurt as desired, and several servings each of fish, poultry, and red meat weekly.

Type 4 patients, moderate sympathetic-dominant metabolizers, were not as extremely vegetarian as the Type 1 patients were. The moderate sympathetic-dominant diet allowed unlimited vegetables, fruits, nuts, seeds, and whole grains as did the extreme sympathetic-dominant diet, but a smaller proportion of the food needed to be raw, about 60 percent. Fish and poultry could be eaten several times each week, along with eggs and dairy products daily. But red meat needed to be restricted to no more than once a week.

Kelley next identified Type 5 patients, the moderate parasympathetic-dominant metabolizers, who required somewhat less red meat than the extreme parasympathetics. The moderate parasympathetic patients did best with one to two servings of fatty red meat a day, fewer servings of organ meats, and a more varied intake of vegetables—though the diet still forbade leafy greens. Moderate parasympathetics, like the extremes, did well with cruciferous and root vegetables. Patients could have a single serving of fruit a day, but again, no citrus. Additional fruit, particularly citrus, Kelley found, would interfere with the progress of the therapy.

The next category, Type 6 patients, were inefficient sympathetic-dominant metabolizers, who, like the Type 1 and Type 4 patients, did best with a primarily plant-based diet, allowing unlimited servings of all the vegetables and fruits. However, nearly all of the food needed to be cooked or taken, in the case of vegetables and fruits, as juices. For these patients, Kelley also recommended nut and seed butters, whole-grain breads and cereals, and brown rice. Patients could eat a moderate amount of animal protein, including eggs and whole-milk organic dairy products, and several servings of fish and poultry a week. Red meat could be eaten only occasionally. The diet emphasized frequent servings of soups and stews, which seemed to help these patients enormously.

Type 7 patients were inefficient parasympathetic-dominant patients, who, like the moderate parasympathetic patients, did well with one to two servings of fatty red meat daily and frequent servings of root vegetables, cruciferous vegetables, and squash, but mostly cooked. As with the other parasympathetic patients, the diet forbade leafy greens. Kelley recommended for these patients frequent servings of soups and heavy stews. Fruit could be eaten once a day, preferably cooked and not raw, but never citrus. The diet allowed cooked beans—as opposed to raw sprouted beans—and cooked grain products such as whole-grain breads and brown rice.

Type 8 patients, moderately efficient balanced metabolizers, like the very inefficient balanced Type 3 group, tolerated and did best with a wide variety of foods. Their diet included all types of vegetables and fruits, as well as nuts, seeds, and whole grains. They also did well with a variety of animal products such as daily servings of eggs and dairy foods, and several servings each week of fish, poultry, and red meat. For these patients, 50 to 60 percent of the food was to be raw, and 40 to 50 percent cooked.

Type 9 patients were moderately inefficient balanced metabolizers. These patients, like the other two balanced groups, did well with all types of foods. However, they required more of it in the cooked form than the Type 8 patients did, but less than for the Type 3 group. For the Type 9 patients, Kelley recommended 60 to 80 percent of the food be cooked.

The rarest type, according to Kelley, was the last type he identified, the Type 10 patients, the very efficient balanced metabolizers. Kelley believed this group made up no more than 3 percent of the US population. These patients did best, as did the other balanced patients, with a variety of foods chosen from all categories. For these patients, Kelley recommended mostly raw food and small meals.

Kelley claimed this group had a very efficient metabolism and could extract maximum nutritional benefit from even minimal amounts of food. These patients seemed so efficient in terms of their digestion and assimilation that they could even derive benefit from "junk food" and refined foods. Kelley rarely saw such patients in his practice because, he believed, they were so uncommon and usually didn't get sick until very late in life.

The dietary needs of Kelley's ten metabolic types are summarized in Table 6.2.

Table 6.2. Kelley Metabolic Types—Dietary Needs

Metabolic Type	Diet
1 Extreme Sympathetic Dominant	80 percent raw; plant based; unlimited fruit, grains, brown rice, seeds, nuts
4 Moderate Sympathetic Dominant	60 percent raw; unlimited fruit, vegetables, nuts, seeds, grains
6 Inefficient Sympathetic Dominant	mostly cooked; plant based; red meat occasionally; grains, cereals, rice
2 Extreme Parasympathetic Dominant	cooked fatty red meat; root vegetables; occasional fruit; no leafy greens
5 Moderate Parasympathetic Dominant	less fatty red meat than 2; root vegetables; some fruits—no citrus; no leafy greens
7 Inefficient Parasympathetic Dominant	less fatty red meat than 2; root vegetables—mostly cooked; some cooked grains and rice; no leafy greens
10 Highly Efficient Balanced	wide variety (3 percent of population)
8 Moderately Efficient Balanced	wide variety; 50 to 60 percent raw

Metabolic Type	Diet
9 Moderately Inefficient Balanced	wide variety; 20 to 40 percent raw
3 Very Inefficient Balanced	wide variety; mostly cooked

In addition to diet, Kelley prescribed for all his patients supplemental vitamins, minerals, trace elements, and enzymes. Eventually, again through trial and error in his practice, he identified how each of the dietary types responded to various nutrients. Extreme sympathetic-dominant metabolizers such as Kelley himself did best with very large doses of beta-carotene and certain B vitamins, particularly thiamine (B1), riboflavin (B2), niacin (B3), pyridoxine (B6), folic acid, and para-aminobenzoic acid. These patients also thrived on megadoses of vitamin C, fairly large doses of vitamin D, and moderate doses of vitamin E, but they did very poorly with vitamin A and with the B vitamins pantothenic acid, B12, choline, and inositol.

In terms of minerals, these extreme sympathetic-dominant (Type 1) patients did well with very large doses of magnesium and potassium but tended to do much worse with even small amounts of supplemental calcium. This group also required relatively large doses of the trace minerals chromium and manganese but did poorly with any amount of additional zinc.

The moderate sympathetic-dominant (Type 4) patients thrived with the same complement of vitamins and minerals as the extreme sympathetics, but in smaller, more moderate doses. The inefficient sympathetic-dominant (Type 6) patients did well, as did the extreme sympathetic dominants, with very large doses of beta-carotene, thiamine, riboflavin, niacin, pyridoxine, folic acid, and vitamins C and D, but also small doses of nutrients Kelley avoided with his extreme and moderate sympathetic patients, such as pantothenic acid, B12, choline, inositol, calcium, and zinc.

The extreme parasympathetic-dominant (Type 2) group did best with moderately large doses of vitamin A—but not beta-carotene—as well as the B vitamins niacinamide (a particular form of niacin), pantothenic acid, B12, choline, and inositol. This group required large doses of vitamin E but did not tolerate high doses of vitamin C, particularly as ascorbic acid; instead, they did best with moderate doses of the calcium salt of C, calcium ascorbate. The extreme parasympathetic patients worsened with even low doses of vitamin D. In terms of minerals, extreme parasympathetic patients functioned well with large doses of calcium but reacted very poorly—as had Kelley's young allergy patient—to even small amounts of magnesium and potassium. These patients benefited from relatively high doses of certain trace minerals such as zinc and selenium but required only small doses of chromium and manganese.

The moderate parasympathetic-dominant (Type 5) group required the same set of nutrients as did the extreme parasympathetics, but in more moderate doses. The inefficient parasympathetic (Type 7) patients required the same level of nutrients as the extreme parasympathetics did—moderate doses of A; high doses of the B vitamins pantothenic acid, B12, choline, and inositol; and large doses of calcium, selenium, and zinc. However, these inefficient parasympathetic patients also did best with at least small doses of the nutrients Kelley would avoid with his extreme and moderate parasympathetic patients, such as beta-carotene, thiamine, riboflavin, niacin, pyridoxine, folic acid, magnesium, and potassium.

The balanced metabolizers as a group did best with supplements containing the entire range of vitamins, minerals, and trace elements: beta-carotene and vitamin A; all the B vitamins, including thiamine, riboflavin, niacin, niacinamide, pantothenic acid, pyridoxine, PABA, folic acid, B12, choline, and inositol; vitamins C, D, and E; the minerals calcium, magnesium, and potassium; and the trace elements chromium, manganese, selenium, and zinc.

However, for balanced metabolizers, the doses varied considerably, depending on the proportion of raw or cooked food in the diet. For the more efficient types 10 and 8, Kelley prescribed respectively low to moderate doses of the various nutrients. The inefficient types 9 and 3, however, required far greater doses. The Type 3 very inefficient balanced metabolizers required more than double the doses of all the nutrients, as did the most efficient Type 10 patients.

Table 6.3. Kelley Metabolic Types—Supplementation Needs

Metabolic Type	Supplements
1 Extreme Sympathetic Dominant	beta-carotene, B1, B2, B3, B6; vitamins C and D high dose; vitamin E moderate dose; magnesium, potassium, chromium, magnesium; para-aminobenzoic acid
4 Moderate Sympathetic Dominant	same as 1 but more moderate doses
6 Inefficient Sympathetic Dominant	same as 4; add B5, B12, choline, inositol, calcium, zinc
2 Extreme Parasympathetic Dominant	moderate doses vitamin A; niacinamide; B5, B12; choline, inositol; vitamin C high dose; zinc, selenium, high dose; chromium, manganese moderate dose
5 Moderate Parasympathetic Dominant	same as 2 but more moderate doses
7 Inefficient Parasympathetic Dominant	same as 5 but add beta-carotene, thiamine, riboflavin, niacin, pyridoxine, folic acid, magnesium, and potassium
10 Highly Efficient Balanced	full range of supplements and minerals—low to moderate doses
8 Moderately Efficient Balanced	same as 10
9 Moderately Inefficient Balanced	same as 8 and 10 but higher doses
3 Very Inefficient Balanced	same as 8 and 10 but double the dosages

CHAPTER VII:

The Biochemistry of Food

Pottenger spent years investigating the effects of certain nutrients, particularly calcium, magnesium, and potassium, on autonomic function, but his research never really went far beyond these three minerals. And Pottenger had never considered the effect of different types of diet (such as a vegetarian or high-meat diet) on autonomic function. But by the early 1970s, Kelley knew through his work with patients that the sympathetic dominants described by Pottenger did best, whatever their underlying health problem might be, on a largely plant-based, vegetarian-type diet and did terribly with animal protein. The more extremely sympathetic dominant a patient was, the more vegetarian the diet needed to be.

Parasympathetic-dominant patients, Kelley knew from experience, did best with a high-animal protein, high-fat diet, with fatty red meat sometimes recommended three times a day. This group tolerated only minimal to moderate amounts of plant-based foods and did very poorly with leafy greens and citrus fruit. Again, the more strongly parasympathetic dominant a patient was, the more meat the patient needed to eat.

And the balanced metabolizers fell midway between the extremes of sympathetic and parasympathetic dominance. Such patients did best, Kelley discovered, with a varied diet allowing all types of foods from both plant and animal sources.

Kelley began evaluating the various diets he prescribed, in terms of their nutritional content and the effect of these various diets on autonomic function. Kelley knew that a vegetarian diet providing large amounts of fresh fruits and vegetables, particularly leafy greens, contains large doses of certain minerals such as magnesium and potassium. It is magnesium, for example, that gives the green color to leafy greens. Of course, decades earlier, Pottenger had shown that magnesium suppresses sympathetic function, while potassium stimulates parasympathetic activity. Such a diet is also rich in the essential trace minerals chromium and manganese; certain B vitamins including thiamin, niacinamide, pyridoxine, and folic acid (the word *folate* is from the Latin meaning "leafy"); and other nutrients such as beta-carotene and vitamin C. Kelley believed that all these nutrients, whatever else they might do in the body, directly served to either suppress sympathetic tone or stimulate the parasympathetic system into action.

Kelley also believed a vegetarian diet had a profound effect on acid-base balance. Kelley had already learned that his sympathetic-dominant patients tended to be acidic in terms of the environment of their tissues and organs, and this extra acidity promoted sympathetic dominance. He also knew that a largely vegetarian diet is very alkalinizing, and in an alkaline environment, he proposed, sympathetic activity diminishes and parasympathetic activity increases.

When Kelley first suggested in the 1970s that an alkalinizing vegetarian diet might suppress sympathetic and activate parasympathetic function, his ideas were ignored by both orthodox and alternative practitioners. In recent years, however, research studies have confirmed what Kelley claimed thirty years ago. Much of the research relating acid-base balance to sympathetic function comes from the world of cardiovascular physiology and the emergency room treatment of heart attacks. During a heart attack, the heart loses its ability to pump blood efficiently. As a result, waste material such as lactic acid backs up in the blood system. In this situation, the body quickly can become severely acidotic, and this excessively acid state can poison cellular metabolism. Generations of residents were taught that when a patient arrives in the emergency room with a heart attack, assume acidosis and begin administering the antacid bicarbonate in large amounts intravenously to neutralize the presumably dangerous acid.

Though bicarbonate administration had been an accepted part of the lore of medical care for heart attacks, it was not until the 1990s that scientists evaluated this treatment approach in a carefully controlled way. To the dismay of the cardiology world, which for decades had assumed the benefit of this alkalinizing therapy for heart attacks, the studies showed that the overuse of bicarbonate could suppress sympathetic activity to the point that the system could literally shut down. When the sympathetic nerves feeding the heart turn off, wild and often fatal heart rhythm disturbances can occur. Indeed, such experiences have taught us that an alkaline environment does suppress sympathetic function, and in extreme cases, this can lead to disastrous consequences. Kelley appears to have been correct several decades earlier when he claimed an acid tissue environment stimulates, and an alkaline environment suppresses, sympathetic activity.

Kelley also believed—although he didn't know how at the time—that a vegetarian diet also affects levels of neurotransmitters in the brain that control autonomic function. Neurotransmitters are the basic molecules released by nerve endings that produce the desired effect of the nerve—either stimulation of another adjacent nerve, contraction of a muscle cell, or release of a hormone from a gland. In the brain, the release of neurotransmitters allows us to think, to remember, to feel emotion. These molecules allow the nervous system to work.

Scientists have identified several dozen neurotransmitters, and they represent quite a varied group. Some, such as the endorphins and enkephalins, which block pain and produce pleasurable sensations, are morphine-like peptides, protein fragments from larger, parent proteins. Some, such as glutamic acid and glycine, which respectively stimulate and suppress neurons in the brain, are amino acids from dietary sources.

Sympathetic nerves produce two main neurotransmitters, norepinephrine and epinephrine, manufactured from the amino acids phenylalanine and tyrosine. The brain makes serotonin, a major parasympathetic stimulant, from the amino acid tryptophan, and parasympathetic nerves produce their main neurotransmitter, acetylcholine, from the B vitamin choline.

Recently, investigators found that in laboratory animals, a largely plant-based, vegetarian diet increases brain levels of both serotonin and acetylcholine, while reducing norepinephrine and epinephrine. In effect, as Kelley believed thirty years ago, a vegetarian diet—at least in a laboratory model—will suppress sympathetic, and stimulate parasympathetic, activity.

So Kelley learned, through trial and error, that the specific nutrients contained in a vegetarian diet, such as magnesium, potassium, chromium, manganese, pyridoxine, and folic acid, reduce sympathetic activity and stimulate the parasympathetic system. Additionally, through its alkalinizing effect and its impact on levels of the neurotransmitters serotonin and acetylcholine, a plant-based diet further suppresses sympathetic and increases parasympathetic firing. Such a diet can help bring the imbalanced autonomic system of a sympathetic dominant into balance. Kelley, like Pottenger before him, believed a balanced autonomic nervous system led to health.

In contrast to a vegetarian diet, a meat diet contains little magnesium and potassium, but large amounts of the minerals phosphorus and zinc and certain vitamins such as vitamin A; the B vitamins pantothenic acid, inositol, and B12; and vitamin E. And although meat itself does not contain much calcium, Kelley recommended for his carnivore patients bone products such as bone meal or fish soups with bone, as well as supplemental calcium, which he felt should accompany a meat diet. Overall, Kelley claimed, the predominant nutrients present in a meat-based diet, such as calcium and phosphorus, suppressed parasympathetic activity and stimulated sympathetic function.

Red meat is loaded with sulfates and phosphates that in the body are quickly converted into free acids such as phosphoric and sulfuric acids. Physiologists have known for years that one of the quickest ways to acidify the bloodstream is to eat meat. And this acid load in turn stimulates the sympathetic nervous system while suppressing parasympathetic activity.

Furthermore, a meat-based diet contains large amounts of the amino acids phenylalanine and tyrosine, precursors to the sympathetic neurotransmitters norepinephrine and epinephrine. Scientists have recently found in laboratory animals that meat will increase blood and brain levels of phenylalanine and tyrosine, and brain levels of both norepinephrine and epinephrine. In turn, sympathetic activity increases.

Overall, a high-meat diet, loaded with nutrients such as phosphorus and zinc, inositol and B12, the acid-forming sulfates and phosphates, and the neurotransmitter precursors phenylalanine and tyrosine, will reduce parasympathetic activity and stimulate sympathetic firing. This diet can help bring the imbalanced autonomic system of a parasympathetic metabolizer into balance. And in the Kelley model, such balance produced health.

The balanced metabolizer diets provide a wide variety of both plant and animal foods and, in turn, the full spectrum of vitamins, minerals, and trace elements as well as proteins, fats, and carbohydrates, with no particular nutrient present in extreme doses. Such a broad diet includes moderate amounts of the fat-soluble vitamins A, D, E, K, and beta-carotene, along with all the B vitamins such as thiamin, riboflavin, niacin, niacinamide, pantothenic acid, pyridoxine, PABA, folic acid, B12, choline, and inositol. The balanced diet also provides moderate doses of all the minerals including calcium, phosphorus, magnesium, potassium, boron, chromium, cobalt, manganese, selenium, and zinc. In effect, a balanced type of diet contains a range of nutrients that stimulate and suppress both sympathetic and parasympathetic activity. The end result is that both branches of the autonomic system tend to stay in balance, with neither system dominant.

In addition, the balanced diets contain both alkalinizing nutrients such as magnesium and acid-forming nutrients including the phosphates and sulfates. As a result, these diets stimulate production of the sympathetic neurotransmitters norepinephrine and epinephrine, as well as the parasympathetic neurotransmitters serotonin and acetylcholine. This balance in nutrients, in acid-base levels, and in neurotransmitter chemistry prevents either the sympathetic or the parasympathetic system from becoming overly dominating.

Kelley also began to understand more clearly why different types of patients reacted so badly to certain foods. His sympathetic patients reported feeling worse—more stimulated, angry, and irritable, with more digestive problems—after eating red meat. Red meat would only push the already strong sympathetic system into greater activity.

And Kelley could explain the intolerance to leafy greens and citrus reported by his parasympathetic patients. These two foods are loaded with magnesium and potassium and have a very alkalinizing effect on the body, an effect that would push them into greater parasympathetic dominance and worsen problems such as depression and allergies.

Kelley once used the analogy that humans are as variable as animals, for example, cows and bulls compared with lions and tigers. Cows, of course—and bulls—are pure vegetarian, growing and thriving on diets consisting of little more than grass and grains. When you think about it, it is quite a feat for a small calf the size of a dog to grow to a thousand-pound bull, eating rather delicate grass and grains. But cows and bulls have a stomach, a digestive system, a metabolism, a biochemistry, and a physiology uniquely suited for plant foods.

Cows and bulls do very well indeed eating grass, and there isn't a dairy farmer who traditionally would have thought of raising his cow herds on anything but lush grass and grain. Feed a cow nothing but red meat, I have been told, and it will live no longer than several weeks. And add only some animal products to the mixture, even in small quantities—which agri-scientists have tried—and you are asking for trouble, such as mad cows and mad cow disease.

Lions and tigers, of course, in nature eat nothing but red meat, as often and as much as they can catch, and to my knowledge do not cut away the fat. Lions and tigers have a digestive system, a metabolism, a biochemistry, and a physiology uniquely suited for meat. They use protein, fat, and even cholesterol very efficiently. Lions and tigers on their all-meat diet do not suffer cholesterol problems or heart disease or chest pain from too much fat. And if anyone doubts how strong an animal can grow on an all-meat diet, I only suggest one think about climbing into a cage with a lion.

I have read that a lion or tiger will last some six weeks at most eating a grass and grain diet. During the 1920s, when zoos in the United States began to expand and include expensive large cats in their displays, zookeepers tried to feed their prize lions and tigers grains, to cut down expenses. The results were disastrous, and no zookeeper since would think of risking an expensive showcase lion by feeding it a bale of hay. It won't work. Lions and tigers need red meat, raw meat, as much as they want, and they stay healthy and happy with meat.

Kelley used another analogy I always liked. Nutrition, he said, is the fuel that makes the body machine run. Put the perfect fuel in, and the machine runs fine; put in the wrong fuel, and the engine breaks down. And humans, he said, taking the engine analogy a step further, are as variable as Mercedes Benzes and steam engines. With top-quality diesel fuel, a $100,000 Mercedes will run smoothly and efficiently, as it was meant to run. Put distilled water into the tank, and you've just wrecked your engine. However, put diesel fuel into a steam engine, and it's going to explode. With water in the tank, a steam generator runs perfectly fine.

Kelley looked at the autonomic nervous system, and its two branches, as the basic engine, the basic driving system, that ran the body. And though of course humans aren't Mercedes Benzes or steam engines—or lions or bulls, either—we need to look at food as fuel. Without the right fuel, the human engine, the autonomic nervous system, isn't going to work efficiently, and disease is going to occur.

In the Kelley model, as long as we put the right fuel into our bodies by eating the right food for our metabolic type, the autonomic system will be in balance, both branches and the associated organs and glands will function efficiently, the body will work beautifully, and our health will be ideal. However, with the wrong fuel, the autonomic system will go out of balance, it will function less efficiently, the organs and glands will not work well together, and disease follows.

CHAPTER VIII:

The Anthropology of Metabolic Types

Pottenger, in his writings, did not speculate about why different autonomic types should exist. Kelley, however, thought about this question at length and came to believe that the ten metabolic types he had observed were the end product of ecological selection pressures. Each type developed, he believed, in a very distinctive environment, with a physiological makeup ideally suited to the available food supply. He thought, for example, that the sympathetic dominants originated in the countries bordering the Mediterranean, such as Italy, Greece, Spain, the Middle East, and Northern Africa, particularly the areas known historically as the Fertile Crescent of the Tigris and Euphrates rivers.

The Mediterranean and Fertile Crescent regions are notable for a generally mild climate, a long growing season, and fertile soils allowing for a complex agriculture. Here, agriculture as we know it today first began: the land provided a rich supply of grains, vegetables, fruits, nuts, seeds, and dairy products from goats, cattle, and sheep. The large rivers and the Mediterranean Sea served as a source of fish.

The parasympathetic dominants were more northern people, inhabiting the colder regions of Europe, Asia, and the Americas, in climates of extreme cold, long winters, and only a brief growing season. These people survived and thrived on a meat-based diet and only occasionally consumed plant foods. Some "parasympathetic" groups, such as the Eskimos, flourished for generations on a virtually all-meat diet providing no plant products whatsoever.

The balanced types lived in the middle latitude regions of the continents, in ecosystems distinguished by four seasons and a diversity of both fauna and flora. People of these latitudes had access to a great variety of foods, including meat products, fish, nuts, seeds, grains, roots, and fruits. Their diet fell somewhere between the sympathetic and parasympathetic extremes.

For generations, Dr. Kelley believed, the various types lived largely in isolation, separated by natural boundaries and great distances. In today's world, of course, this ecological seclusion no longer holds true. In a country such as the United States, particularly, Dr. Kelley identified all three groups and the various subtypes living together side by side. Because of such mingling and inevitable interbreeding, a certain mixing of genes has occurred.

The anthropological literature clearly supports Kelley's claim that different groups of humans adjusted quite effectively to different types of diets. Perhaps the most definitive documentation comes from the work of the dentist and anthropologist Dr. Weston Price, particularly his classic book *Nutrition and Physical Degeneration*, first published in 1939. Price, like Pottenger, is well known in alternative medical circles, though still ignored by the academic medical mainstream. The books of Drs. Price and Pottenger are both available from the Price Pottenger Foundation in San Diego. The book *Traditional Foods Are Your Best Medicine* by the naturopath Dr. Ronald Schmid contains a nice summary of Dr. Price's life and work.

Born in Canada in 1870, Price graduated from dental school in 1893. Early in his practice, he observed that his younger patients suffered significantly more dental caries and crowded, crooked teeth, along with other health problems such as allergies, than their parents and grandparents. He began to suspect that some change in dietary habits explained the trend. He noticed in his younger patients a shift from the largely unrefined, unprocessed diet of fresh plant and animal foods—the rich American "farm" diet of their parents and grandparents—to a diet with more modern foods—white sugar, refined grain products, refined fats and oils, and canned goods rather than fresh.

Price suspected that this "modern" diet lacked certain nutritional factors that might explain the health problems in the younger generation of his patients. He then decided to perform a very unusual study. For seven years, from 1931 until 1938, he and his wife traveled the world seeking out groups of people on all inhabited continents still living on their traditional diets. His travels led him from mountain valleys in the high Swiss Alps, to the Outer Hebrides of Scotland, to the Eskimos still living the hunter's life, to the Masai in Africa, to Peruvian Indians in the high Andes, to the Maori of New Zealand.

He assessed their teeth but also their overall health. He then compared these groups with people of the same culture living on the foods of civilization—refined grains, sugars, and canned and processed foods. He systematically categorized the health and disease levels of each group, often with the help of local medical personnel.

Price made several basic observations, explained in great detail in his classic book. First, he found that traditional human groups subsisted and thrived on a variety of diets ranging from the pure meat and fish diet of the Eskimos, with no plant foods, to the largely cow blood and milk diet of the Masai, to the seafood, root, and fruit diet of the Polynesians. Price realized, throughout his travels, that no traditional group lived on an exclusively plant-based diet; all these groups, even those with access to plant foods, included at least some animal products in their diets.

Most significantly, Price also discovered that as long as these groups followed their traditional diets of natural foods, they enjoyed excellent health. In all traditional populations, from the Eskimos to the Polynesians, he found virtually no cavities, a perfect dental arch with no crowded teeth, and virtually no degenerative diseases. He met one physician who in thirty years tending to Indians and Eskimos in Northern Canada had never seen a single case of cancer in those following their ancestral diet. However, as soon as members of these cultures incorporated civilized foods into their eating such as white sugar and refined grain products, their health deteriorated.

In such people, Price documented rampant levels of the diseases of civilization such as diabetes, heart disease, and cancer. Their children suffered malformed dental arches and large numbers of dental caries. Though Price's findings created enormous controversy when first published, his lengthy book is filled with photographs comparing the dental arches and teeth of those people following a traditional diet to those eating civilized foods. The pictures and documentation are impressive.

Price's exhaustive experiment in nature can never be repeated. The isolated groups he found around the world seventy years ago, following traditional natural diets, no longer exist. The civilized way of eating has invaded even the remotest parts of the remotest continents.

Other scientists working during the first half of the twentieth century confirmed what Price had discovered. One of the most colorful of these was the adventurous American anthropologist Vilhjalmur Stefansson. Of Scandinavian descent, Stefansson grew up on a ranch in North Dakota during the closing decades of the nineteenth century. His childhood was spent in the plains and mountains of the American West, surrounded by wilderness and wildlife.

After graduating from the University of North Dakota, Stefansson studied anthropology at Harvard. Restless with the confines of academic life, he decided he really wanted to go into the field—the remoter and more untouched by civilization, the better. After some thought, in 1905 he chose to visit and live with the Mackenzie River Eskimos of the Canadian Arctic, a group who at the time had rarely interacted with whites or their "civilization." In fact, when Stefansson first went to the Arctic Circle, no scientist had ever spent any time among these northern peoples. The academic Western world knew, in fact, very little about the Eskimo.

Between 1905 and 1915, for ten full years, Stefansson lived with Eskimos who still followed their traditional hunter life. Of all the aspects of Eskimo life, their diet most perplexed Stefansson when he first arrived in the Arctic. Eskimos, Stefansson quickly learned, lived on nothing but fatty red meat and fatty fish. The diet included no fruits, no vegetables, no nuts, no seeds, and no grains. This shouldn't have been surprising, because the Arctic Circle region is subjected to the most extreme climate on Earth, with a ten-month winter, a two-month summer, and a soil unsuitable for agriculture as we know it.

Quite simply, in the Arctic Circle region where Stefansson came to live and work, there were no fruits, no vegetables, no nuts, no seeds, and no grains to eat. Plant life is limited to lichens, shrubs, and flowering plants that can quickly grow and bloom during the brief summer. But the lichens on land, and the rich plankton populations in the sea, form the basis of a complex ecosystem and food chain that supports large populations of vertebrates such as polar bears and caribou on land, and whales, seals, sea lions, and fish in the sea. The only foods available to the Eskimos were these fish and animals, and this is what they ate.

Early on in his sojourn, Stefansson calculated that the Eskimo diet was actually a high-fat diet, consisting of approximately 80 percent fat and 20 percent protein. The Eskimos told Stefansson that an all-meat diet with less fat would make them sick, that the diet required such a high fat content for optimal health and strength. They knew precisely how to plan their eating to obtain these proportions, but such proportions went against everything Stefansson had learned in his biology courses at Harvard. First, he had been taught that no human could live on an all-animal food diet, that carbohydrates and sugars were necessary to produce energy in our cells. Furthermore, by the turn of the last century, academic scientists already perceived fat as being toxic to the human body, and Stefansson went to the Arctic believing no human could survive on a diet containing more than 40 to 50 percent fat.

Yet here was a group of humans surviving in one of the most rigorous environments on Earth, on an all-meat diet consisting of mostly fat. Not only did the Eskimos survive on such a diet, but they seemed to thrive. Stefansson observed that as a group the traditional Eskimos enjoyed excellent health, with none of the degenerative disease already epidemic in Western society such as cancer, diabetes, and heart disease.

The personality of the Eskimo particularly impressed Stefansson. Though they lived a difficult life in one of the most isolated, harshest regions of the world, they seemed to him perpetually happy and at peace with their world. As Stefansson documented in his books, they lived in a cohesive and cooperative society, centered on the family unit. The Eskimos didn't even have a word for depression; they did understand mourning, after the death of a loved one, but not clinical depression as described by Stefansson. They thought the idea of unhappiness for no reason preposterous.

Stefansson himself originally arrived in the Arctic Circle with a limited supply of provisions in the form of packaged and canned goods. He expected to have his stores replaced yearly by visiting ships. However, when the supplies were late in arriving after his first year, he reluctantly went on the Eskimo diet and eventually lived on an all-meat, high-fat diet for most of his ten years in the Arctic.

After he returned to the United States in 1915, he documented his experiences with the Eskimos in more than fifteen books that made him rich, very famous, and a much-sought-after lecturer. But when Stefansson first wrote of the Eskimo diet, and the good health enjoyed by the Eskimo, fellow academicians and scientists attacked his writings as fraudulent. Civilized academic scientists knew that no human could live on an all-meat diet, especially a high-fat diet, and they discounted Stefansson as a huckster, a charlatan, an adventurer with a vivid imagination. To Stefansson, the attacks from the armchair scientists who had never been to the Arctic seemed bizarre, particularly because common sense would dictate the Eskimos had no food available but fatty red meat.

However, some scientists did take Stefansson seriously. Finally, after years of debate, in 1926, Stefansson and a colleague from his expeditions agreed to go into a locked ward at Bellevue Hospital in New York under the direction of a group of eminent scientists from Cornell University Medical College and other institutions. In that locked ward, under close supervision, he and his associate would live on an all-meat, 80 percent fat diet. The project generated extensive debate and media attention, and scientists predicted Stefansson would last no more than a week or two on such a diet.

However, after two months, Stefansson was thriving on a diet consisting of large quantities of organ meats such as liver and brains, fatty steaks, and bacon. At that point, the scientists agreed to let Stefansson return to his apartment in New York, though he continued to live on an all-meat diet for the full year as he had promised. Periodically, he returned to Bellevue for evaluations, which all confirmed the excellent state of his health. His cholesterol during this time ran in the range of 130–150, a level surprising to all involved.

The scientists in charge of the project eventually published a series of papers in the major peer-reviewed medical journals documenting their observations of Stefansson and his Eskimo diet. Stefansson published his own version of the adventure at Bellevue, as well as his earlier adventures with the meat diet among his Eskimo friends, in his book *Not by Bread Alone*, published in 1949.

Spurred on by Stefansson's claims, between 1929 and 1934, McGill University Medical School sent a group of researchers to the Arctic to study the traditional Eskimos and their diet. As Stefansson had claimed, the scientists found that indeed the Eskimos lived on an all-meat, high-fat diet and enjoyed excellent health. Among this group, the McGill team could find little evidence of cancer, diabetes, or heart disease. However, as soon as the Eskimos settled in the white towns and adopted a Western diet with less fat, dominated by processed and refined foods, white refined sugar, sodas, alcohol, and processed fats, their health quickly deteriorated. Even during Stefansson's time, the health of Eskimos living among Westerners was already in critical decline.

Kelley found in the writings of people such as Price and Stefansson support for what he had observed in his own practice, that humans varied greatly in their dietary and nutritional needs. One size, indeed, did not fit all.

More recent investigations have confirmed what Price and Stefansson described. In an article entitled "Paleolithic Nutrition" appearing in the January 31, 1985 issue (312 [5]: 283–89) of *The New England Journal of Medicine*, Drs. S. Boyd Eaton and Melvin Konner reviewed more recent attempts to analyze the eating habits of "primitive" peoples around the world. They reported great variation in the composition of traditional, non-Western diets, ranging from the plant-based diet of the hunter-gatherers in Africa and Australia, with only 20 percent of the food derived from animal sources, to the near-total meat diet of the traditional Eskimos, with virtually no plant-based food. Interestingly, they describe no pure vegetarian groups anywhere.

CHAPTER IX:

Why People Get Sick

In Kelley's model, as long as we follow the appropriate diet for our type, our autonomic nervous system will be in balance, and our health will be ideal. However, Dr. Kelley proposed this balance can be disrupted in a number of ways. We can follow the "right" diet for our type but use refined, synthetic, or otherwise nutrient-depleted foods—the types of foods Price warned of sixty years ago.

An extreme sympathetic dominant might be on a plant-based diet but rely on vigorously cooked canned fruits and vegetables instead of raw, fresh produce and refined white flour products instead of natural whole grains. He or she might consume large amounts of white sugar daily, instead of natural sugars from fruits. A parasympathetic might be on a meat diet but consume processed, chemically treated meat, from animals raised with hormones, antibiotics, and less-than-optimal feed. The proportions and amounts of many nutrients, Kelley claimed, will differ considerably from the proportions and amounts in meat raised under more natural growth conditions.

In these two cases, metabolic equilibrium cannot be maintained, or even attained. Over time, both the strong and weak branches of the autonomic system will deteriorate. This decline may be gradual, but according to Dr. Kelley, it will inevitably occur.

We might also follow a diet suitable for another metabolic type. A sympathetic dominant might eat red meat two or three times a day; a parasympathetic might become a vegetarian. In this situation, we provide our bodies with excess amounts of those nutrients that support the strong system and further suppress the weak. Autonomic imbalance only worsens.

Dr. Kelley recognized gradations of "wrong" diet. Many people follow the right diet for their type some of the time, and alternate wholesome with nutrient-depleted foods. Overall, the more we stray from the ideal diet, the further we move from metabolic equilibrium. If the imbalance is not corrected with proper nutrition, overt disease can develop.

Dr. Kelley associated very specific symptoms and illnesses with each of the three types as they move through autonomic inefficiency and autonomic imbalance. A sympathetic-dominant patient following a plant-based diet but eating nutrient-depleted, refined, synthetic foods will gradually become less and less efficient, declining along the vertical efficiency axis. Both the sympathetic and the parasympathetic systems deteriorate, with the sympathetic always somewhat stronger.

Such patients initially experience emotional ups and downs and a lack of endurance. They might develop chronic indigestion, heartburn, and esophageal reflux because of declining parasympathetic function. As they become more inefficient, Kelley claimed, these sympathetic patients suffer severe mood swings, significantly diminished endurance and energy, and worsening chronic digestive problems. They become victims of frequent bacterial infections. Illness such as diabetes, rheumatoid arthritis, ulcers, and migraine headaches can occur.

Sympathetic-dominant patients who follow a high-red-meat diet will be pushed into stronger sympathetic dominance, with weaker parasympathetic activity, and their symptoms and problems correlate with this worsening autonomic imbalance. Initially, patients might experience impulsive behavior, mild anxiety, mild insomnia from overproduction of adrenaline, and mild constipation. As they move into stronger sympathetic dominance, these individuals can suffer chronic anxiety, irritability and temper outbursts, severe insomnia, and severe constipation. As the sympathetic system turns on full bore, they can develop dangerously high blood pressure and strokes and fatal cardiac arrhythmias.

A parasympathetic dominant who follows a high-red meat but nutrient-deficient diet will, like the sympathetic patient on depleted foods, tend to collapse along the vertical efficiency axis. Initially, such patients develop persistent weakness and fatigue, particularly severe in the morning, associated with depression and a lack of motivation and ambition. Sex drive and sexual function become significantly affected. These parasympathetic patients often develop frequent viral infections, such as persistent herpes or chronic Epstein-Barr. As they deteriorate still further, the parasympathetics suffer chronic exhaustion, poor concentration and memory, and suicidal depressions. In the final stages of decline, severe hypoglycemia, osteoarthritis, congestive heart failure, and massive heart attacks can occur.

A parasympathetic dominant who follows a largely plant-based diet will be pushed further into parasympathetic dominance, and corresponding sympathetic weakness, along the horizontal axis. Initially, these individuals might experience an increased need for sleep, allergies, mild asthma, and low-grade chronic diarrhea. As they move further into parasympathetic dominance, such patients require even more sleep; they experience debilitating asthma and allergies and chronic skin conditions such as eczema and psoriasis. They often become obese due to weakening sympathetic and thyroid function and can develop lupus and other autoimmune diseases because of strong parasympathetic stimulation of the immune system.

Patients born with a balanced autonomic system can experience syndromes associated with either sympathetic or parasympathetic decline. Such individuals who follow a varied diet but eat nutrient-depleted foods decline vertically, along the efficiency axis. They can experience problems associated with both sympathetic and parasympathetic failure, such as mood swings, diminished endurance, chronic indigestion, bacterial infections, diabetes, fatigue, depression, weak sex drive, chronic viral infections, hypoglycemia, and heart attacks. Balanced patients following a largely meat-based diet can move into sympathetic dominance and develop problems identified with an overly strong sympathetic system including anxiety, irritability, insomnia, and constipation. A balanced patient following a strongly vegetarian diet can be pushed into parasympathetic dominance and develop chronic sleepiness even after a full night's sleep, allergies, asthma, skin problems such as psoriasis, and autoimmune diseases.

In his model, Dr. Kelley described the pathophysiology of cancer in particular detail. From his experience with thousands of cancer patients, Kelley associated the common "hard tumors," the malignancies of the internal organs such as lung or colon cancer, with sympathetic nervous system dominance.

Kelley agreed with Beard that primitive trophoblast cells, holdovers from our fetal development, lie dormant in every tissue and organ in our bodies. Kelley believed these trophoblast cells—or what more contemporary scientists would call stem cells—were not in tissues by random chance, but served to replace damaged or defective cells. However, as Beard had said decades earlier, control of trophoblast (stem cell) growth required adequate amounts of pancreatic enzymes. In a situation of enzyme deficiency, the stem cells could grow uncontrollably and without direction; they could become cancer cells.

Researchers as far back as Pottenger knew that the sympathetic nervous system, when active, suppresses the production and release of pancreatic enzymes. In general, sympathetic-dominant patients in the Kelley model will have a weak, inefficient pancreas, incapable of a large enzyme output. Furthermore, the sympathetic system, when active, creates an acidic environment in the blood, the intracellular fluids, and the cells and tissues. Pancreatic enzymes, however, work most efficiently in an alkaline environment: acidity inhibits their activation and function. If sympathetic dominants follow the wrong diet for their type and ingest considerable red meat, the nutrients in the meat, as well as its acid-forming effect, will further turn on the sympathetic system, turn off the pancreas, and reduce the manufacture and release of the pancreatic enzymes needed to protect against cancer.

To make things even more serious, a high-protein–high-meat diet requires large amounts of pancreatic proteolytic enzymes for digestion, making them less available for cancer surveillance. And the acidic environment will suppress what few enzymes make their way into the bloodstream. Kelley believed that a sympathetic dominant on a high-protein diet was inviting disaster and was at risk of developing one of the classic hard tumors, such as cancer of the breast, lung, stomach, colon, prostate, uterus, or ovaries.

Parasympathetic dominants, according to Dr. Kelley, have a durable, efficient pancreas capable of producing copious amounts of all the digestive enzymes. Furthermore, in their bloodstream and tissue spaces, these patients run on the alkaline side, ideal for proteolytic enzyme activity. Consequently, this type tends to be protected against the hard "sympathetic" malignancies. But parasympathetics, despite an abundance of circulating enzymes, are susceptible to the soft tumors; these are the cancers of the white blood cells of the immune system, including leukemias, lymphomas, Hodgkin's disease, and multiple myeloma.

Kelley believed thirty years ago that the parasympathetic nervous system activates many aspects of immune function, a hypothesis now confirmed by more conventional physiologists. Scientists have identified receptors for acetylcholine and serotonin, the main parasympathetic neurotransmitters, on cells in the thymus and spleen, the two major immune organs. Furthermore, lymphocytes, one of the major families of immune cells that produce antibodies to protect against viral, bacterial, and fungal infection, have on their cell membranes receptors for these parasympathetic neurotransmitters. They also release a host of cytokines—chemical messengers that serve to activate a cascade of immune reactions.

In the Kelley model, parasympathetic dominants have an efficient, strong immune system. If a parasympathetic patient follows the wrong diet for the type, such as a largely plant-based diet, the parasympathetic system can turn on even more strongly. A vegetarian diet, as we have seen, is rich in nutrients such as magnesium and potassium and B vitamins such as thiamine and B6, which suppress sympathetic and stimulate parasympathetic activity. Plant foods also tend to be alkalinizing and raise the levels of the parasympathetic neurotransmitters.

All this is guaranteed to increase parasympathetic function. If parasympathetic firing becomes too strong and too dominant, the immune system can go out of control and malignancies such as leukemia and lymphoma can result. In these patients, effective treatment requires that the parasympathetic system be turned down; pancreatic enzymes alone will not control these immune cancers. Sympathetic dominants, however, have a weak parasympathetic and, in turn, weak immune system. Consequently, they rarely develop these types of malignancies.

In general, balanced metabolizers develop cancer much less frequently than either the sympathetic or the parasympathetic types. But if they follow the wrong diet for their type, these individuals can end up with either the hard sympathetic or the immune parasympathetic tumors. A balanced individual who follows a largely animal protein, animal fat diet is at risk of becoming too acid and too sympathetic dominant. In such a situation, hard tumors can result. A balanced metabolizer on a strict plant-based vegetarian diet, however, can end up over time too alkaline and too parasympathetic dominant, and prone to the parasympathetic immune cancers such as leukemia and lymphoma.

Interestingly, twenty years ago Kelley warned that the near-universal promotion of low-fat, low-animal-protein diets emphasizing fruits, vegetables, whole grains, and other plant-based foods as the "healthy diet" for all humans would lead to an increase in lymphomas and leukemias. Well-meaning parasympathetic metabolizers who follow such a diet will only push themselves into being more alkaline and more parasympathetic dominant; balanced patients on a vegetarian diet could also end up too alkaline and parasympathetic dominant. With a national trend away from red meat and toward more alkalinizing plant-based foods, an increase in parasympathetic immune system cancers would be, in the Kelley model, inevitable. Such an increase has occurred, to the confusion and consternation of more orthodox researchers.

So, by the careful use of diet, Kelley claimed that he was able to effect major changes in autonomic function and bring about balance in a dysfunctional nervous system. Further, as the autonomic system comes into greater harmony and balance, when the autonomic branches are equally strong, all systems—from immunity to cardiovascular function—work better regardless of the underlying problem. In terms of cancer specifically, long experience had taught Kelley that it was not enough to load patients with pancreatic enzymes to achieve optimal results. Enzymes alone might work sometimes, but Kelley believed that by using diet and nutrients to manipulate autonomic function, his success with patients improved dramatically.

Part II:
Some Science

CHAPTER X:

Digestion, the Pancreas, and Pancreatic Enzymes

Digestion actually begins with the sight of food—or even its image in our mind. The thought, smell, or look of food immediately sends signals to the brain, which then activates the glossopharyngeal nerve, the main parasympathetic nerve that controls the salivary glands. The salivary glands when activated begin manufacturing and secreting large quantities of mucus-laden saliva, containing the digestive enzymes amylase and lipase. The mucus helps lubricate the food bolus, to aid in chewing and to help the food move more easily along the mouth and esophagus. The amylase family of enzymes begins breaking down carbohydrates such as starches, complex arrangements of sugars linked together, into simpler fragments. The lipases begin the process of breaking down triglycerides, a major dietary fat, into their fatty acid components.

The presence of food in the mouth stimulates the vagus nerve, the parasympathetic nerve that controls the upper part of the digestive system from the esophagus to the mid-colon. Branches of the vagus nerve activate two different types of cells, the parietal and chief cells, in the body of the stomach. Even before food makes its way from the mouth into the stomach, the parietal cells are producing and releasing hydrochloric acid, and the chief cells secrete the enzyme precursor pepsinogen. When the food bolus itself makes its way into the stomach, secretion of both hydrochloric acid and pepsinogen increase significantly and begin the gastric phase of digestion. In addition, the cells lining the stomach secrete a thick mucus coating that protects the stomach from the acid and pepsin.

Pepsinogen is actually the inactive parent molecule for the active digestive enzyme pepsin. The chief cells of the stomach manufacture and store pepsin as pepsinogen to prevent autodigestion of cellular components. In its inactive state, pepsinogen will not attack proteins, including the proteins of the cells that make it. Once secreted into the main body of the stomach, hydrochloric acid then cleaves off a terminal forty-four-amino-acid segment of pepsinogen, leaving the active enzyme.

Pepsin itself is active only in a very acidic environment, which hydrochloric acid provides. In such an environment, pepsin begins the process of breaking down complex food proteins into simpler fragments. Pepsin is very specific in its digestive capability and breaks only protein linkages containing certain amino acids—tryptophan, phenylalanine, tyrosine, methionine, or leucine.

The presence of food stimulates the vigorous contraction of the muscles of the stomach wall. These contractions enhance the mixing of food particles with the digestive juices. As the gastric phase of digestion reaches completion, these contractions also push the now semidigested semiliquid food into the duodenum, the first part of the small intestine, where digestion continues.

Digestion in the duodenum is a complex process, regulated by both the nervous system and hormones, and it is in this intestinal phase of digestion that the pancreas and its enzymes become active. The pancreas in the adult is about 10–15 cm in length (5–7 in.), with a widened head, a narrowing body, and a tapering tail. The head of the pancreas fits snugly in the C-shaped duodenum, the first part of the small intestine. In one of my lectures, I once described the pancreas as looking like the head of a seagull, or tern, with the head and the gradually tapering beak.

Microscopically, the tissue of the pancreas consists of two distinct cell types: the endocrine, or hormone-secreting cells, and the exocrine, or digestive-enzyme-producing tissue. The endocrine cells are scattered in clusters, the islets of Langerhans, throughout the pancreas. The islets consist of three basic cell types: alpha cells, beta cells, and delta cells, which are very distinctive under the microscope. Alpha cells produce and secrete glucagon, which the pancreas releases in response to low blood sugar levels. Glucagon circulates in the bloodstream and stimulates both the muscle and liver cells to break down glycogen, a storage form of sugar, into glucose, which is released into the bloodstream to serve as a source of cellular energy.

Beta cells of the pancreas secrete insulin in response to high blood sugar levels, as occurs after a meal. Traditionally, scientists believed that insulin served to drive glucose, the main blood sugar, into muscle and liver cells, where it can be stored as glycogen. In recent years, scientists have learned that insulin is a far more complex hormone than originally thought, involved with processes other than sugar metabolism. Cancer researchers, for example, now believe insulin is a growth factor that in excess can stimulate certain tumors to grow uncontrollably.

Delta cells of the pancreas produce and secrete somatostatin, a complex hormone that is also produced by cells lining the intestine as well as certain neurons in the brain. In the pancreas, somatostatin can inhibit the release of either glucagon or insulin, to help maintain blood sugars in a very narrow range. Scientists do not know how one hormone, somatostatin, can inhibit either glucagon or insulin release, to drive blood sugar levels up or down as needed by the body.

These endocrine cells of the pancreas—the alpha, beta, and delta cells—are dispersed in clusters throughout the entire pancreas, like stars in the sky. They release their hormone products directly into the bloodstream, for action at distant sites such as the liver and muscle.

The cells of the exocrine pancreas, which produce the various digestive enzymes, are arranged in a very distinctive pattern. These cells cluster in what are called acini; these resemble cul-de-sacs of a housing development, with a single layer of elongated cells forming the house lots around a common space that leads into a duct—the equivalent of a roadway—for secreted pancreatic enzymes. The cells lining this common opening are very active cells, producing copious amounts of enzymes needed by the body each day.

In Beard's day, scientists had identified the three basic pancreatic digestive enzymes: the proteolytic, or protein-digesting, enzyme trypsin; the starch-digesting enzyme amylase; and the fat-digesting enzyme lipase. We now know that the pancreas produces many enzymes in each of these three classes. For example, several dozen proteolytic enzymes have been identified now in addition to trypsin, such as chymotrypsin, carboxypeptidase A, carboxypeptidase B, elastase, aminopeptidase, dipeptidases, tripeptidases, and another form of pepsin, the enzyme also produced by stomach cells.

Each of these enzymes has a very specific and precise function. Trypsin will break down a protein only at amino acid linkages containing either arginine or lysine. Chymotrypsin attacks proteins only at points with tryptophan, phenylalanine, or tyrosine. The dipeptidases break down protein fragments consisting of two amino acids, and tripeptidases cleave three-amino-acid fragments.

The acinar cells also secrete multiple lipases and esterases, both fat-digesting enzymes with very specific target molecules. And the family of pancreatic amylases, like those released with saliva in the mouth, break down starch into simpler sugar linkages.

The proteolytic enzymes such as trypsin and chymotrypsin are very powerful molecules and will attack any protein—including the protein of the pancreas itself. This problem has been neatly resolved in the acinar cells, which produce the various proteolytic enzymes in inactive or, technically, precursor forms. For example, the acinar cells manufacture trypsin initially as trypsinogen, which is completely inactive with no digestive ability whatsoever.

Trypsin is itself, like all enzymes, a protein, consisting of 255 amino acids arranged in a very complex three-dimensional pattern. Trypsinogen is trypsin with an additional six amino acids, added to the end of the molecule like a tail. These six amino acids make the difference between an active and a totally inactive enzyme. Chymotrypsin is initially produced in the acinar cells as chymotrypsinogen, and carboxypeptidase A and B are manufactured as procarboxypeptidase A and B—all inactive precursor forms of the enzymes.

The acinar cells store the inactive precursors in little sacs, or vacuoles, in the cytoplasm, until they are needed for digestion. As long as these pre-enzymes remain in their inactive form, they pose no threat to the pancreas cells themselves.

The body has a remarkable mechanism for signaling the acinar cells of the pancreas to begin manufacturing as well as secreting stored precursor enzymes. First, the presence of food in the mouth and in the stomach stimulates the vagal nerve to release its neurotransmitter, acetylcholine. All the pancreatic acinar cells have on their membranes receptors for this parasympathetic neurotransmitter. When the acetylcholine from the vagus attaches to these receptors, the acinar cells begin releasing the stored pre-enzymes into the common space of the cul-de-sac.

In addition, when digestive products of the stomach make their way into the duodenum, the presence of food stimulates the cells lining the duodenum to secrete the hormone cholecystokinin into the bloodstream. This hormone, like the vagal nerve, stimulates the acinar cells to produce and release stored enzymes. After the cells secrete the precursor molecules, these pre-enzymes then make their way down the small ducts, or enzyme roadways, until they reach the main pancreatic roadway, the duct of Wirsung, which traverses the length of the pancreas and then joins the bile duct to empty into the duodenum at the ampulla of Vater.

When these pre-enzymes such as trypsinogen and chymotrypsinogen first make their way into the small intestine, they are still in their inactive form and useless for digestion. But the body has a very efficient process for activating the digestive enzymes. The cells lining the small intestine produce a proteolytic enzyme called enteropeptidase, whose function is specifically to cleave off the six-amino-acid tail of trypsinogen, leaving the very active and very powerful trypsin. Trypsin itself can then activate other trypsinogen molecules, as well as chymotrypsinogen and the other proteolytic enzymes. Scientists describe this process as a cascade, which speeds up as more trypsin molecules are produced.

But there's an added complication. The semiliquid food boluses that make their way from the stomach into the small intestine are extremely acidic, from all the hydrochloric acid secreted by the stomach to start the digestive process. But pancreatic enzymes such as trypsin and chymotrypsin can perform their digestive function only in an alkaline environment. In the presence of acid, even the active forms of the enzymes do nothing.

To solve this problem, when the lining cells of the small intestine sense the acid load of the incoming food, they release yet another hormone, secretin, into the bloodstream. Secretin stimulates the cells lining the ducts of the pancreas to produce copious amounts of bicarbonate-rich water that quickly empties along with the enzymes into the duodenum by the duct of Wirsung. Bicarbonate is a powerful antacid, known commonly as baking soda. The bicarbonate very quickly neutralizes the acid products coming into the duodenum from the stomach. Now, the activated enzymes have the ideal environment in which to begin their digestive work.

If the major pancreatic ducts become blocked—by a tumor, a gallstone, or scarring from drugs or infection—the pancreas, and its owner, are in serious trouble. In response to the usual stimuli—such as the sight or smell of food—the acinar cells continue to secrete the inactive enzyme precursors into the smaller pancreatic ducts, and the lining cells of the duct of Wirsung and other ducts will continue to secrete bicarbonate. But if the ducts obstruct, the enzymes will sit there unable to move, in an ideal alkaline environment. With time, trypsinogen will spontaneously convert into trypsin, and the activation cascade can proceed very rapidly. The enzymes then begin to attack the pancreas tissue itself, producing pancreatitis, which can be a life-threatening emergency. In addition, as the enzymes back up, the small blood vessels that circulate through the gland begin absorbing the overflow of enzymes; physicians routinely monitor blood levels of the two major pancreatic enzymes—lipase and amylase—to assess progress, or the lack of progress, with pancreatitis.

In recent decades, the embryological development of the pancreas has been worked out in great detail, confirming much of what Beard claimed one hundred years ago. As he proposed, the pancreas itself begins to form very early in fetal life, during the fourth and fifth week after conception. The pancreas actually develops in two parts. The larger dorsal (back) part of the pancreas, which ultimately forms the main body section of the pancreas, grows as a bud off the primitive foregut, the simple tube-like structure that eventually matures into the intestinal tract. A small nub, the ventral or frontal portion of the pancreas, forms from primitive liver tissue, then migrates 180 degrees over a period of several weeks to connect and eventually merge with the dorsal section of the pancreas.

During the initial weeks of fetal life, the cells of the primitive pancreas appear very undifferentiated, and each has the potential to develop into either hormone-secreting islets or enzyme-producing acini. The key to the differentiation process lies in the connective tissue, or mesenchyme, that forms the basic ground material of the pancreas. All organs have, as their basic foundation, fibrous connective tissue made up of long strands of collagen that holds the organs together. I visualize connective tissue as the woven straw that gives a basket—in this case, an organ—its shape.

Until recently, scientists believed connective tissue to be fairly inert. We now know that connective tissue is actually very metabolically active, particularly during embryological growth, when it can determine the destiny of specialized cells in each of our organs. In the pancreas, if the developing cells as they migrate through the primitive pancreas physically come into contact with the developing mesenchyme connective tissue, the cells become exocrine, enzyme-producing cells. If the primitive pancreatic cells do not actually touch the connective tissue, these cells will become endocrine. It appears that accessibility to mesenchyme determines the fate of the primitive pancreatic cell, again showing how intricate the process of differentiation can be.

Even in the earliest stages of pancreatic formation, when the acini begin to form, these cells produce enzymes. As the pancreatic tissues become more differentiated, enzyme production speeds up, during the seventh and eighth week of fetal growth. Beard, indeed, was correct when he claimed that the pancreas begins producing proteolytic enzymes early in life.

CHAPTER XI:

The Making of an Enzyme

In 1857, the French chemist Baron Corvisart first isolated a powerful proteolytic enzyme in an extract of animal pancreas. The enzyme seems initially to have attracted very little attention, and it languished on laboratory shelves until 1867, when the German scientist W. Kuhne began to investigate this very potent molecule. Kuhne named the enzyme trypsin, from the Greek "I wear away"—an apt description, Kuhne felt, in view of its powerful digestive ability.

By the end of the nineteenth century, physiologists knew a lot about trypsin, which they extracted for research purposes from the pancreas glands of animals slaughtered for meat. They had discovered that the pancreas produced trypsin as a precursor that had to be activated before it could perform its digestive function, that trypsin worked only in an alkaline environment, and that it was inactive if exposed to acid. They had also learned that trypsin was unstable once activated in an alkaline liquid solution at body temperature, because in such an environment the enzyme would tend to self-destruct, or autodigest, very quickly. Furthermore, all physiologists of that time believed that trypsin and related enzymes would actually be destroyed in the presence of acid, such as in the stomach.

By 1900, a very simple but accurate assay of trypsin activity had been developed by an English chemist. Though this might seem like so much scientific esoterica, in fact this test was to prove very important in the development of trypsin products for pharmaceutical use. In this assay, the amount of milk protein, casein, that was coagulated by the enzyme over an hour would be measured. A milligram of trypsin that digested twenty-five times its weight, 25 milligrams, of casein in an hour would be considered to have one tryptic unit of strength. A milligram of trypsin that digested fifty times its weight, 50 milligrams, in an hour would have two tryptic units of strength, and so on. Laboratories today still use this basic assay, and these same units of strength, to assay proteolytic pancreatic enzyme preparations.

Researchers other than Beard began to consider trypsin for use in a variety of medical conditions. For such purposes, trypsin needed to be available systemically, in the bloodstream and ultimately throughout the body, not just in the digestive tract, where it is normally found. It was believed at the time that the only effective way to administer trypsin for this use was as an intramuscular injection. Oral formulations of the trypsin, or of any pancreatic enzyme, researchers thought, would be useless because they would be destroyed by hydrochloric acid in the stomach.

Even if trypsin survived acid attack in the stomach, the alkaline small intestine presented another major barrier. Here, trypsin would quickly autodigest and essentially self-destruct. However, there was yet another, and perhaps more profound, obstacle to the absorption of trypsin from the gut. Scientists in Beard's day knew trypsin was a very large, complex molecule, and by the dogma of the time, such large molecules, even if they arrived intact into the duodenum, could never be absorbed through the lining of the small intestine. It was thought that there was simply no possible way oral preparations could be useful to treat systemic problems.

The first successful use of injectable trypsin was in the treatment of diphtheria. This was long before the advent of antibiotics, and at the time, diphtheria was a very prevalent scourge throughout Western Europe and the United States. The diphtheria bacillus killed by producing a tough membrane in the throat that could lead to suffocation. In an experimental model, an injectable preparation of trypsin appeared to dissolve very effectively this deadly membrane in animals infected with bacteria. When tested in humans, trypsin worked equally well as in animals, and by 1900, two pharmaceutical companies, Merck and Fairchild, began to consider the commercial production of trypsin for human use.

The large-scale manufacture of trypsin for injectable use, however, was not an easy prospect, and it immediately presented a series of difficult problems. First of all, any commercial venture required large amounts of trypsin. However, there was no possible way at that time to produce trypsin, or the other two known pancreatic enzymes, lipase and amylase, synthetically from scratch. Trypsin particularly is a large molecule with a very intricate three-dimensional shape. Chemists, though they knew the basics of its structure, simply didn't have the tools necessary to determine the amino acid sequence of this complex molecule. Only during the final decades of the twentieth century did sophisticated amino acid sequencers enable scientists to decipher the amino acid content of proteins.

But even if scientists in Beard's day had known the structure of trypsin, there would have been no way to manufacture such a protein. Currently, drug companies can produce large quantities of synthetic proteins for pharmaceutical use through the application of molecular biology and gene technology. Complex proteins such as insulin are now commercially manufactured from genetically modified bacteria, into which the human gene for insulin production has been inserted.

Such technology wasn't even a dream in 1900. The Merck and Fairchild chemists working on the problem of trypsin manufacture had no choice but to rely on extracting the enzyme from the glands of animals such as beef cattle slaughtered for meat. But trypsin, under slaughterhouse conditions, was a very unstable molecule: during butchering, the freshly extracted pancreas, still warm, was swimming in its own very alkaline juices, and in this environment the precursor trypsinogen molecules would spontaneously and rapidly activate and then begin digesting one another. Within several hours, no active enzymes would remain.

This problem was, theoretically, easy enough to solve: if the pancreas glands were quickly removed and placed on ice, and transported to the factory on ice, the enzyme content, in its inactive form, would largely be preserved. But this of course required the close cooperation of the slaughterhouse personnel, because the glands needed to be iced almost as soon as they were extracted. Any delay would mean loss of enzymes. And delays seem to have been quite the rule.

Furthermore, the pancreas is not a simple sack of active enzymes waiting to be extracted. The pancreas is a complex blend of both cellular components, including the vacuoles containing the trypsin in its inactive form, and noncellular constituents such as fibrous tissue, arteries, veins, and stored fat. But an effective injectable preparation required a concentrated solution of pure, active trypsin. To their credit, the Merck and Fairchild scientists developed a procedure for activating and then extracting trypsin from the organ in a reasonably controlled manner. If the glands were minced into a slurry and allowed to sit for a number of hours at close to freezing temperatures, the precursor trypsinogen molecules would convert to trypsin, though very slowly.

Through trial and error, these scientists learned approximately when maximum activation had occurred. At this point, the resulting mix would be soaked in solutions of water or, more commonly, water and alcohol. Because proteins, such as trypsin, are soluble in water and alcohol, the pancreatic enzymes would separate out into solution from the surrounding tissue and fat. The solvent, containing the active trypsin, would then be poured off. However, this was an inexact science: throughout the entire extraction process, there would be loss of considerable amounts of active enzyme, as the trypsin molecules would tend to attack each other. But it was the best they could do at the time.

Though the Fairchild and Merck chemists had come a long way, the final product—a vial of fairly pure, active trypsin in solution, or of trypsin, lipase, and amylase together—was very unstable, even when refrigerated. The activated trypsin molecules enthusiastically attacked, and digested, each other, as well as molecules of lipase and amylase. There really was no way, a hundred years ago, to stabilize such a volatile mix, and no one seems to have tried to provide the enzymes in powder form, which could be put into solution just before use. The Merck and Fairchild enzyme preparations were simply not very reliable.

By the time Beard presented his first papers on the trophoblastic theory of cancer and the proposed anticancer effect of pancreatic enzymes in the years 1902–1905, the Merck and Fairchild formulations were already in production. Beard was very aware of these preparations, and as the controversy, discussion, and debate swirled around him, he decided to test his theory in the single animal model for cancer available at the time, the Jensen mouse sarcoma model. Careful scientist that he was, he believed that such animal work should precede any experimentation in human patients.

Cancer researchers of Beard's time had looked for years to develop an animal system that could be used in the laboratory to evaluate anticancer agents. Scientists had already begun breeding mice and rats for experimental purposes, and they had already learned that such inbreeding at times produced animals that showed an increased tendency to develop certain tumors, such as breast cancer. But the tumor occurrence was still too sporadic and unreliable for any practical laboratory application, so scientists began to transplant tumors from one laboratory animal to another, sometimes even between animals of different species. Invariably, the animal receiving the transplant would reject the tumor, as it would any foreign tissue.

However, Dr. Jensen found one particular sarcoma in one particular mouse that, when transplanted to a mouse of the same species, grew without restraint. Cancer researchers finally had the animal model they had long sought. And Beard could test his trypsin therapy in a controlled laboratory experiment.

Beard in his writings seems to have been somewhat unhappy with the available trypsin formulations, but he believed based on his own research that the Fairchild product was the most potent and the most stable. In his animal experiments, he used the Fairchild preparation with apparent impressive results despite his legitimate concerns. In the *British Medical Journal* on January 20, 1906, Beard reported his first successes with the trypsin therapy, discussing the repeated death of tumors in the Jensen mouse tumor model. His work, even by the standards of twenty-first-century science, seems impeccable, flawless, and appropriate. And of course, Beard's work was viciously attacked.

Though the Jensen mouse tumor had been accepted by academic researchers as a legitimate laboratory model for testing cancer treatments, when Beard reported his first positive results, critics—instead of accepting Beard's results—questioned the model. In an article in the *Medical Record* on January 5, 1907, Beard took on his critics, particularly one vocal opponent, a well-respected London surgeon, W. Roger Williams:

> But the original question, raised by Mr. W. Roger Williams, touches much graver issues. He denies that this tumor is a cancer at all! If this conclusion be right, it is not very flattering to the scientific acumen of any one of all the investigators of cancer, who have used or still employ this neoplasm in their work. . . . What is the criterion for the statement that this mouse-tumor is not a cancer? Scientific reasons are not contained in the original report of his lecture in London or in his letters to the medical papers. The criterion for his

judgment is simply his authority. The Jensen mouse-tumor is not a cancer because—he says it is not! (Beard 1907, 24)

Despite such criticism, by late 1905, Beard's lectures, papers, and animal work and, basically, his dogged persistence had generated sufficient interest that physicians and researchers in England, continental Europe, and America wanted to start using the enzymes on human patients. Despite the success in animals, however, Beard believed the Fairchild formulation to be too weak for use in human cancer patients. By 1906, he seems to have carried enough clout that the Fairchild chemists were willing to work with him to improve the quality and the strength of the trypsin product. Beard himself visited the London slaughterhouses where the butchers extracted the glands for Fairchild and meticulously observed every step in the manufacturing, from the arrival of the pancreas glands on ice, to the addition of the final product to the vial. Beard insisted each lot be assayed to guarantee consistent strength in the product. He also strongly recommended that lots intended for cancer treatment should never be more than several days old, because the product deteriorated so quickly.

Beard himself supervised the first use of the injectable enzymes in patients suffering advanced cancer. Because the enzymes had never been used in humans before, Beard calculated doses based on his experiences with the mouse model. And indeed, he had learned quite a bit from his animal experiments. He observed that if he injected too much trypsin into animals with the Jensen sarcoma, the mice would die sooner than the animals that had no cancer. But when Beard injected the same dose into healthy animals without cancer, the animals would continue to live quite happily.

Beard began to suspect that if the dose of trypsin were too high, the tumor would die very quickly, releasing enormous amounts of toxic debris into the animal. It was, Beard believed, the toxic debris from the dead tumor that overwhelmed and killed the mice. Beard tried a variety of doses and a variety of dosing schedules, and he ultimately discovered that the trypsin worked best if, after several days of treatment, he then stopped the trypsin for several days before resuming the enzyme injections. With such cycling, the life-threatening toxic symptoms could be kept under control.

Beard also learned that if in the cancerous animals he followed each course of trypsin injections with injections of pure amylase for several days, or if he gave amylase concurrently with the trypsin, the animals could tolerate higher doses of trypsin for a longer period of time. The amylase, which he never suspected had any direct anticancer action, seemed to break down the deadly waste from the dissolving tumor into less toxic fragments. Amylase, from that point on, became an essential component of his treatment.

Beard seems very quickly to have determined an effective dosage schedule for humans. He recommended the Fairchild preparation, approximately one thousand units of trypsin and two thousand units of amylase, both given in intramuscular injections into the buttocks daily. The physicians who worked with Beard, using the right preparation from Fairchild and following his dosage schedule, reported very good results, even with terminal patients. Unfortunately, these successes reported in the scientific literature during the years 1906–1910 caused a mad rush by other drug companies to market their own enzyme products as a treatment for cancer, without Beard's input or approval. Analytical laboratories hired by Beard tested a number of these formulations and found them worthless, totally devoid of any significant proteolytic activity; only the Merck and Fairchild preparations, as unstable as they were, provided any level of active trypsin.

Not surprisingly, physicians using preparations other than the Fairchild product had little if any success. And physicians who did use the Fairchild enzyme but who ignored Beard's dosing schedule and his warnings about the need for amylase had no success at all. Beard's opponents used these failures effectively in their attacks against him, to his great frustration.

In an article appearing in the *Medical Record* on January 5, 1907—the same article in which he attacked Mr. Williams, the surgeon who had discounted his results with the Jensen model—Beard railed at scientists who had tested his hypothesis using an improperly prepared enzyme product. In this long article, he wrote the following:

> Certain British surgeons and others have obtained only negative results. Why have they not reported them? The reason for their failures would then have been apparent. Some of them tell patients that they have tried trypsin and found it "useless in cases of cancer." How do they know that they were using trypsin? Have they ever tested, as a chemist must do his reagents, the injection as to its ferment [enzyme] powers? Are they sure they were not using something little, if any better than glycerin and water? . . . I and others have tested all the injections advertised, and I have seen the results of assays. The finds are astounding. My published scientific work lays down that the injection should be "the secretion of that important digestive gland, the pancreas," that is to say, be prepared from the fresh gland direct, that this injection should contain all the ferments, that, generally speaking, it should be given for not a very great number of weeks. . . . When in 1903 I wrote of the secretion of the pancreas gland, do those who have failed imagine that I really meant the dispensing in a chemist's back shop of somebody's trypsin in powder just as though it were so much blue pill? There is only one set of preparations now on the market which satisfies the above requirements. (Beard, 1907, 25)

In his book *The Enzyme Treatment of Cancer*, Beard wrote about his experiences with Fairchild and his difficulties in getting physicians to use the right form and the right protocol:

> I knew of no better ones on the market—indeed, for a very long time, of none as good: and, in addition to other advantages, they had for my purposes the very great recommendation that through agents they could be obtained in

almost every part of the world, at the Cape, in Australia, India, Italy, Spain, etc. Thus, no single correspondent had to be told that reliable injections of trypsin and of amylopsin [amylase] were out of his reach. Moreover, these injections had active ferment powers in whatever part of the world they happened to be purchased, a thing which cannot be said of certain other injections. . . .

Many physicians and surgeons have "tried the treatment" with either (1) injections so weak or inert as to be no better than glycerine and water or (2) weak injections of almost pure trypsin, fortunately as a rule in very small doses. For, as I have more than once warned the medical profession, trypsin alone is about the most deadly remedy for cancer which could possibly be devised. . . . Again, trypsin with no amylopsin has been used (London), and amylopsin alone (Geneva and Paris) and pepsin alone (Glasgow), and lastly, anything with the label "trypsin," the medical men concerned not knowing or troubling to find out whether they were using trypsin, or amylopsin, or both, or something else, or neither the one nor the other. At times, as I found, the general directions for the use of genuine preparations of trypsin and amylopsin were being employed with preparations which would have been quite useless even as a cure for corns. (Beard 2010, 195)

During the years 1906, when the enzymes were first used in human patients, until 1910, 126 physicians working at forty-three hospitals, including several that specialized in cancer, used trypsin to treat patients with advanced cancer. Very few seemed to have followed Beard's instructions or heeded his warnings about appropriate preparations, proper dosing, and the use of amylase. As a result, very few reported good results. Yet always, those physicians who followed Beard's protocol to the letter reported successes.

When I reviewed the historical documents from the time, I realized the international level of debate Beard's work generated. Pharmaceutical companies continued to follow the battle. The August 1909 edition of E. Merck's *Annual Report of Recent Advances in Pharmaceutical Chemistry and Therapeutics* (Vol. XXII) discussed the ongoing controversy surrounding Beard's work:

The mode of action and the value of pancreas preparations in cancer has not yet received a wholly reliable explanation. Great difficulties are encountered because the preparations used by the various investigators differed greatly in respect to their chemical properties, their purity, and in the amount of active substances they contain, and often these factors are not fully known to the student of the literature, or to the physician who has used them and describes their action. . . . [A]nd how shall we gauge the action of pancreatin and trypsin ampullae whose mode of preparation and whose composition is not mentioned in the original paper, neither is there any mention made of their sterility or the method by which they have been sterilized? We need not wonder, then, to find that one author has never seen local inflammation follow the injection, while another reports severe local irritant effects. (Merck 1909, 340–41)

But such statements and Beard's more vocal warnings seemed to have been largely ignored. Greedy firms, seeking to cash in on the potential cancer cure, continued to produce useless preparations. Beard's critics continued to use failures with these products to attack Beard, radiation became the hope of the cancer research world, and Beard passed into near oblivion.

During the 1920s, when Dr. Morse in St. Louis rediscovered Beard's work, he developed his own injectable formulation of trypsin and amylase, which he used with great success. Dr. Frank Shively, a surgeon working in Dayton, Ohio, during the 1950s and 1960s—at the same time as Kelley, though the two didn't appear to know of each other's work—also independently rediscovered Beard's book and results. Shively got a local Ohio drug company to manufacture, for his own use only, small batches of injectable trypsin and amylase, which he used on advanced cancer patients with some very impressive results. Interestingly, Shively found the preparation worked even more effectively when he added chymotrypsin—another pancreatic proteolytic enzyme that was unknown in Beard's day—as well as lipase. He believed based on his own clinical results that the broader range of enzymes gave significantly better results than the old Beard formula.

Shively described his results with 192 patients with a variety of advanced and terminal cancer in a self-published monograph in 1969. Though all these patients were by my reading terminal or near-terminal patients who had failed all orthodox treatments, twelve appeared to have been cured, and a large number partially responded to the therapy. Yet despite Shively's success, in 1969 the U.S. Food and Drug Administration issued an edict outlawing the manufacture and use of injectable pancreatic enzymes, and Shively resumed a more orthodox surgical practice. Since then, injectable pancreatic enzymes have not been available in the United States. However, with interest in enzyme therapy again on the rise, injectable formulations are being manufactured and used in a number of European countries, particularly Germany.

CHAPTER XII:

More Making of an Enzyme

Beard knew of only three pancreatic enzymes: trypsin, the main proteolytic enzyme; lipase; and amylase. In his writings, he never referred to the endocrine component of the pancreas, which at the time was largely a mystery to scientists. They knew there was some sort of hormone produced that controlled sugar metabolism, but they didn't know much more. It wasn't until the year of Beard's death in 1923 that scientists began to unravel systematically the complicated array of pancreatic endocrine and exocrine secretions. In that year, the Canadians Banting and Best isolated insulin from the pancreas of a dog, and shortly thereafter, injectable insulin extracted from the glands of animals was available for the treatment of diabetes.

Insulin, like the pancreatic enzymes, is a protein, and scientists soon learned that each species of animals produced an insulin unique to that species that differed in amino acid structure (sometimes slightly, sometimes considerably) from the insulin of other species. As demand for insulin escalated, pharmaceutical chemists learned that of all the potential sources of the hormone, the pig pancreas provided insulin most similar to the human molecule, which worked very efficiently in human patients with diabetes. In fact, until the wide-scale production during the 1990s of genetically engineered human insulin from bacteria, pig insulin was the mainstay of diabetes therapy.

This was the first effective treatment for the disease, which previously had a relentless and rapidly deadly course. The discovery of insulin, and its successful application in clinical medicine, made front-page news around the world. Banting and Best shared the Nobel Prize, and their work spurred intensive research into pancreatic function, both endocrine and exocrine. The hormones glucagon and somatostatin were isolated and identified. Physiologists and biochemists began to realize that the pancreas didn't produce just one proteolytic enzyme, or one lipase, or one amylase, but perhaps dozens of enzymes in each class. By the 1940s, scientists had identified many pancreatic enzymes, including, in addition to trypsin, chymotrypsin, carboxypeptidase, ribonuclease, deoxyribonuclease, guanase, and guanosinase: an array of fat-digesting enzymes including an entire family of lipases as well as cholesterol esterase and lecithinase and a family of amylases.

As knowledge of the pancreas grew during the 1930s and 1940s, drug companies in the United States began to consider marketing tablets and capsules of pancreatic enzymes for oral use. These products were not intended as a cancer treatment, because Beard's work had been forgotten, but rather as a simple digestive aid in syndromes of pancreatic insufficiency such as occurs with pancreatitis and cystic fibrosis. Cystic fibrosis is a complex genetic disease affecting many organ systems, particularly the lungs and the pancreas. In patients with the illness, the cells lining the pancreatic ducts lose their ability to produce and secrete water and bicarbonate, both necessary for activation of pancreatic enzymes in the duodenum. In their absence, the pancreatic enzymes accumulate in the ducts and gradually activate, eventually destroying the pancreatic tissue itself. As a result, patients with cystic fibrosis ultimately develop a severe deficiency of pancreatic enzymes, which can be countered by oral supplementation.

The manufacturing process for pancreatic enzymes hadn't changed much from Beard's day, even though the product was intended for oral, not injectable, use. All commercial methods up until 1950 were designed first to activate the precursors, and then to extract the enzymes from the rest of the pancreas tissue. Fresh pancreas glands from butchered animals would be minced, mixed with water, and then allowed to sit at near-freezing temperatures. The mincing, mixing, and standing would allow the conversion of the precursor forms to active enzymes, but the cold temperatures slowed, theoretically at least, autodigestion and loss of product.

The thick mixture would then be pressed to separate out a crude solution of enzymes from the pancreas tissue, which would be discarded. The remaining solution would then be mixed with absolute (pure) alcohol, which caused the enzymes to precipitate out of solution. The enzymes would then be filtered and dried at low temperatures in a vacuum, leaving a concentrated, active enzyme powder. Once in dry, powder form, it was thought, the enzymes would be stable at room temperature for many months.

The large-scale commercial production of pancreas products required literally tons of pancreas, so an inexpensive, readily available supply was critical. This limited options to animals commonly used in the meat industry, such as cattle, sheep, and pigs. In Beard's day, the glands of beef cattle seemed to have been the primary source of pancreatic enzymes. But in subsequent decades, pharmaceutical chemists were to learn that insulin from pigs was most similar to human insulin in terms of effect. Similarly, during the early 1940s, it was found that enzymes from the pig pancreas were very similar to human enzymes, in terms of composition and activity.

Importantly, the pancreas from pigs appeared to be loaded with enzymes; glands from other commercially raised animals, however, had a very low proteolytic enzyme content. Cows, for example, have an extra stomach, where most digestion occurs through a complex process of bacterial fermentation. These animals have little need for pancreatic digestive enzymes, and the pancreas glands of these animals have a very low enzyme content. The pancreas of sheep, another herbivore, also has a lower enzyme output than that of pigs. For all these reasons, by the early 1940s, most commercially available enzyme products were derived from the pig pancreas.

The biochemist Ezra Levin, working out of Champagne, Illinois, during the 1940s, was very familiar with the enzyme manufacturing methods commonly used in industry and in fact held several patents related to refinements in the standard technique. He was a very hardworking scientist, a perfectionist who was not at all pleased with the quality of the enzyme products marketed at the time—even though he had helped develop some of the manufacturing steps. From his own research, he knew that the industrial process for extracting digestive enzymes from animal pancreas tissue was very inefficient, leaving up to 75 percent of viable enzymes in the discarded residue. This was, to Levin, an intolerably inefficient process.

Levin also learned through his own testing that the extraction method itself, despite the use of low temperature, caused an additional significant loss of enzyme activity. Levin suspected that the rough handling of the pancreas tissue during manufacture—the mincing, pressing, and alcohol extraction—caused destruction of much of the enzyme content. The enzyme material itself, once put into tablet form, also seemed to be very unstable, despite improvements in processing. Levin suspected that the tablets still contained too much water, and the liquid environment allowed the enzymes to continue attacking one another. When tested by Levin, a number of pancreas products being sold at the time had no enzymatic activity whatsoever. They were worthless, as worthless as many of the preparations being marketed during Beard's day.

Levin was driven to find a better way of making pancreatic enzymes, a method to produce enzymes exclusively in their activated, not precursor, form without causing degradation during manufacturing. And he wanted a final product with a long shelf life.

Levin first tackled the problem of activation of the precursor enzyme molecules. Manufacturers knew that if they let the freshly butchered pancreas glands sit around at room temperature, within hours most of the precursor molecules would be activated. A crescendo of enzyme activation, similar to what occurs in the duodenum during normal digestion, would occur. A few molecules of trypsinogen would first be converted spontaneously to trypsin, and these trypsin molecules would then activate other trypsinogen molecules as well as other inactive proteolytic enzyme precursors such as chymotrypsinogen.

Initially, there would be very few active trypsin enzymes in the mix, and proportionally many more inactive precursors, so the probability was greatest that an active trypsin would collide with an inactive precursor. This was fine, and it led to more active enzymes in the solution. But as the cascade proceeded, and as the percentage of active trypsin molecules increased, the probability of an active trypsin hitting another active trypsin would also increase.

When two active proteolytic enzymes collide, they digest each other, leaving a coagulated and inactive protein. When most of the precursors became active, the likelihood was greatest that an active enzyme would collide with another active enzyme. At that point, the mixture would convert very quickly from a soup of high enzymatic content to a collection of useless amino acids and protein fragments. Of course, chemists in Beard's day had already learned that if the process occurred at near-freezing temperatures, the activation would proceed slowly, and degradation could be more easily controlled. Nonetheless, even at low temperatures, Levin found the loss of product was substantial.

Scientists in Beard's day already knew that there was some critical point, some specific time in the process at which maximum activity would be achieved. If the material were allowed to continue sitting beyond this time, rapid degradation of enzyme potency would follow as the activated enzymes furiously digested one another. But this point of maximal activity, prior to Levin's research, had never been precisely determined, though drug companies had been making pancreatic enzymes for fifty years. Levin, through trial and error, found that if he took the pancreas glands from freshly killed animals, minced the glands, and then let the resulting tissue mush sit at 30 degrees Centigrade for exactly twenty-four hours, he would obtain maximum activation of the precursor.

But the problem of stopping continued enzyme action proved very difficult to solve. Levin experimented with a number of approaches. He discovered, somewhat serendipitously, that certain low-molecular-weight solvents containing a halogen molecule—that is, a molecule of chlorine, bromine, or iodine—could stop enzymatic activity without denaturing the enzymes themselves. The enzymes would be chemically frozen, inactive but undamaged. Of all the solvents he tested, Levin discovered that ethylene dichloride worked most efficiently. This was exactly the answer he had been looking for; when added to a mixture of activated minced pancreas, ethylene dichloride would stop enzymatic action almost immediately, without damaging the proteins. Essentially, the solvent put the enzymes into a type of suspended animation. A fifty-year problem had been solved.

But Levin still faced the enormous problem of separating the activated, though suspended, enzymes from the pancreas tissue itself, the most inefficient step in the traditional manufacturing process. Levin approached the problem by, first, looking at the pancreas itself and its chemical composition. The pancreas, like any other tissue, consists mostly of water, at least 60 percent by weight. The gland also contains a fair amount of fat, perhaps 25 percent by composition, either as stored fat dispersed with the connective tissue, or as the lipids that make up the cellular components such as cell membranes. The protein component contains all the stored digestive enzymes, the enzymes used by the cells for their own metabolism, the structural proteins of the cell, and the surrounding fibrous tissue, which is itself mostly protein.

The Fairchild chemists had approached the problem by first activating the proteases, solubilizing them in water or alcohol, and then washing them off in solution. As Levin studied the pancreas, he began to suspect that he needed to approach the problem of isolating the enzymes from a completely new direction—in fact, from the opposite direction. Instead of solubilizing the enzymes and pouring them off, as was still done in industry, he considered dissolving and washing away the unneeded components—primarily water and fat—from the pancreas and pouring these off, leaving behind the entire enzyme-rich protein compartment of the gland. All the enzymes would be preserved in the protein residue. The water and fat would be thrown away.

However, this approach seemed initially very complicated. The water and lipid components of the gland had completely different physical characteristics and would require, Levin reasoned, completely different methods of extraction. Furthermore, though there were many known hydrocarbon solvents routinely used in industry that could dissolve fat, most of these solvents also denatured proteins, such as trypsin. Levin's process required a solvent that would emulsify fat but not change or damage the protein enzymes.

The removal of water posed another potential roadblock. The easiest and most direct way of removing water from a mixture is heating the mixture to speed evaporation. But Levin knew that many of the proteolytic enzymes of the pancreas would denature and become completely useless at temperatures above 60 degrees Centigrade. This precluded boiling or standard distillation, which require heating water to 100°C. Water would evaporate slowly at low temperatures, but the process took so long that even in the presence of ethylene dichloride, the active enzymes would eventually start digesting one another.

Levin knew that there are mixtures of certain solvents with water, called azeotropic mixtures, that allow both the solvent and water to boil off at much lower temperatures than would be required for either alone. He also learned, through trial and error, that ethylene dichloride—the very solvent that he knew would stop enzymatic activity—did form an azeotrope with water. In fact, under low pressure, water could be distilled off at considerably less than 60 degrees. And, fortuitously, ethylene dichloride, a classic hydrocarbon solvent, very nicely dissolved fat without denaturing protein. With one ideal solvent, ethylene dichloride, he had solved all his problems.

Levin quickly perfected his method. He would mince the pancreas from freshly slaughtered pigs and allow the pancreas to sit at 30 degrees for twenty-four hours. This provided maximum activation of most if not all the precursor enzymes. At the point of maximum enzyme potency, he added ethylene dichloride, which at once stopped enzyme action and autolysis, dissolved the fat, and created an azeotrope with water. The water could then quickly be distilled off at a low temperature under pressure, without causing any denaturing of the protein enzymes, and in the next step, the ethylene dichloride, with all the fat dissolved in it, would simply be poured off. Any residual solvent could quickly be distilled off, again at a low temperature.

The procedure worked beautifully. Levin had a process that salvaged virtually all the enzymes from the pancreas in an active form, with very little loss from processing. The final powder was almost completely dry, and it lost very little potency even after months at room temperature.

Levin's accomplishment was not simply an esoteric adventure in science. An enormous and potentially profitable demand for proteolytic enzymes, above and beyond their use in medicine, developed during the 1940s. Industrial chemists had learned that proteolytic enzymes such as trypsin were valuable in such diverse processes as leather tanning and improving the texture of chocolate. But previously, enzyme manufacturing was so inefficient no company could produce a reliable, cheap product to meet industry needs.

With Levin's approach, all that changed. Not only was the process very efficient, with little loss of potency, but with Levin's method a concentrated enzyme product could be extracted from the pancreas of animals such as sheep and cattle, which had traditionally been relegated to dog food because of the low proteolytic content. Levin also successfully isolated and concentrated good-quality trypsin and other enzymes from fish intestine, previously a useless byproduct of the fishery industry. Levin's method, with its valuable ethylene dichloride solvent, revolutionized enzyme manufacturing around the world.

In 1950, Levin patented his method for activating and extracting enzymes and then created his own company, Viobin, which used his processing methods. Because Viobin owned the patent, the company quickly cornered the market for both pharmaceutical and industrial pancreatic enzyme products. Today, Viobin is a subsidiary of a Canadian drug company and still makes enzymes using Levin's methods.

When Kelley was in the depths of his illness in 1961, he knew nothing of John Beard or Ezra Levin, and very little about pancreatic enzymes. He did know he had a very serious problem. The large tumor sitting in his pancreas blocked the major pancreatic ducts. Every time he tried to eat, his pancreatic cells would start pumping out enzymes, but the enzymes would sit in the ducts in the alkaline pancreatic juices, unable to pass into the duodenum to do their digestive work. The inactive precursors would begin to activate and start digesting his pancreas—a very painful process.

The pain was so excruciating, Kelley would cry out in agony. And without enzymes in the duodenum, the partially digested contents of the small intestine would sit like a rock. He had terrible problems with bloating, reflux, nausea, and vomiting. He lost some 70 pounds, going from 210 to 130, on a big 6' 3" frame. One of his four children—the reason why he would fight so hard to stay alive—told me he would scream at times from the pain.

In desperation, Kelley approached his pharmacist friend for some kind of help. His friend astutely suggested he start taking pancreatic enzymes, and in large doses, with each meal. The enzymes would certainly help with digestion, the pharmacist explained, and the presence of enzymes in the duodenum would turn off the nervous and endocrine signals that were stimulating the pancreas to release enzymes with every bite of food. This would help with pain.

The pharmacist specifically suggested he use Viobin enzymes, which in his mind were the best on the market. There were other brands, he told Kelley, but none as effective as Viobin. These are the enzymes Kelley bought by the case. The enzymes worked wonderfully: his digestion improved after the first dose, and his pain gradually resolved. He began gaining weight, and his tumors began to dissolve. And, as a very nice side benefit, he didn't die.

Had this pharmacist, whoever he may have been—I never did learn his name—recommended a less potent, less stable, less well-designed brand of pancreatic enzymes, Kelley would have died. Though Levin knew nothing about Beard's theories about cancer, his obsession to make the best enzyme product possible saved Kelley's life.

Kelley could not believe that he was the first human to observe such an effect from pancreatic enzymes. When he felt strong enough, he began reading through the medical literature and learned of John Beard and his trophoblastic theory. Kelley was surprised to learn Beard believed that only injectable forms of pancreatic enzymes would be effective against cancer. As he reviewed Beard's work, Kelley suspected Beard was right about most things, but wrong about the need to use injectable enzymes. His own experience had shown him this.

At the time Kelley first began using enzymes on himself in 1963, pharmaceutical chemists assumed—as Beard had assumed—that oral formulations of pancreatic enzymes, such as the Viobin product, could have no possible systemic effect. The oral formulations might help with digestion, but they still believed that most of the pancreatic enzymes would largely be denatured by stomach acid. Any enzymes that survived the acid assault would then eventually be shattered into fragments during the digestive process in the duodenum. Even if any enzymes survived this second battleground, there was no way such big protein molecules could be absorbed.

But Kelley observed, whatever the academic dogma might be, that when he took large doses of enzymes by mouth, he felt changes in his tumors within half an hour. Within days of beginning his enzyme regimen, Kelley observed that tumor growth slowed and then stopped. Eventually, the tumors began to regress.

Because all these changes occurred only after he added pancreatic enzymes to his nutritional program, he could only assume that the enzymes were absorbed in an active form into the bloodstream and had a powerful effect on cancer. As an experiment to prove this to himself, at one point Kelley stopped taking the enzymes. After a week, the tumors started to grow, and grow rapidly once again. He resumed the enzymes, and tumor growth stopped; he felt it within a day. Kelley needed no further proof.

Kelley went back to the medical literature. He was surprised to learn that during the 1940s, as oral preparations of pancreatic enzymes became more commonly available, a number of physicians had experimented with large doses of orally ingested enzymes in patients suffering a variety of diseases that ostensibly had nothing to do with digestion. Although none of the researchers at the time seemed aware of Beard's work, and none reported using the enzymes to treat cancer, they did discuss impressive improvement in problems such as allergies, asthma, psoriasis, and severe arthritis.

These physicians and researchers began to rethink the issue of absorption. We know—and scientists knew then—that there are only two basic mechanisms for absorbing nutrients after digestion has been completed in the small intestine. Fats such as triglycerides and cholesterol, and the fat-soluble vitamins such as vitamins A, D, E, and K, enter the lymphatic channels surrounding the intestinal lining. The various lymphatic channels of the body form a circulatory system parallel to the blood circulatory system. Eventually, lymph flow enters the venous system in the chest, where the large lymph vessel, the thoracic duct, connects to the superior vena cava, the large vein of the chest that carries blood to the right side of the heart.

Eventually, the blood carries these fats and fat-soluble nutrients to the liver. Most other nutrients, including sugars, most vitamins and minerals, amino acids, and protein fragments—and presumably, whole proteins—are absorbed from the small intestine into small blood capillaries, which eventually merge into the large portal vein that feeds into the liver directly. If whole pancreatic enzymes were being absorbed and were circulating throughout the body, they would be circulating in the blood vessels, not the lymphatic channels.

These researchers then conducted a number of studies in a variety of laboratory animal species. The animals were fed large doses of pancreatic enzymes orally for various periods of time, and then blood and urine levels of enzymes would be monitored. Interestingly, no matter how large a dose the animals took, and regardless of how long, the blood levels invariably remained constant. However, after a number of days, large amounts of enzymes in their active form would begin appearing in the urine. Eventually, the urinary output matched oral intake, as if a steady state had been reached.

This was a perplexing situation. Clearly, the appearance of active pancreatic enzymes in the urine seemed to prove that these large proteins not only survived digestion in the gut, but were indeed being absorbed, were circulating, and were eventually excreted. But the stable blood levels, which didn't change even after weeks of oral intake, were a puzzling finding.

The researchers began sacrificing animals at different stages of the experiments, to try to find where the enzymes went. They found that shortly after the animals began ingesting large doses of enzymes, enzyme levels in the pancreas increased. Apparently, the body has a mechanism to recycle and reuse pancreatic enzymes for digestion.

This made sense, because physiologists had known for some time that the body has an elaborate method for recycling other essential digestive components such as bile salts. Bile salts are produced in the liver, stored in the gall bladder, and released into the small intestine during digestion. There, these salts aid in the emulsification of fats. In the last segment of the small intestine, bile salts are then reabsorbed into the capillaries, and eventually they are extracted by the liver for reuse.

To their astonishment, these researchers learned that pancreatic enzymes were also sequestered in a number of organs besides the pancreas, such as the liver and spleen, that were not thought to contain such enzymes. It seemed that the body had an elaborate storage capability for pancreatic enzymes: once this capacity was full, any excess of enzymes would be dumped by the kidney into the urine for excretion. Only after several days of enzyme supplementation did the organs become saturated, and until that point, the urine contained no enzymes. Throughout this entire process, blood levels would remain steady. Apparently, the various storage organs would very quickly extract enzymes from the blood, preventing blood levels from increasing. This is not an unusual phenomenon; the body maintains blood levels of many substances critical for life in a very narrow range.

For example, potassium, one of the major salts, or electrolytes, in the blood, is essential for normal heart and nerve function. The body maintains blood levels of potassium within a very narrow range, and even slight excess or deficiency can result in serious cardiac rhythm disturbances. In cases of excessive potassium intake, the mineral will be quickly pushed into cells for storage and the remaining excess will be excreted by the kidneys. In the case of a potassium deficiency, cellular stores will be used to maintain blood levels, and the kidney will efficiently reabsorb potassium from the urine for reuse.

Scientists also performed enzyme absorption studies on human test subjects (minus, of course, the evaluation of organ stores). Just as in the animals, after several days of oral ingestion, enzymes appeared in the urine. All the while, blood levels would remain constant. Clearly, contrary to all that had been previously believed, these large proteins were surviving acid in the stomach and digestion in the small intestine and were being absorbed in their intact and active form into the blood.

During this period of intensive enzyme research, scientists first documented that pancreatic enzymes circulated in the blood of normal test subjects who were not taking pancreatic enzymes orally and who had no history of pancreatic disease. Subsequently, analytical laboratories developed simple assays to measure blood and urine levels of the major pancreatic enzymes trypsin, amylase, and lipase. A proposed normal range for the pancreatic enzymes was calculated and has been used ever since as a guide to monitor pancreatitis. But no one seemed to question why these enzymes would be in the blood in the first place.

Despite this extraordinary flurry of research activity during the 1940s, by 1960, most of this research had been forgotten. I think it was simply a case of dogma over data. Physiologists continued to preach that orally ingested pancreatic enzymes would largely be destroyed by stomach acid, and any surviving enzymes would then be digested, like any protein, in the duodenum. And, finally, dogma stated unequivocally, as if the elegant studies from Levin's day had never happened, that pancreatic enzyme molecules were so large they could never be absorbed through the intestinal lining. Nonetheless, from the beginnings of his cancer practice in the early 1960s, and despite the dictates of academic physiologists, Kelley used only an oral preparation of pancreatic enzymes.

During the 1970s, there was a resurgence of interest in pancreatic enzymes. In 1975, Drs. Liebow and Rothman published an interesting study in *Science* (189: 472–74), a highly respected international research journal. These two scientists looked at the fate of proteolytic enzymes secreted by the pancreas into the duodenum. They conducted a series of elaborate experiments confirming, at least in laboratory animals, that enzymes secreted by the pancreas into the duodenum would be reabsorbed intact through the lining of the intestinal tract.

Rothman, in a series of subsequent experiments, demonstrated that in animals, the absorption of pancreatic enzymes through the intestinal lining is a very complex process. The cells lining the small intestine seemed to have specialized receptors specifically for pancreatic enzymes such as trypsin and chymotrypsin that enabled the enzymes to get into the cells. Once absorbed, the enzymes would make their way to the opposite end of the cell that borders the small capillaries that transport nutrients away from the gut. The enzymes would then be secreted into the bloodstream and would circulate around the body until they arrived at the pancreas. There, the circulating enzymes would be picked up and repackaged in the cells for reuse. Clearly, these enzymes must be very important, to warrant such elaborate conservation systems.

The research of scientists such as Liebow and Rothman led to a series of articles during the 1970s and 1980s confirming that pancreatic proteolytic enzymes such as trypsin and chymotrypsin are not destroyed in the intestinal tract after being secreted during digestion. Instead, after doing their job, the enzymes are largely reabsorbed and ultimately reconcentrated in the pancreas for reuse (though no one, since the earlier experiments in the 1940s, has reconsidered the issue of enzyme storage in other organs).

Then in 1980, a group of Russian scientists in Leningrad decided to test the dogma that proteolytic enzymes such as trypsin are heat and acid sensitive. They performed a very simple experiment, which they repeated a number of times. They took pure trypsin and boiled it in concentrated hydrochloric acid for an hour. To everyone's surprise, when these enzymes were subsequently placed in an alkaline environment, there was no loss of proteolytic activity whatsoever. Trypsin proved to be resistant not only to acid, but also to prolonged high temperatures. While proteolytic enzymes may not be active in an acid environment, contrary to what gastrointestinal physiologists had believed for a hundred years, trypsin is not destroyed in acid.

All this work culminated in a major conference held in Munich in 1993 entitled "Absorption of Orally Administered Enzymes." At the conference, researchers from around the world presented data confirming that orally ingested pancreatic proteolytic enzymes are not destroyed by stomach acid, are absorbed into the bloodstream, and can have very potent systemic actions—including actions against inflammation and possibly cancer.

CHAPTER XIII:

Dr. Kelley and Ethylene Dichloride— One Era Ends, Another Begins

In 1981, the year I first met Dr. Kelley, the Food and Drug Administration of the United States issued an edict forbidding the use of ethylene dichloride in pharmaceutical processing. A number of animal studies had indicated that the solvent, in extraordinarily high doses taken for prolonged periods of time, might be carcinogenic, and this was enough to prohibit its use.

In his patent, Levin stated that a number of solvents could be used in his azeotropic method, and Viobin began using alternatives. But Levin always believed that ethylene dichloride for many reasons was the most effective. Kelley agreed, and after the manufacturing change, he felt his program was simply not as effective. Of course, Viobin manufactured enzymes strictly as digestive aids; Kelley used these enzymes for his own purposes, to treat cancer, and he believed the newer solvents did not extract as potent a product. During the years I knew him, he was continually frustrated by what he believed were problems with the anticancer efficacy of the available enzymes.

During my review of Kelley's records, I did notice that after 1981, the effectiveness of his program seemed to diminish. There were patients, including the one with pancreatic cancer I discussed in my Kelley report, who had begun in 1982 and seemed to do well. But as far as I could see from the records themselves, after 1982, his program simply did not work as well, and the miracle cases were few and far between.

Of course, there were a number of variables. After the Steve McQueen episode in late 1980, Kelley had largely withdrawn from direct patient care. He turned over his patients to the community of counselors he had trained over the years. These counselors came from all walks of life; some were physicians, but most were former patients who had taken a number of training seminars Kelley offered during the 1970s and early 1980s. The counselors worked directly under Kelley's supervision, and a number of them, even though they lacked formal medical training, seemed to manage his program quite well. Several of the patients in my research monograph had actually been treated by these counselors, under Kelley's supervision.

Kelley felt the counselors weren't the problem, and neither did I, because they had been managing patients effectively for some years before 1981; several had large "Kelley Program" practices. But clearly, after 1982, something significant had changed. I could see this from the records. Kelley himself, from the reports from his counselors, and from my own documentation, knew his program wasn't working the way it once had, and the failures tortured him. And of course, as more patients failed, the counselors themselves became discouraged. I knew of several former Kelley patients whose lives he had saved, and who had worked with him for years, who began discouraging patients from beginning the program.

To Kelley, the problem was without doubt the new methods that were being used to make pancreatic enzymes. Kelley tried enzymes from different manufacturers but felt the alternatives were generally useless against cancer. Finally, after a year of enormous frustration, in 1986 Kelley decided to close his Dallas office.

I remember so well the last time I visited Kelley in Dallas, shortly before he moved to Pennsylvania. It was in the spring of 1986, when I was finishing my fellowship with Dr. Good, in Florida, and was still optimistic that I would be able to publish my monograph and get funding for clinical trials. Despite the opposition, and the disappointments, I had been able to finish my project, as I had promised Dr. Kelley I would do.

I didn't realize, until I visited with Dr. Kelley, how badly he was doing. He was living in his office, sleeping on the couch. The once frenetically busy place that I had first come to in July of 1981 was eerily empty. Most of the furniture was gone, except for a few folding tables and chairs and the couch where Kelley slept. Packed cardboard boxes were piled everywhere, containing office records, the mementos of the past years. He had one part-time secretary, who came in to answer the phone and the mail. All the other staff had been let go. The counselor network had collapsed, and Kelley was taking no new patients. I didn't know how he was paying for food.

I tried to be upbeat and positive, and indeed he was very pleased when I showed him the final draft of the research monograph. At one point, the phone rang, and Kelley himself answered. Kelley didn't identify himself at first, then announced that he was the janitor, Jack, and quickly got off the phone, saying he "didn't know where Dr. Kelley was." I suspected the caller was a bill collector. Kelley became very morose, as we sat on folding chairs in his empty, ghostlike office.

When I came to New York in 1987, I knew that to salvage Kelley's work, I needed to identify a suitable supply of pancreatic enzymes. Without a suitable source, there was no therapy. I began to rethink all I had learned about enzymes over the past six years from Dr. Kelley and from my readings. I studied the Ezra Levin patent from 1950 (#2,503,313) for hours at a time, trying to understand why Dr. Kelley's program, which had produced such extraordinary results during the 1970s, ended up in ruins.

I began to understand why Levin believed ethylene dichloride was a perfect solvent in so many ways. I also began to fear, as had Kelley, that without an equivalent, a good anticancer enzyme supplement would be difficult to make.

I knew there had to be an answer. I also didn't have a lot of time to find one. But I gave myself the leisure of several weeks to think about the problem: if I couldn't come up with an answer, I would have to start thinking about doing something else.

I began to study and analyze each step of Levin's patent. Levin argued, as a primary assumption, that the ideal pancreatic product should contain the entire enzyme component, not just select enzymes such as trypsin. Though Levin's purpose was completely different from Kelley's—Levin wanted to design the best digestive aid possible and Kelley wanted to treat cancer—I suspected that the original Levin product worked so well against cancer because it contained the full protein complement of the pancreas, including all the known enzymes. I thought it possible that this product also contained enzymes that had not yet even been identified, or perhaps peptides and smaller proteins that might serve as activation factors, protective factors, or stabilization factors for the major enzymes. Perhaps some of these unidentified cofactors might even have powerful anticancer effects. I suspected that all these various components might work synergistically together, producing a greater effect than any single purified, isolated enzyme.

From my readings, I knew that many nutritional and herbal substances work best as part of complexes, as found in nature. For example, during the 1940s, many individual members of the B complex became identified and available for experimental purposes. Scientists began administering large doses of individual B vitamins, such as thiamin, to laboratory animals as well as human volunteers. They learned that a lab animal—or a human volunteer—fed large doses of a single B vitamin would very quickly, sometimes in a matter of weeks, develop deficiencies in other B vitamins. We now know, of course, that the many B vitamins work together as a complex.

Many well-known herbal remedies contain a variety of known but also unknown factors that are all required for maximum effect; oftentimes, a highly processed product supposedly containing the main active ingredient has proven to be less useful. A recent, highly publicized example is the herb St. John's wort, widely used for decades in Europe and now in the United States to treat depression. Clinical studies, particularly in Germany, have documented that the herb is effective in the treatment of mild depression. These positive studies invariably relied on extracts of the whole herb, containing a variety of active ingredients, some identified, some not.

Pharmacologists recently isolated what they believe to be the main active ingredient in St. John's wort, hypericum. However, clinical tests using just hypericum have shown very little effect. The lesson? Nutrients and natural therapeutic products from herbs tend to work best as part of a complex, not as isolated components.

Why should the situation be any different with pancreatic enzymes? I decided as a start that any product I would use had to contain the entire complement of pancreatic proteins, as the Levin product did, not just a few of the major enzymes.

But the other assumptions in Levin's patent—which Kelley always accepted—I began to question. Levin, from his earliest research, sought to make a maximally potent product, with all the precursors in the activated state. He never once doubted that such a preparation would be the best. Kelley, in my many conversations over the years, always believed that such a product, with no precursors present, was the most efficient against cancer. He never once expressed any doubts about this at all.

But why should this be true? I knew Beard required an active product because he was using the enzymes injectably, and presumably there would be no way for precursors to activate in the bloodstream. But Levin and Kelley were using enzymes orally, and the body had a system for precursor activation in the small intestine that worked very quickly and very efficiently. Even if much or most of an oral pancreas product were in the precursor form, activation should proceed very rapidly in the small intestine and the end result would be as good, perhaps, as starting with a fully active oral preparation. As I thought about the problem, I began to believe that a pancreas product that was only partially active might work even better.

Certainly, based on what I knew, such a product should be stable through the processing even without ethylene dichloride, with fewer active enzymes around to cause trouble. With a lower concentration of active enzymes, I thought, the capsule or tablet would also be stable, with a lower probability of an active enzyme colliding with another active enzyme. Such a product might be ideal in the digestive tract; the precursors should be even more stable to acid in the stomach than the fully active enzymes. In the alkaline duodenum, the active trypsin would work with the duodenal enterokinase to start the activation cascade, quickly converting the remaining precursors.

I suspected that in the alkaline duodenum, a fully active preparation such as Levin's would ultimately leave fewer viable enzymes than a partially activated product would, because the probability of an active enzyme colliding with another active enzyme, denaturing one another, would be much greater. With a partially active product, enzymes such as trypsin would be as likely to collide with, and in turn activate, a precursor—an ideal situation.

Perhaps Kelley—and Levin—were wrong in their belief that a fully activated product was the best! I could see no rationale for not trying a partially activated product. And such a product would not require ethylene dichloride to prevent active enzymes from destroying one another during processing. If many or most of the enzymes were in the precursor form, this would not even be an issue. Levin's process needed a solvent such as ethylene dichloride only because he sought to produce a maximally active preparation.

Levin also believed without ever expressing a doubt—as did Kelley—that the ideal product would not only be maximally activated, but would also be fat-, or lipid-, free. Kelley had never in my years of discussing enzymes with him questioned this premise, but this was another assumption that made less sense the more I thought about it—and the more I studied fats.

CHAPTER XIV:

Fats and the Pancreas—A Closer Look

Both physicians and laypeople tend to think of fats as inert padding in the body, with no greater purpose than to make our lives cosmetically difficult. But lipids, or fats, are a very complex and critically essential biochemical component of the body, affecting processes ranging from inflammation to heart rhythm. Without certain fats, the brain and eyes will not develop normally, our lungs will fail, and our cells will simply collapse.

Lipids as a group differ considerably in their molecular structure, biochemical properties, and physiological effects. Technically, all lipids are organic compounds: this means simply that their backbone structure consists of carbon atoms, linked together either in simple chains or in more complex ring structures, with additional hydrogen and oxygen atoms attached to each carbon atom as well.

Proteins and carbohydrates (sugars) are also organic compounds made of carbon, hydrogen, and oxygen; lipids differ from the other two groups in certain basic properties. Carbohydrates and proteins tend to be soluble in water and insoluble, or immiscible, in oils and solvents such as benzene. Lipids tend to be insoluble in water but readily soluble in oils and benzene.

Lipids with a high melting point will be solid at room temperature, such as the fat in a marble steak. Other lipids, with very low melting points, including oils such as olive or flaxseed oil, are liquid at room temperature. The wide differences in melting point among the lipids depend on the linkages of the basic carbon atoms and the number of what are called double bonds between adjacent carbon atoms. The more double bonds in the lipids structure, the lower the melting point is.

Lipids can be divided into four major categories: 1) fatty acids, 2) neutral fats or triglycerides, 3) phospholipids and related compounds, and 4) cholesterol.

Fatty acids are simple chains of carbon atoms linked together with an acidic, or carboxylic, group at one end. Fatty acids are the basic unit of all lipids: both triglycerides and phospholipids contain fatty acids bound to glycerol, itself a three-carbon alcohol.

Cholesterol, though far more complex in structure than the other lipids, is made in the body from fatty acid components linked together.

Our bodies can use fatty acids, as well as carbohydrates, to produce the energy required to maintain life. In the mitochondria of the cell cytoplasm, fatty acids are gradually broken down two carbons at a time with the release of large amounts of chemical energy. This energy is stored in the high-energy phosphate bonds of adenosine triphosphate (ATP), the basic energy source for all reactions in our cells, tissues, and organs. In addition, each two-carbon unit cleaved off the fatty acid can then be shunted into the citric acid cycle within the mitochondria for the production of more high-energy ATP.

Fatty acids are defined as either unsaturated or saturated, terms that relate to the presence or absence of double bonds between carbon atoms in the fatty acid chain. Bonds between atoms, such as carbon atoms in fatty acid molecules, are the linking of two atoms through the sharing of electrons in the outer electron orbits of each. These shared electrons keep atoms bound together, hence the term *bond*. In a single bond, two adjacent carbon atoms share only two electrons, the minimum required to produce a chemical link between atoms. In a double bond, two carbon atoms share four electrons.

Saturated fatty acids are defined as fatty acids without any double bonds between their carbon atoms, while unsaturated fatty acid carbons share one or more such double bonds. Polyunsaturated fatty acids have multiple double bonds in their carbon chains. Fatty acids with multiple double bonds are subdivided into two basic groups, depending on the location of the first double bond counting from the nonacidic carbon end. Omega-6 fatty acids have the first double bond at the sixth carbon from the nonacidic carbon. The omega-3 fatty acids, which have been receiving considerable publicity because of their effect on nerve and cardiac function, have the first unsaturated bond at position 3.

The length of the fatty acid chain, as well as the number of double bonds in the molecule, helps determine the chemical and physical properties of fatty acids. The longer the fatty acid, the higher the melting point, and the greater the number of double bonds, the lower the melting point. A long-chain saturated fatty acid such as behenic acid, with twenty-two carbons and no double bonds, is a solid fat up to 80 degrees Centigrade, well above room temperature (100 degrees Centigrade is the boiling point of water). A highly unsaturated long-chain fatty acid, such as docosahexaenoic acid, with twenty-two carbons but with six double bonds, is a liquid well below freezing (0 degrees Centigrade).

In the frigid waters of the Arctic, plankton, the single-celled algae that are the basis of the entire Arctic food chain, produce large amounts of the long-chain polyunsaturated fatty acids eicosapentaenoic (EPA, twenty carbons, five double bonds) and docosahexaenoic (DHA, twenty-two carbons, six double bonds) acids, both omega-3 fatty acids. These fatty acids have very low freezing points because of their multiple double bonds and function as a cellular antifreeze, preventing the algae from solidifying in the ice-cold waters of the Arctic seas. These two fatty acids accumulate in the fish that feed on the plankton and protect the fish from freezing as well. The whales, seals, and polar bears that eat the fish, and the Eskimos who traditionally ate them all, will in turn concentrate these two lipids. Not only do EPA and DHA function as antifreeze in plankton and fish, but in humans, these fatty acids reduce inflammatory reactions of the immune system, lower blood levels of cholesterol and triglycerides, reduce platelet stickiness, and in turn affect blood clotting.

Inflammatory reactions can occur in any tissue of the body as a protective response to injury, whether the result of an invading microorganism, a toxic substance such as an allergen, or physical trauma. With tissue injury, damaged cells release a series of biochemical products such as serotonin and histamine, which cause capillaries to become leaky. Fluid collects around the damaged tissue, immune cells from the bloodstream arrive, and platelets—the cell-like components from the blood responsible for blood clotting—begin forming fibrous clots. As a result of these events, the damaged area becomes walled off from the rest of the body, preventing the spread of infection and of potentially toxic waste from injured cells.

An uncontrolled inflammatory response can lead to serious tissue damage, and researchers now believe that inflammatory reactions in blood vessels are the first step in atherosclerotic heart disease. In an area of vascular injury, after the initial inflammatory response, the body begins depositing cholesterol and triglycerides, both blood fats, in the damaged area. Then fibrin and platelets collect, forming enlarging clots over the injured vessel walls. If this process continues over time, an atherosclerotic lesion can form in the artery, with a blood clot superimposed—all an invitation to disaster.

The anti-inflammatory, cholesterol- and triglyceride-lowering, and platelet-blocking action of the omega-3 fatty acids EPA and DHA explain, at least partially, why Eskimos living on a traditional high-fat Arctic diet rarely if ever developed significant atherosclerosis or suffered heart attacks.

Interestingly, recently scientists discovered that high levels of fatty acids in the blood—as invariably occurs with a high-meat, high-fat diet—effectively stimulate the sympathetic nervous system into action. In the Kelley model, for the meat-eating parasympathetic dominants with their weak sympathetic nervous system, such an effect would be ideal.

In our normal metabolic processes, our cells use some several dozen different fatty acids, ranging from the four-carbon butyric acid, which the lining cells of the intestinal tract convert to energy, to the long-chain polyunsaturated docosahexaenoic acid, with twenty-two carbons and its cardioprotective action. Nearly all of these can be manufactured in our bodies with the exception of two, linoleic and alpha-linolenic acid, both eighteen-carbon polyunsaturated fatty acids. Linoleic acid is an omega-6 fatty acid with two double bonds; alpha-linolenic acid is an omega-3 fatty acid with three double bonds. Linoleic and alpha-linolenic acid are classified as essential fatty acids, because they must be supplied by the diet and are required for normal growth and development. Infants deficient in either of these lipids fail to grow normally and develop anemia, dry scaly skin, and hair loss. Deficiency in adults also results in anemia, chronic eczema, and hair loss.

Both of these essential fatty acids are critical components of all cell membranes, including the outer membrane surrounding the cells as well as the membranes of the small subcellular organelles, such as the mitochondria and cell nucleus. The essential fatty acids help control membrane fluidity and, through electrostatic forces produced by their double bonds, help anchor cell membrane proteins. These membrane proteins serve as gatekeepers, regulating the entry of needed nutrients and preventing admission of unwanted toxins and infectious agents such as viruses.

Most importantly, the essential fatty acids are required for the absorption of oxygen by the lung alveolar cells, the transfer of oxygen to red blood cells, and the release of oxygen from the red cells to the target tissues. Without essential fatty acids, oxygen transfer occurs very inefficiently.

In addition to their role in cell membranes and as oxygen transporters, both linoleic and alpha-linolenic acid are converted into other fatty acids and fatty acid derivatives. The enzyme delta-6-desaturase transforms linoleic acid to gamma-linolenic acid (GLA), and in turn, the enzyme fatty acid elongase adds two carbons to GLA, converting it to dihomo-gamma-linolenic acid, with twenty carbons and three double bonds. The enzyme delta-5-desaturase then adds another double bond to dihomo-gamma-linolenic acid, converting it to arachidonic acid, a twenty-carbon omega-6 fatty acid with four double bonds.

Alpha-linolenic acid, the starting point for the omega-3 fatty acid series, converts first to eicosapentaenoic acid (EPA), a twenty-carbon, omega-3 fatty acid with five double bonds. The elongase enzyme then adds two carbons to EPA, forming docosahexaenoic acid (DHA), the twenty-two-carbon omega-3 fatty acid, with six double bonds.

Importantly, dihomo-gamma-linoleic acid, arachidonic acid, and eicosapentaenoic acid are in turn converted into hormone-like derivatives called the prostaglandins, which control biochemical reactions ranging from hormone secretion to inflammation. Scientists have identified more than thirty different prostaglandins, all of which consist of twenty carbons and a ring structure at one end. The prostaglandins were first isolated in prostate tissue, hence the name.

Scientists divide the prostaglandins into three series, depending on the fatty acid starting point. Series 1 prostaglandins derive from the omega-6 fatty acid dihomo-gamma-linolenic acid. Series 2 prostaglandins derive from arachidonic acid, also an omega-6 fatty acid. Series 3 prostaglandins develop from the omega-3 fatty acid eicosapentaenoic acid (EPA).

The series 1 prostaglandins have an overall anti-inflammatory effect, blocking the release of mediators of inflammation such as serotonin; reducing platelet stickiness, thus preventing clots; and improving circulation. The series 1 group also reduces cholesterol synthesis and may prevent cancer cells from dividing. Members of the series 2 prostaglandins have a distinctly pro-inflammatory effect; they stimulate the release of mediators of inflammation such as histamine, enhance platelet stickiness and clot formation, and cause salt and water retention in the kidneys.

The series 3 prostaglandins from eicosapentaenoic acid (EPA) are strongly anti-inflammatory; members of this group block release of inflammatory products, reduce platelet stickiness and blood clotting, and cause the kidneys to lose salt and water. The pronounced antiplatelet effect of the series 3 prostaglandins further helps explain the low levels of heart disease in the Eskimos consuming their traditional all-meat, high-fat diet. The high levels of EPA in this diet in turn lead to high levels of the circulating series 3 prostaglandins and a lowered tendency of the blood to clot. Less clotting translates into fewer heart attacks.

Arachidonic and eicosapentaenoic acid are also the starting points for another class of compounds, the 4 and 5 series of leukotrienes, respectively. Leukotrienes, first isolated in the white blood cells, or leukocytes, are another class of inflammatory mediators found most commonly in the various immune cells such as leukocytes and mast cells, as well as platelets and the cells lining the blood vessels of the lungs and heart. The 4 series leukotrienes from arachidonic acid are powerfully pro-inflammatory; they strongly contract smooth muscles in the bronchi of the lungs, producing bronchoconstriction and wheezing. The 4 series leukotrienes cause blood vessels to leak, resulting in edema, and attract white blood cells to areas of injury. This strong inflammatory response is countered by the 5 series leukotrienes from eicosapentaenoic acid, which reduce smooth muscle contraction, reduce blood vessel leakiness, and block the chemo-attractant effect of the series 4 group.

All this shows how complex fatty acid metabolism is. Not only do the fatty acids serve as a primary energy source in the cells, but both directly, as the essential fatty acids, and indirectly, through their prostaglandin and leukotriene derivatives, they affect a range of metabolic processes including inflammation, the immune response, circulation, and respiration as well as salt and water balance.

The second category of lipids, the triglycerides, is a storage form of fat. These lipids consist of a three-carbon glycerol backbone, with a fatty acid linked to each of the three carbons. Animal products are the only dietary source of triglycerides, because plants do not make this type of fat. Dietary triglycerides are absorbed from the small intestines into the lymphatic vessels as part of chylomicra, which are basically fat carriers made up of protein. Eventually, the dietary triglycerides reach the liver, where they are extracted and either broken down for energy or packaged in lipoproteins, another fat carrier produced in the liver itself.

If the triglycerides are not needed for immediate energy production, the lipoproteins, with the excess triglycerides, are released by the liver cells into the bloodstream. The fat cells, or adipocytes, then extract the triglycerides from the circulating lipoproteins for storage. Adipocytes quite efficiently store triglycerides and can accumulate up to 80 to 95 percent of their total cell volume with lipids.

Our livers can also manufacture triglycerides from the breakdown products of sugar, protein, and fat metabolism. We store excess calories, whatever the food source may be, primarily as triglycerides. After production and processing in the liver, newly created triglycerides circulate in the blood just as those from the diet, as part of lipoproteins, which eventually make their way to the adipocytes.

In times of starvation or caloric restriction, adipocytes, through a complex series of hormonal and neurological signals, break down triglycerides into the component glycerol and fatty acids, which are then released into the bloodstream. The fatty acids make their way back to the liver, where the fatty acids are broken down to acetoacetic acid and beta hydroxybutyric acid, both containing four carbons, and acetone, with three carbons. These three compounds—known as ketone bodies—are released into the bloodstream, where they can be picked up and used for energy by virtually all cells of the body.

On an all-meat diet, with no carbohydrate source available, ketone bodies become the major energy source for all our cells. The cells of traditional meat eaters, such as the Eskimos, are very adept at using ketone bodies. In addition, the presence in the bloodstream of acetoacetic and beta hydroxybutyric acid, both very strong organic acids, pushes the blood to be more acidic. This increased acidity in turn stimulates sympathetic nervous system activity—an ideal effect for Kelley's meat-eating parasympathetic-dominant patients.

The third category of lipids, the phospholipids, has a similar structure to triglycerides, with a three-carbon glycerol backbone. And as in triglycerides, fatty acids link up to the first two carbons of the glycerol molecule. However, phospholipids differ at the third carbon position. Here, instead of another fatty acid linkage, the carbon connects to a phosphate group, consisting of the element phosphorus and four attached oxygen molecules. The phosphate group gives phospholipids electric polarity because of the electrons in the oxygen molecules; such polarity is lacking in the triglycerides.

In phospholipids, one of these oxygen molecules attached to the phosphorus atom then links to a non-fatty acid molecule, such as the B vitamin choline, producing phosphatidyl choline, part of the lecithin complex. Other molecules that can bond at this phosphate position include inositol, or serine, producing phosphatidylinositol and phosphatidylserine, respectively, both important for nerve cell function. In clinical trials, in fact, phosphatidylserine has been shown to improve memory loss associated with aging, even in patients with Alzheimer's disease.

Phospholipids are the foundation of all membranes of all cells in all living organisms, from single-celled paramecia to the cells of elephants and those of the giant redwoods. Without phospholipids, cell membranes, and life, could not exist. Biological membranes actually consist of two layers of phospholipids, with the polar phosphorus groups on the outside and the fatty acid chains pointing inward. This polarity of the phospholipid molecules allows stable membrane structures to form and remain intact.

The membranes surrounding cells keep all cells together, as individual identities, separated from the environment and other cells. Furthermore, phospholipids, working with membrane proteins, regulate the entry and exit of molecules into and out of cells. Cell membranes selectively block the entrance of noxious materials but allow the transport of essential nutrients and oxygen into cells and the removal of waste products out of cells.

Membranes also encapsulate many organelles within the cell interior, such as the nucleus and the energy-producing mitochondria. In addition, membranes form much of the manufacturing machinery within the cells, such as the endoplasmic reticulum and the Golgi complex—where pancreatic enzymes, for example, are actually manufactured—and separate the products of their work into vacuoles. In such vacuoles, the pancreatic acinar cells store the potentially deadly proteolytic digestive enzymes until needed in the duodenum.

The specific fatty acid composition of phospholipids determines how fluid, or how solid, a particular cell membrane will be. Usually, the middle carbon of a phospholipid links to an unsaturated fatty acid, such as linoleic acid, to allow fluidity in the membrane, while the first carbon links to a saturated fatty acid, to provide some stability and strength. Slight changes in the fatty acid composition of phospholipids, because of dietary deficiency of the essential omega-3 or omega-6 fatty acids, can gravely disrupt membrane function and cellular health.

Cholesterol, the last major lipid category, is a complex molecule consisting of three six-carbon ring structures and a five-carbon ring linked together, with a long carbon chain attached to the five-carbon ring. The four ring structures make up the steroid nucleus of cholesterol.

The typical American diet provides anywhere from 0.3 to 0.8 grams of cholesterol per day, entirely from animal sources such as red meat, eggs, and dairy products. Plant cells manufacture sterols that are similar in structure to cholesterol, but they do not make cholesterol itself. Although over the past thirty years, much has been made of dietary cholesterol and its proposed relationship to atherosclerosis and coronary artery disease, our bodies manufacture at least one gram of cholesterol a day, more than we ever take in from food. Our liver cells, the hepatocytes, are the main source for circulating cholesterol, but all cells of all tissues can make cholesterol for their own use. In fact, with increased dietary intake, cholesterol production in the liver and other cells falls; with decreased intake, production increases.

The starting point for cholesterol production in cells is the two-carbon molecule acetate, the end product of both sugar and fatty acid metabolism. In cholesterol synthesis, acetate molecules successively link to one another, eventually producing the complex cholesterol molecule. A diet high in sugars can actually lead to increased serum cholesterol levels, because sugar not used for immediate energy needs is broken down to acetate, which the liver can then convert to cholesterol.

Although we have been taught to think of cholesterol as a great evil with no purpose other than to clog our arteries and cause disease, this lipid is absolutely essential for health and well-being. In the liver, up to 80 percent of manufactured cholesterol is further transformed into bile salts; these salts are first stored in the gallbladder and then released into the intestinal tract to aid in fat digestion. Absorption of the soluble vitamins such as vitamins A, D, E, and K requires bile salts.

Cholesterol is also the starting point for the manufacture of all steroid hormones in the body. These include the various hormones produced by the adrenal cortex, such as the glucocorticoids, which help provide a steady stream of glucose and fatty acids in the blood to meet the energy needs of all our cells. After a meal, as fatty acids, cholesterol, and glucose flood the bloodstream, the adrenal cortex secretes only minimal amounts of the glucocorticoids. However, levels of both glucose and fatty acids can drop if the time between meals becomes unusually extended, or if the pancreas produces too much insulin, which drives sugars and fats out of the blood into the cells of the muscles and liver. Low blood sugar, or hypoglycemia, can result. This is a potentially serious situation because the brain, which uses 25 percent of energy produced in the body, prefers glucose as its primary energy source.

As the blood sugar and blood fatty acid levels drop, specialized cells in the hypothalamus, the autonomic nervous system center of the brain, become activated. These cells in turn send signals activating the sympathetic nervous system. The outflow of the sympathetic hormones norepinephrine and epinephrine stimulate release of stored sugars and fatty acids from the liver and muscle cells. In addition, the hypothalamic cells signal the anterior pituitary, which sits right underneath the hypothalamus in back of the brain, to secrete the hormone ACTH—adrenocorticotropin hormone. This peptide circulates in the blood, stimulating the release of glucocorticoids from the adrenals. These hormones, along with the sympathetic neurotransmitters, cause release of sugars and fatty acids from the liver and prevent a potentially dangerous depletion of energy supplies to the brain and other organs.

Adrenal cortex hormones also protect against uncontrolled inflammation, by blocking immune cells such as mast cells from releasing mediators of inflammation, including serotonin and histamine. DHEA, widely touted as a "youth hormone," is actually a precursor to the glucocorticoids and, again, is made in the adrenals from cholesterol.

Another class of adrenal cortex hormones, the mineralocorticoids such as aldosterone, help regulate fluid balance in the body and, in turn, blood pressure. Aldosterone particularly helps prevent the potentially serious effects of excessive fluid loss, as can occur with rapid bleeding or severe dehydration. Such situations can be life threatening, because with significant fluid loss, blood volume and blood pressure drop, reducing the amount of blood circulating to the vital organs, including the brain and heart. Stroke, heart attacks, and death can result. But as blood volume and blood pressure drop, the brain mounts a very aggressive response.

First, pressure-sensitive cells in the hypothalamus send signals to the brain centers that control the sympathetic nervous system, which rapidly activates. The sympathetic firing increases the rate and strength of heart contractions. This in turn produces increased cardiac output, to help compensate for the reduction in blood volume. Sympathetic activity also selectively directs the flow of blood to critical areas such as the brain and heart to guarantee an adequate supply of oxygen and nutrients. The vessels feeding the entire digestive system, including the liver and the pancreas, constrict so that no more than the minimum amount of blood necessary for tissue survival flows through. Digestive function, including enzyme production and bile flow, basically shuts down. The vessels to the skin constrict as well, but the arteries to the brain and the heart itself open wide, to help ensure adequate blood flow to these essential organs.

The sympathetic activity then signals the outer layer of the adrenal cortex to secrete aldosterone into the bloodstream. Aldosterone specifically stimulates the kidney tubules to reabsorb both salt and water, an effect that helps offset the potential damage from excessive fluid loss. Decreased blood volume that occurs with dehydration or blood loss also stimulates pressure-sensitive cells in the kidney, the juxtaglomerular cells. In response to dropping blood pressure, these cells release renin, an enzyme that helps convert the plasma protein angiotensinogen ultimately to angiotensin II. This latter peptide is a very powerful vasoconstrictor that, along with the sympathetic activity, fights to keep blood pressure from dropping to dangerous levels.

Angiotensin II also stimulates aldosterone release from the adrenals. In times of fluid excess, the whole process reverses: sympathetic firing slows, renin secretion diminishes, and ultimately aldosterone production and release from the adrenals falls to minimal or nonexistent levels. The efficiency of this intricate system of fluid control fundamentally depends on cholesterol; without cholesterol, there would be no aldosterone, and our ability to survive even minor fluid crises would be severely compromised.

Cholesterol is also the basic unit for the manufacture of the sex hormones, including the various estrogens and progesterone produced in the ovaries of women, and testosterone, made in the testicles of males. In fact, without cholesterol in the diet, sex hormone production falls; women on very low-fat diets as well as women who are bulimic or anorectic can be so cholesterol deficient that estrogen and progesterone production is too low to support the normal monthly menstrual cycle.

Along with the phospholipids, cholesterol is a critical component of all cell membranes and helps regulate membrane fluidity. Cholesterol serves as a membrane foundation, and without this lipid, membranes would be so fluid they would literally fall apart. Furthermore, the epidermal cells of our skin secrete large amounts of cholesterol into the outermost skin layer. There, cholesterol prevents evaporation of water from the skin, which would otherwise be excessive and even life threatening. Burn patients, for example, whose skin barriers are not intact, can lose quarts of water a day from evaporation. The cholesterol also prevents absorption of many water-soluble chemicals through the skin that could be toxic to the body. Cholesterol is very resistant to the action of many solvents, including salts, acids, and bases, that might otherwise, without a cholesterol coating, literally dissolve away the surfaces of our bodies.

The pancreas is itself a lean organ, with very little storage fat around or in it. The fat content, which Levin with great determination sought to remove, consists of the phospholipids and cholesterol in the cell and organelle membranes, and some minimal amounts of stored triglycerides in the cells themselves. The vacuoles of pancreatic acinar cells containing the precursor proteolytic enzymes are encapsulated within such a lipid membrane.

When I thought about the Levin process, I could understand why he wanted to remove as much water as possible, because in a watery environment, the active enzymes would quickly set off the cascade ending in denaturation and enzyme destruction. But I didn't understand why he was so sure the best enzyme product would have no fat. In the acinar cells, most of the lipid would be in the membranes, including the membranes around the enzyme vacuoles. These vacuolar membranes are there to keep the enzymes, or their precursors, isolated and inactive, separated from the rest of the cell; to my thinking, intact membranes, with the enzymes isolated in their vacuoles, would be an asset, not a detriment.

The more I thought about the functions of the lipids in the pancreas, the more certain I was that the best manufacturing process should leave the lipids and, hence, the cell and organelle membranes intact. A pancreas enzyme product with all its lipids, including cholesterol, to me would most likely be the most resistant to degradation during processing and the most stable in the capsule. Furthermore, fatty acids are such a complex group of compounds with so many biochemical and physiological effects, I began to wonder if the lipids in the pancreatic cells might not work with the proteolytic enzymes synergistically.

Ultimately, I decided that the best anticancer pancreatic enzyme should be only partially, not maximally, activated and contain all its fat. Only the water should be removed.

But this, I knew, was all theory, and even if I was right, I still didn't have a source of enzymes to use in practice. I thought about my options. I knew that the major pharmaceutical companies that manufactured enzymes either used variations of the Levin approach, as did Viobin, or still used the old extraction techniques that Levin had found so inefficient forty years earlier. However, because I was completely unknown in both the mainstream and alternative medical world, and because I was not yet in practice, I knew I could not get a major manufacturer to work with me to test out my theories. I could only hope that some company already manufactured a pancreatic enzyme supplement that at least came close to what I felt would work best.

I spent several weeks trying to locate a source of acceptable enzymes. I started off by calling a number of pharmaceutical companies that I knew had begun making pancreatic enzymes. I talked about their source of animals and their manufacturing methods. All of these companies used animals from the Omaha feed lots, and all used solvent extraction methods. A number of these companies sent me samples of product, for testing.

I tracked down a former colleague of Ezra Levin, who was retired and living in California. We spent hours on the phone, trading ideas and information. I was relieved when he said I might be on to something with my ideas, but he knew of no enzyme that would meet my specifications. All currently available products, he thought, were solvent extracted and lipid-free. The Ezra Levin patent, he said, had dominated thinking in the "enzyme industry," as he called it, for years.

One day, in mid-August, I went to Willner Chemists, a well-known nutritional pharmacy, in mid-Manhattan. I had a long talk with Mr. Willner himself, who at that time still ran the pharmacy. I explained what I was looking for, a minimally processed enzyme product that was not lipid-free. He immediately recommended the enzyme supplement from a company, Allergy Research Group (ARG), whose products, I already knew, were used by many alternative physicians. This company made an entire line of animal glandular products, such as thymus, liver, and adrenal, which alternative doctors often used in their treatment.

All these animal products, including the enzymes, Willner explained, were minimally processed: the owner of the company, Stephen Levine, PhD, a molecular biologist by training, believed firmly that processing destroyed too many active and important factors. These supplements, Willner further explained, were all in capsule form, not in tablets, because Levine believed that even the pressure of tableting an enzyme would cause loss of potency. All this seemed almost too good to be true. I immediately pulled several bottles of the ARG enzyme supplement from the shelf. To my relief, they were pork enzymes, from animals raised in New Zealand—the country that I had already come to believe had the strictest standards in the world for animal husbandry.

I brought half a dozen bottles back to my mother's home and immediately emptied several capsules on my tongue. From my years with Kelley, I had come to know what a good enzyme product should taste like—meaty, producing a tingling on the tongue because of the enzyme activity. The ARG product passed the test; at least it tasted like a well-made enzyme. I also felt the supplement had a slightly greasy taste, an indication that it contained some fat. I then gulped a number of capsules down. I knew that an appropriately made pancreatic enzyme supplement should not produce any digestive distress; in the months before Kelley closed his practice, he continually reported that all the enzyme products he tried with patients created enormous digestive problems even when taken in small doses.

The ARG enzymes caused no problems. They had passed the two basic but important clinical tests. Now, I had to consider the actual potency of the supplement. Enzyme assays done by analytical laboratories are quite expensive. Because our resources were so limited, I developed my own assay to determine the activity level of the pancreas enzyme product. In this simple test, I compared the amount of Knox gelatin—which is pure protein—digested over time by the ARG product compared with the amount digested by the Viobin enzyme. The assay, while crude, cost only a few dollars to set up and run in my mother's kitchen.

The ARG enzyme supplement had approximately 2–3X strength, which meant it was partially, not completely activated—exactly what I had been looking for. I called the president of the company, Dr. Stephen Levine, in California, to discuss his supplements and his production capabilities—because if these enzymes really worked in practice, I was going to need a steady and large supply.

Although I was a total unknown in the alternative medical world, he was very gracious and answered questions I had about his products. He confirmed that the enzymes were minimally processed and did contain at least some fat. Water was extracted through freeze-drying, a method in which the pancreas glandular material is frozen and then subjected to vacuum distillation to remove water. He believed no chemical solvents were used to make the enzymes at any point in the manufacturing. When I explained why I wanted the enzymes, he said he would help in any way he could to guarantee a steady supply.

My life changed because of the kindness of friends. Within several weeks, I had a room to see patients in the Park Avenue office of my old physician friend, from my journalism days, and his doctor wife. Although an orthodox physician by training, he had always been interested in new ideas, and after reading my Kelley manuscript, he felt I might be on to something. I now had a place to work and potentially good enzymes; I just needed patients.

I had also come to know Dr. Robert Atkins during my journalism days. Atkins was already famous as a diet doctor and increasingly well known as the leading alternative doctor in New York. He had best-selling books, his own radio show, and a thriving nutritional practice on East 56th Street. Dr. Atkins had followed my career through medical school—and at one point he came to speak at Cornell as part of a lecture series on alternative medicine that I had set up.

When he heard I was back in New York, he invited me to dinner with his fiancée and asked me to bring a copy of my Kelley manuscript. During dinner, I discussed my struggles to find a good supply of enzymes for my treatment. Several days later, after reading the study, he suggested I come by his office to see what he was doing. The following day, after a morning sitting at his side as he worked with patients, he offered me a job in a clinic, with a salary beyond my expectations, a support staff, and a steady supply of patients. He would also do anything he could, he said, to guarantee a supply of whatever supplements I needed.

But after several days in Dr. Atkins's office, I realized that I needed to be on my own, doing things my own way. I turned down his very generous offer, but he still invited me on his radio show to discuss my work with Kelley. I did go on, and because of that show, I got my first patients. I remember very well my first cancer patient, a very nice fifty-five-year-old woman from Long Island, with widely metastatic pancreatic cancer. She had been diagnosed several months earlier and was already in the advanced stages of the disease, with multiple tumors in her liver and lungs. Nonetheless, she wanted to try my "enzyme treatment." I designed a full program for her, with large doses of enzymes to be taken around the clock. She and her husband were very grateful for the opportunity to try the treatment, because her doctors had already told her nothing could work.

She responded exactly as Kelley had taught me patients should respond. She tolerated the enzymes without initial difficulty, but after several days she became increasingly fatigued and anorectic and developed severe pain in the midabdominal region—right in the area of the pancreas. She said the pain was particularly worse half an hour after each dose of pancreatic enzymes. She also complained of muscle aches and pains and a low-grade fever. I knew from my days with Kelley that as the enzymes attacked and destroyed a tumor, very often patients complained of pain right in the tumor area. Kelley said this was a direct effect of the enzymes doing what they were supposed to be doing, killing tumors.

In addition, large quantities of toxic waste would be released into the blood system from the dying tumor cells, just as Beard had warned eighty years earlier. This tumor debris would be primarily processed in the liver and then excreted via the intestinal tract. As more and more cancer cells died, the waste could overload the liver's processing capability and remain backed up in the blood. At this point, patients could then develop a flu-like illness, with low-grade fevers, muscle aches, and malaise—exactly what this patient described. Dr. Isaacs and I celebrated; the enzymes seemed to be working fine.

At one point, after about a month on the program, this patient passed a large, egg-shaped tissue mass with tentacles, like an octopus. Her husband, suspecting this was one of the tumors that had invaded her duodenum, put it in alcohol and brought it in to me. My doctor colleagues and I all believed it was a tumor that the body had thrown off. Unfortunately, several weeks later, this very determined woman, who had a history of heart disease, died suddenly of a pulmonary embolus, a blood clot in the lung.

Her husband expressed nothing but gratitude and only regretted that my therapy had not been available sooner. He believed—as did I—that the enzymes were indeed attacking and destroying her tumor. We had other failures, but we also began having successes—some still alive today. And these initial responses convinced me that we could salvage the enzyme therapy and keep the program alive.

But I never did stop obsessing about pancreatic enzymes. Over the next two years, I continued to study enzyme manufacturing, and in 1989, I began to work directly with a company in New Zealand, Waitaki, which specialized in manufacturing active biologicals for the pharmaceutical industry.

Dr. Isaacs and I would work closely with the staff at Waitaki over the next nine years, striving to produce what we thought would be the ideal anticancer pancreatic enzyme preparation. Largely through constant rethinking, and with ongoing experimentation, we eventually learned precisely what percentage of the pancreas material should be in the active form, and what percentage should be left as precursor for the best therapeutic action. We learned how to activate the product to exactly this point—and then the scientists at Waitaki found a compound that could stop further enzyme action, in a manner similar to ethylene dichloride, to produce a stable preparation.

We also learned, after years of constant research, the ideal fat content of the material that allowed for maximum stability and maximum therapeutic effect. As the pancreas supplement evolved over the years, Dr. Isaacs and I could see the improved clinical results. Although the first enzyme preparation I had used in 1987 worked, the later generations of pancreatic products worked better. By 1998, just as the National Cancer Institute approved funding for our large-scale controlled clinical trial, Dr. Isaacs and I believed that, working with Waitaki, we had perfected the manufacturing process. The problem that had haunted Beard one hundred years ago, and more recently Levin and Kelley, we felt had finally been solved.

Part III:
Case Report

CHAPTER XV:

The Case of Mort Schneider

I remember very well the first time I met Mort Schneider. It was a dreary, rainy mid-December day in 1991. I still worked in the office I sublet from my doctor colleagues on Park Avenue at 71st Street on the East Side of Manhattan. This seemed like an unlikely location for me to have ended up in, on one of the most elegant avenues in the most expensive part of Manhattan. And ironically, Memorial Sloan Kettering Cancer Center at the Cornell Medical Center, where I had enthusiastically first discussed Kelley's work with Dr. Robert Good, was only five blocks directly east. But those days when I was a medical student seemed so far away that Sloan Kettering might as well have been at the other side of the universe.

I lived at the time on East 51st Street right off the East River, and oftentimes, I would walk to work north up York Avenue. The Cornell-Memorial complex began at about 66th Street and York, with the park-like grounds of Rockefeller University, off the East River to the right. There, at Rockefeller, scores of eminent scientists from all over the world did their work. Across the street from Rockefeller was the imposing façade of Memorial Hospital, between 67th and 68th streets. Behind Memorial, west toward First Avenue, stretched the elaborate complex of buildings making up the Sloan Kettering Research Institute, where Good had once reigned.

Mort was the last patient of a very long day, but with an interesting story. He was seventy years old at the time and living outside of Orlando, Florida, with his wife. I already knew from his initial intake interview with our staff and my review of his medical records before the first visit that he had a history of metastatic pancreatic cancer to the liver, a very deadly disease with usually a rapidly terminal prognosis.

He came to my office alone that first day because his wife, he explained, was too sick herself to travel—she had a history of breast cancer and irritable bowel, and just couldn't make the trip. Despite his own diagnosis—and apparently a very ill wife—I still remember not feeling sorry for Mort at all. He lacked any trace of self-pity—though he had a condition where survival is measured in months.

Mort was a retired bookkeeper, he told me, in a simple, straightforward way. He struck me immediately as a man with little pretense; I liked him at once.

In Mort's case, there was considerable cancer in the family. His father had died of an aggressive sarcoma, a type of connective tissue malignancy. Mort's sister had died from breast cancer, and a second sister had died quickly, he reported, from an aggressive brain tumor. Mort himself had smoked cigarettes for about twenty years, having quit some fifteen years earlier. Prior to developing cancer, he had been in good health, except for hypertension and atrial fibrillation (a type of heart rhythm disturbance).

His current problems had begun in late July of 1991, when he had had a fainting episode and had been brought to a local emergency room near his home in Florida. Heart disease was ruled out, but a routine chest X-ray revealed a mass in the upper right lung. Mr. Schneider was thought stable enough to go home, with plans to continue evaluation of the lung lesion. A subsequent CT scan of the chest on August 20, 1991, showed a solitary right 6-mm upper lobe nodule that was consistent with lung cancer. In addition, the radiologist reported several large lymph nodes in the central chest, or mediastinal region, that indicated potential metastatic disease. A bone scan done on the same date showed "abnormal activity of the right hip and right shoulder suggestive of metastatic disease."

In addition, a CT of the abdomen done September 6, 1991, demonstrated considerable evidence of spread, including four tumors in the right lobe of the liver, a tumor in the right adrenal gland 2 cm in size, and a 4.5-cm mass in the head of the pancreas "suspicious for metastatic disease." At that point, the radiologist suggested an abdominal ultrasound, which can often help differentiate between benign and malignant lesions. An ultrasound done September 24, 1991, documented, as the official report states, "areas consistent with metastatic involvement of the liver, the largest of which is approximately 3.4 to 4 cm maximal dimension."

Mort's doctors needed a tumor sample for a diagnosis, and they decided the lung tumor was most accessible. On September 24, 1991, Mr. Schneider was admitted to Winter Park Memorial Hospital in Winter Park, Florida, and the day after his admission, he underwent chest surgery for removal of the right lung tumor. This proved to be infiltrative moderately differentiated adenocarcinoma, a type of cancer that can originate from a number of sites, including the lung, pancreas, or large intestine. Because of the pancreas tumor seen on the earlier CT scan, his physicians assumed the lung lesion was most likely metastatic disease from the pancreas. At the time, Mort's primary physician summed up the situation by describing in his notes, "At some point, I suspect he will require oncology and radiation medicine consultation for what is most likely a pancreatic carcinoma with multiple metastatic lesions."

After the surgery, the Schneiders together met with an oncologist, who told Mort he had a terminal disease for which chemotherapy and radiation would not be useful. The oncologist told Mrs. Schneider later in private that he might have six to eight weeks to live. She was understandably devastated; they had been married for thirty-seven years, and Mort had helped nurse her through her own illnesses.

Mrs. Schneider, a retired English professor, was determined that Mort should not die. She had an interest in nutrition and immediately started her husband on an aggressive supplement program that included high-dose vitamin C, vitamin E, calcium, magnesium, trace minerals such as selenium, and other antioxidants. Despite the terminal prognosis, Mr. Schneider seemed to hold his own. Then, some weeks after he was diagnosed, Mort's wife learned about me from an article written about my work that had appeared in an alternative journal. She quickly called my office and made an appointment.

Mr. Schneider began my therapy with great determination and an enormously supportive wife who helped Mort stick to the program. Clinically, he seemed to improve month by month, with improved energy, stamina, and appetite. Despite the terrible prognosis, months passed, and he didn't die.

Because he was feeling so well on his treatment, initially neither Mort nor I thought follow-up testing with CAT scans to be necessary. First, Mort wasn't going to change his therapy regardless of what the tests showed, and I wouldn't treat him any differently. As far as we both knew, there was no other treatment that could offer him a better chance for prolonged survival than the enzyme therapy. And the ultimate test of the treatment would be his survival.

When he visited my office for a return visit in December 1992, he was already fifteen months from diagnosis and was doing, to use his word, "great." He really had no problems, so we had the time to talk about things other than pancreatic enzymes and carrot juice. I learned there was more to Mort than bookkeeping. He had a master's degree in archeology and had studied art at the Sorbonne in Paris. He was an expert in nineteenth-century French Impressionist painting and had started leading tours as a volunteer at the local art museum in Orlando. He was a deacon in his local church. Even though he had a terrible disease and dire prognosis, and even though he still needed to tend to his chronically ill wife, he seemed to be happy and enjoying his life.

His worst complaint was about the dullness of the diet: in fact, although he seemed religiously compliant with the supplements and the detoxification procedures such as the coffee enemas, he sheepishly admitted he had been cheating in terms of food. His main weakness at that time—at other times there would be other weaknesses—was lox and white-flour bagels that he bought at a local delicatessen. I gave my usual stern lecture about the need to be absolutely vigilantly compliant; I talked about the severity of his disease and the standard prognosis, all of which he already knew.

In February 1993, when Mort was eighteen months from his original diagnosis of terminal cancer, his local physicians decided to repeat the CAT scans to assess the state of his disease. I had mixed feelings about the tests, because in my experience, the fact that he was alive and feeling well was the best indication of how he was doing. The average survival for patients with metastatic pancreatic adenocarcinoma with multiple lesions in the liver is three to five months, and virtually none lives a year. He had passed the most important diagnostic test I knew: he was alive, not dead.

In addition, at times with patients such as Mort, tumors do not change for years. Sometimes, tumors can enlarge, even in patients who ultimately do well. I didn't want a "worse" test report to undermine his confidence. I have had patients who clinically were doing well long after they were supposed to be dead, who became traumatized after CAT scan reports showed a "bigger" tumor.

The CAT scans were done February 4, 1993, and showed some change. The radiologist now identified five liver tumors, instead of four—though it was possible the fifth lesion simply had been present but not clearly identified on the original scans. The other four were about the same size. The pancreatic tumor was actually larger, now measuring 5.5 cm, increased from the 4.5 cm in largest diameter. The large tumors of each adrenal were again noted, as well as enlarged lymph nodes around the pancreas. The radiologist summed up the findings as the following:

> THERE ARE LIVER LESIONS, PORTAL AND PERIPANCREATIC LYMPH NODES THAT ARE ENLARGED AND BILATERAL ADRENAL MASSES, ALL CONSISTENT WITH METASTATIC DISEASE. AS FAR AS I CAN TELL FROM THE PREVIOUS REPORT, ALL THESE LESIONS WERE IDENTIFIED BEFORE.

When we discussed the results of the scan on the phone, Mort was completely unfazed. He told me I had warned him that the tumors might not change, that the tumors might actually increase in size, and he trusted me. He felt fine, and he was doing great. He was trying to cut down on the bagels and lox—and cream cheese—but the effort had not been particularly successful.

In July of 1993, Mort was one of the patients I discussed at my National Cancer Institute presentation in Bethesda. At that time, Mort was twenty-two months from his original diagnosis and had been on my therapy for nineteen months. I brought to the meeting the actual CAT scan reports from 1991 when he was first diagnosed, as well as the films from February of 1993. Although the most recent scans showed no improvement, and perhaps slight enlargement in the main pancreatic tumor, I thought his excellent clinical status and nearly two-year survival remarkable.

I knew, at the time, the National Cancer Institute had very stringent and well-defined criteria for determining a response to treatment of a patient such as Mort. The NCI defined a complete response as total regression of tumor that lasted at least four weeks, and a significant partial response as at least 50 percent tumor regression lasting at least four weeks. In the NCI cosmology at that time, clinical status and survival did not count. The emphasis was completely on tumor regression—even if the patient ultimately died. As odd as it might seem, a patient such as Mort who had already enjoyed unusual survival and an excellent quality of life would not by these criteria be considered a responder because there was no tumor shrinkage!

At the meeting, I did discuss a number of my patients who had obvious tumor regression in accord with the NCI standard for response. However, I very deliberately presented several patients such as Mort who by all accepted criteria had terrible disease with an obvious poor prognosis, yet had survived prolonged periods of time in good health, even though the tumors may not have changed or may have actually increased in size. In Mort's case, I emphasized his good clinical status and his unusual long-term survival, even though there was no "improvement" by CAT scan studies.

I suggested to the assembled scientists that we might need to change our thinking about cancer, and to approach the disease the same way doctors approach diabetes, as a chronic ailment that can be managed effectively for years, even if never cured. This really wasn't my idea at all: Kelley had frequently, in his discussion of his approach to patients, used the analogy of diabetes. Diabetes, if uncontrolled, can be a debilitating disease, leading to blindness, heart disease, kidney failure, and premature death. Before the discovery of insulin by Banting and Best, diabetes was as rapidly deadly as many cancers. But with proper dietary management and with insulin, most diabetics can live a normal, productive lifespan. Diabetes may never be cured, but it can be managed for many decades.

Kelley believed that cancer is like diabetes, a deadly disease if untreated, but a disease that can be controlled, for years and even decades, with appropriate diet and, instead of insulin, pancreatic enzymes. In Kelley's mind, it wasn't necessary to kill every cancer cell or destroy every tumor to have a patient survive a terrible prognosis and lead a productive life. This was one of the hardest lessons for me to learn, coming as I did from a very orthodox research orientation; I suspect this lesson was even harder for Dr. Good, who found much of Kelley's approach contrary to all he had been taught about cancer biology.

At the NCI presentation, I referred to a very interesting, though often ignored, study published in 1980 in the *Journal of the National Cancer Institute* by Stanley and colleagues. Stanley and his group studied more than five thousand patients with inoperable lung cancer over a ten-year period in an effort to assess what factors best determined survival in poor-prognosis patients. The scientists evaluated seventy-seven different characteristics, including tumor size, the histological type of cancer, and clinical status, technically referred to as "performance status." Surprisingly, Stanley and his group found that of all the many criteria considered, the single most important factor was not the size or cell type of the tumor, but the performance status of the patient—basically, how the patient felt.

Patients who felt better, and who could do more things for themselves, did better than those who felt worse and did less. Tumor size and histological type had only a "minor" effect on survival. I argued that in view of documentation such as this from the literature, as well as my own experiences in practice, survival needed to be considered, not just tumor shrinkage for four weeks. For a cancer patient, survival and the quality of life were what counted.

Although the NCI meeting began with the standard criteria for response in place—a 50 percent reduction lasting four weeks—by the end of the meeting, when Dr. Freidman suggested I pursue a pilot study, he discussed survival only as an end point. Increasingly, in the years since, the NCI has begun to look at issues of quality of life and survival and not purely tumor reduction as end points. In fact, the FDA approved the use of the drug Gemzar for the treatment of pancreatic cancer based primarily on improvements in quality of life, rather than survival or tumor shrinkage.

In recent years, I have read articles in the orthodox oncology journals by eminent researchers who now say we need to change our orientation about cancer and modify our belief that a good outcome requires every last cancer cell be destroyed. Cancer, I have read in such articles, needs to be approached as a disease that can be effectively managed as a chronic illness, like diabetes, and patients can live for many years even if not completely cured. I find it remarkable when, once again, Dr. Kelley is proven ahead of his time.

After the 1993 scans, Mort decided to forgo any testing for his cancer for a number of years. He continued on his program and continued returning to New York every six months to meet with me. He remained determined, compliant, and optimistic and continued to lead a full life. At one point, he needed a hip replacement because of severe osteoarthritis, but otherwise he did well. Eventually, in 1995, his wife became a patient of mine, and Mort at times seemed more concerned about her health than his own.

In July of 1998, Mort's local physicians prevailed upon him to have repeat CAT scans. At that point, he was seven years out from his original diagnosis. The scans were done July 15, 1998. The radiologist's summary speaks for itself:

> PRIOR STUDIES FROM 1991 AND 1993. . . READING THE REPORT FROM THE 1993 STUDY IT SOUNDED LIKE THE PATIENT HAD OBVIOUS METASTATIC DISEASE AND THE LARGEST STRUCTURE BEING A LARGE PORTAHEPATIS AND PERIPANCREATIC MASS. NO SUCH MASS IS SEEN TODAY. THERE IS NO ADENOPATHY. THE ADRENALS ARE PROMINENT AND THERE ARE TWO VERY SMALL LIVER LESIONS THAT CANNOT BE CHARACTERIZED BECAUSE OF THEIR SMALL SIZE.

This time, the scans indicated near-total resolution of his once widely metastatic disease.

Today, in late 2001, Mort is ten years from diagnosis. He remains generally very compliant except for occasional dietary indiscretions. At seventy-nine years of age, he is in excellent health with no complaints and continues to lead a very active life. He still leads tours at the art museum; he still is active in his church. He still eats occasional lox and bagels—and cream cheese.

Why did Mort do so well? Of course, I am happy to take credit for his success, and I could easily say it's all very simple: Beard and Kelley were right; pancreatic enzymes kill tumors, even aggressive big tumors. Mort's improvement and long-term survival prove this. Of course, all aspects of the program, with the large doses of pancreatic enzymes, the organic carrot juice, the individualized diet, and the aggressive detoxification routines are all critical. But they aren't enough.

Over the years, I have come to recognize certain intangible qualities that I invariably see in my successful cancer patients. These include an enormous capacity for faith, a quality of trust, fearlessness even in the face of death, and gratitude. I believe I have seen these four qualities in every single patient I have treated who did well.

From the moment I met him, Mort seemed to have absolutely no doubt that he could get well, despite what his doctors had told him. He had, quite simply, enormous faith: faith that he was going to survive, faith that I could help him, faith that my program could work. It was unspoken, but very real and evident right from the first minutes in my office.

Mort is a very educated, very smart man. He knew what the score was, from the first day he was given his diagnosis. He had advanced, metastatic adenocarcinoma of the pancreas, a rapidly progressive deadly disease that does not respond to any form of orthodox treatment, not chemotherapy, not radiation, not bone marrow transplantation or interferon. Survival is measured in months. Mort knew and understood all of this. But what impressed me about Mort—and what always impresses me about patients like him—is that not once in the nine years I have been treating him has he expressed doubt that he was going to do well.

It wasn't that he was in denial; he was told he was going to die by very competent doctors he trusted, and he certainly understood what that meant. But though he always has spoken of his doctors with great respect, he just didn't believe they were right. It's as if he heard what they said, let it register, and then decided he would find a solution. He had faith he could find a better way. I have known many patients like Mort, and I don't know where they get their faith or how it happens, but when it's there it could not be more obvious.

Mort was, in fact, quite a happy man when he arrived in my office for his first visit; we could have been discussing Impressionist art in his or my living room—not the battle for his life. Of course, I met Mort nearly three months after he was diagnosed, and I am sure there were some sleepless nights before he made his way to my office, and times when the gloom of his situation must have consumed his mind. But somehow, he had gotten beyond the fear and anxiety. Perhaps it was the article he had read about me, or what his wife might have heard about my therapy from their local health food store owner. Obviously, something had clicked in his mind. I don't know why he had such faith, but it was there, and a relief to me.

If Mort had faith he was going to do well, he also, from the first minute, seemed to have total trust in me. He seemed to believe that I would do the very best I could to help him. He never once asked where I went to medical school, what my training was, or whether I had ever treated anyone like him before. He didn't ask for the names of three patients "with the same condition" he could speak to, for confirmation he was making the right choice. I wasn't on trial; he didn't want me to prove myself. He just wanted my help.

I admit, even today, I don't know where his trust in me came from, just like I don't know where his faith came from. Certainly, there were many reasons then, and many reasons today, why he should have had no faith or trust in me whatsoever. Yes, I have attended three Ivy League schools, and yes, I have been mentored by some of the best orthodox and unorthodox physicians and scientists. But at the time Mort met me in 1991, I had no pilot study or Nestlé grant; I had no published report or NCI support. I had no hospital affiliation, no evidence of respect from my colleagues. I was an alternative practitioner largely perceived to be on the fringes of the medical world, widely scorned by orthodox physicians who perceived me as a quack, a delusional charlatan.

Nine years later, I am well known, have my published study and NCI grant, and have increasing academic support, but I have also been investigated for years by the medical board and sued twice. Indeed, there are many reasons not to have faith in me or trust what I do today, just as there were many reasons nine years ago. But faith and trust, I have learned over the years battling in the trenches with cancer patients, don't operate by reason. From our first moments together, Mort seemed to believe that my only motivation was to help him. In fact, even when I have been attacked in the press, Mort is often the first patient on the phone, expressing his anger and disgust with the media. The hatefulness of others toward me does nothing to shake his faith, or his trust.

Patients who have such faith, and who operate out of trust, to me seem fearless. I never, in nine years of treating Mort, have ever sensed fear or anxiety in him. His fearlessness wasn't because he was too ignorant to understand his "true" condition. He had gotten through it, and by the time I met him, if there had ever been fear, it was gone. His faith had overcome whatever fear may have been there.

Life hasn't been easy for Mort, in recent years. He and his wife struggle financially. In addition, Mrs. Schneider's own health is very tenuous. At times, she is housebound, so that Mort must tend to the shopping and errands.

He could be very angry, resentful, and bitter for the hand life has dealt him. But in the nine years I have treated Mort, I have not once seen in him even a trace of anger, resentment, or bitterness. In fact, all I've ever felt with Mort is gratitude toward me, and the treatment, and for what he thought I was trying to do for him. When the CAT scans showed near-total resolution of the tumors, he cried on the phone with appreciation. I suspect that even if my therapy had failed and he had died, on his deathbed he would have been grateful for my efforts. And despite the enormous real stresses in his life, he continues, at age seventy-nine, to lead tours at the local art museum. He is that kind of man.

Part IV:
The Hypothalamus and the Autonomic Nervous System

CHAPTER XVI:

Revisiting the Sympathetic and Parasympathetic

We take for granted just how complex, how extraordinarily complicated, life really is. It is indeed very fortunate that we are able to ignore the intricate details of our lives, at least in a biological sense, on a day-to-day basis and still function as well as we normally do.

To use myself as an example, the past five minutes of my own life, as I prepared to write these words, would hardly seem to be unusual, momentous, or in any way spectacularly different from the thousands of five-minute periods that fill my life. Five minutes ago, it was five minutes before six in the evening. I had finished with my last appointment and was sitting at my desk, winding down from a long day with very sick patients. My mind, which had been racing over the intricate details of the last case, was starting to calm down: the patient was doing well, and I could for a moment turn off the labored thoughts of cancer and the battle against it. I felt satisfied that I now had a chunk of time to work on my book, an endeavor that has helped get me away from the trench warfare of cancer medicine. I was moving from a state of enormous mental activity to a feeling of relaxation.

In such a state of tranquility—as short lived as it might be—my sympathetic system, the stress nervous system, was toning down, and my parasympathetic system, the system of repair, of rebuilding, the system of calm, was in control. I felt warm almost; my face felt flushed—a predictable reaction, because as the parasympathetic nerves of the body fire, the blood vessels of the face dilate as blood rushes in, creating the sensation of warmth. I felt a little lazy, not a surprising reaction because in a state of parasympathetic activity, we tend to feel very calm. Motivation, aggression, and action are complicated phenomena, neurophysiologically, but ultimately they are carried out by the sympathetic nervous system. As I sat at my desk, drifting into a quiet state, the sympathetic part of my nervous system was itself very quiet.

My thoughts drifted randomly, inevitably focusing on the book and the writing I had promised myself I would do. Immediately, as I remembered how much difficult work writing always involves, with the deadlines, pressure, and stress, the sensation of warmth left my face. I could feel, within milliseconds, the muscles of my arms and legs tensing as I became aware of my heart pumping. My sympathetic system, the stress nervous system, with no more stimulus than a thought about a book I am writing, turned on full blast.

With such sympathetic activity, the neurotransmitter norepinephrine and the hormone adrenaline poured into my body. I felt no longer calm, but increasingly anxious. I couldn't sit at my desk, thinking lazy thoughts. My abdominal muscles tightened, and I felt the need to move into the next room, where I keep my computer and the research materials essential for the writing project.

Without a further thought, I stood up at my desk, intending to walk—and walk quickly—the steps out of my office, down the hall, and into the workroom that adjoins my patient consultation room. Calm thoughts were completely gone.

It's extraordinary, from a biological, neurological point of view, just how complicated on so many levels the simple process of standing up really is. First, I made the conscious decision to do so, a decision that happens in the "thinking brain," the cerebral cortex, the outer layer of brain tissue that is so highly developed in humans. Here, we think, we make decisions, we move with direction. Here we are conscious, in a very distinctively human way.

Then just the thought of a specific movement, such as standing up at a desk, even before the first slight motion occurs, begins a cascade of physiological events. First, the idea of standing comes to life specifically in the frontal part of the cortex. From here, neurological signals travel to an area in the midcortex known as the motor strip, the region that controls willed movements.

This motor cortex in turn sends instructions via neuronal axons down the brain, into the spinal cord. These impulses then activate specific motor nerves with their cell bodies in the spinal cord itself and with axons that travel out of the spine to connect to the specific muscles required for the particular movement—in this case, standing up from my desk. For this motion, the extensors at the front of the leg must shorten to bring the calves and thighs into a straight line, and the flexors, which bring the lower part of the leg into a right angle with the upper leg, must relax. When we stand, we want the legs to be straight, not flexed.

While I am still seated, before I have even begun my first upward movement, the posterior flexors of the leg begin to relax, and the anterior extensors begin contracting, in a choreographed sequence of muscle action. In a sense, the muscles begin acting appropriately to start the process, just with the thought in the cortex, before I have even started to stand.

As the extensors start contracting and the flexors begin to relax, something else happens while I am still seated. Blood vessels under the control of the sympathetic nervous system dilate in the contracting muscles and only in these muscles, allowing for increased blood flow and, with it, an enhanced supply of nutrients and oxygen that the muscles will need as they prepare for action. All this transpires, remarkably, with just the thought of movement, before I've begun to stand. It's interesting that the sympathetic nerves can regulate blood flow so precisely, dilating vessels only in those muscles that will be contracting to fulfill the proposed motion, which at this point is still only a thought.

However, if I were to suddenly switch gears and instead of standing decide to return one more phone call, before I even reach for the phone, the appropriate flexor muscles in my left arm, which is my phone arm, would start contracting and the opposing extensor muscles would start relaxing. The leg extensors would then relax and blood would be shunted where it needs to be, and only where it needs to be, in the arm. The activity in the legs would come to a quick halt until I finished the phone call, and until my thoughts returned to the book I am writing and the need to move myself to the next room.

Let's say I've decided not to return any more calls, but to start getting up. As the extensors of the leg contract, as the flexors relax, the muscle fibers themselves start sending nerve impulses back to the spinal cord and to the brain, to let the brain know what is going on. These impulses originate in microscopic organelles known as proprioceptors that are located in each muscle fiber, and that relay the state of contraction or relaxation of the leg muscles to the spinal cord, then up to an area at the back of the brain and at the bottom of the skull known as the brainstem. From here, nerve impulses move upward to a small region at the top of the brainstem, the hypothalamus, which is in charge, ultimately, of the autonomic nervous system. As a result of the signals originating in the proprioceptors of the muscles, the hypothalamus becomes aware that the legs are starting to move.

Any movement, no matter how commonplace—such as blinking your eyes, for example—or how majestic—such as running the 660 in the Olympics—activates the posterior hypothalamus, which is the control center specifically for the sympathetic nervous system. Not only movement itself, but the thought of a proposed movement—be it blinking the eyes or running a race—does the same, in a sense priming the autonomic pump. Both the anterior hypothalamus, which regulates the parasympathetic nerves, and the posterior hypothalamus are very precise in their control; in this specific example, that of me thinking about standing up, the posterior hypothalamus instructs the sympathetic nerves that regulate blood flow into the extensors of the leg to turn on, an effect that further increases blood flow.

The conscious thought of moving in the cerebral cortex starts a series of events that lead to the contraction and relaxation of the leg extensors and flexors. The sympathetic nerves to the vessels in the flexors—and only in the flexors—begin to fire. Then the extensor muscles send signals back to the spinal cord and ultimately to the posterior hypothalamus, which then turns on the sympathetic system more strongly, to allow an even greater blood supply to the appropriate—but only the appropriate—muscles. The thought of standing has already created a whirlwind of neurological activity at all levels of the nervous system.

Standing is a particularly complicated maneuver because of the problem of gravity. Gravity is trying to pull you down from the moment you starting moving upward. That's the way life on Earth is. Fortunately, certain areas in the brainstem continuously monitor our position in the environment relative to gravity and send the appropriate instructions for the muscles in the legs and along the spine. Once you're standing, the extensors need to stay contracted and the flexors relaxed, while the long spinal muscles all contract. All this activity will allow us to stay straight and not fall down like Sir Isaac Newton's apple to the ground. No conscious thoughts or willed instructions from the higher cortex are needed for this motion; it happens automatically.

Standing is a problem for another reason, because as we stand, gravity tends to pull blood away from the brain, sitting as it does at the top of the body. Though it might weigh a mere 2.5 pounds, perhaps one-seventieth of the weight of an adult male, the brain is a very metabolically active organ, using up generally 25 percent of the body's total energy production and 25 percent of all inhaled oxygen. The brain cells take blood sugar, that is, glucose, which they break down in the presence of oxygen to produce ATP—the fundamental energy source of all cells in the body, including those of the brain. Even slight reductions in available energy sources to the brain cells, or reductions in oxygen supply, can result in diminished concentration, diminished memory, and a sensation of spaciness; more severe deficiencies in blood glucose or oxygen lead to confusion, erratic behavior, eventually unconsciousness, and even, in the more extreme situation, seizures. Of course, the brain receives the glucose and oxygen it needs in one way only, from the blood supply to the brain: cut the blood supply, and within two minutes irreversible damage occurs.

Standing up isn't so simple because gravity works against the heart as it tries to keep an ideal blood supply up to the brain. Fortunately, the thought of movement has already turned on the posterior hypothalamus, which knows exactly what to do about the gravity-blood problem. The posterior hypothalamus activates the specific sympathetic nerves that connect to the heart; these nerves start firing strongly, and in turn the pulse increases and the heart muscles contract more strongly with each beat. This sympathetic effect increases cardiac output, or simply put, the amount of blood pumped out of the heart per unit of time. When you stand, that's a good thing, to increase the amount of blood that's leaving the heart and the force with which it leaves. This helps somewhat, to override the powerful effects of gravity.

However, raising the cardiac output isn't enough. Even if more blood leaves the heart with greater force, with standing, blood would normally tend to collect in the abdomen, in the extensive collection of arteries and veins that fan out into the small and large intestines, the liver, and the spleen. These vessels, when dilated, can hold a lot of blood, all very far from the brain. It's great that the heart is pumping more strongly, but if blood pools in the gut and not in the brain, there is no benefit. But the posterior hypothalamus, and its minion, the sympathetic nervous system, won't let this happen.

As the sympathetic system becomes more active throughout the body—including in the abdomen—the arteries and arterioles feeding into the stomach, intestines, pancreas, etc., constrict, reducing the inflow. The veins that carry blood away from these organs also constrict, in effect pumping blood back to the vena cava, the great vein of the abdomen, and eventually back toward the heart. At the same time, as the sympathetic system fires, the vessels in the skin constrict as well, while the carotid and vertebral arteries that flow into the brain remain open. With the major circulatory routes in the gut and skin shut down, blood diverts where it is needed, to the brain, to keep the glucose and oxygen supply flowing.

If the sympathetic system happens to be weak, as occurs in syndromes known as autonomic failure, the simple act of standing up can lead to fainting, as the heart rate and stroke volume decrease, blood pools in the gut and skin, and the brain becomes instantly and dramatically starved for both glucose and oxygen. Increasingly, many cases of chronic fatigue syndrome may be a milder form of autonomic failure that may not lead to fainting but that can result in persistent terrible fatigue, clouded thinking, and depression, all of which worsen with even minor activities—such as standing up and walking into another room.

What amazes me is how very precise the sympathetic system can be. It can fire very locally, for example limiting its influence to the blood vessels in a small region, such as those that feed the extensor muscles of the legs. It can also operate globally, affecting every area from the skin at the top of the skull to the plantar surfaces at the bottom of the feet, and everything in between. In my own case, as I progress from the thought of standing up to walking quickly into the next room, sympathetic influence has itself evolved from a very mild local firing in the legs to a rather strong full-blown systemic process: increasing heart rate and cardiac contraction; constricting the myriad of blood vessels, both arteries and veins, in the gut; constricting the vessels of the skin; dilating the pupils; and so on. All within seconds.

By the time I have taken my first steps toward the adjoining office, my sympathetic system is firing away, from top to bottom. My thoughts are racing, and I feel the beginnings of anxiety. I need to write a note to my editor and send a copy to my agent; I am not sure I know where the next chapter is going. I wonder how I am going to distill thousands of pages of scientific information into an understandable explanation of the autonomic nervous system, without losing the extraordinary sense of importance it has. All this during the first step.

Neuroscientists teach that the cerebral cortex, the outer layer of our highly developed human brains, is the center for all thought. What this ignores is how the autonomic nervous system—perceived as a more primitive system, found in vertebrate animals such as mice and birds, which do not have a particularly impressive cortex—influences the cortex and the nature of our thoughts, the nature of our emotions, and the way we view the world.

When the sympathetic system is on, it sends impulses not only "lower down," to the tissues and organs of the body, but through connections in the brainstem and the hypo-thalamus, it sends signals "higher up," right into the sophisticated intellectual and emotional centers of the cortex. There, the main sympathetic neurotransmitter, noradrenaline (also known as norepinephrine) exerts a very direct stimulatory effect throughout the cortex. When the sympathetic system fires, we think more quickly and more confidently, even aggressively. Initially we might feel somewhat indestructible, even euphoric, but if the nerves release enough norepinephrine, we can become quite angry very quickly, taking no prisoners. My advice is always to avoid anyone in a state of sympathetic overdrive.

Physical movement, even walking a couple dozen steps, and the process of thinking require increasing amounts of glucose. I am walking fast, my thinking is fast, and my muscles and brain are hungry. I'm in luck because the sympathetic system is building up a head of steam. Heart rate and cardiac contractility increase still more, and blood continues to shift from the gut and the skin to the muscles and the brain, to support the demands of increasing physical and mental activity. In addition, the sympathetic neurotransmitters noradrenaline and adrenaline stimulate the liver to start breaking down glycogen, a complex form of stored sugar, into the simpler six-carbon glucose, which the brain uses so efficiently as its primary fuel. The liver also begins releasing stored fatty acids that can be used in a pinch as an energy source.

As I continue walking through the hall toward the room adjoining my office, and as the sympathetic nerves fire strongly and more strongly, the centers in the anterior hypothalamus that regulate the parasympathetic system become increasingly quiet. This phenomenon is known as reciprocity, or reciprocal inhibition, so fundamental to understanding the autonomic nervous system. As one of the two branches becomes active—in the case of my walking into the other room, the sympathetic—the other—in this case, the parasympathetic system—turns off. A spiral ensues, with more intense sympathetic firing further blocking the parasympathetic nerves.

A lot has happened, neurologically, since I sat at my desk just minutes ago, calmly thinking about my last patient. When I reach the workroom, I am not in a storm, but I am clearly not relaxed. I see the chair in front of the computer, but I ignore it and instead walk to the windows of the office, which overlook a lovely garden in the courtyard below. It is very green, with trees and lush bushes, a stone path from one end to the other, a Japanese-style arbor, and a wooden bench. It is immediately very calming, in the late afternoon light, and I know I must get some calm back before I try to write. Writing requires some degree of calm.

One of the reasons I like my office so much is because of this garden, which sits between the building that houses my office and the back of the apartment house opposite. The many-floored structures block any street sound, so even though I am three or so blocks from the Empire State Building in the center of Manhattan, it is very quiet, as well as very green. Birds routinely make the garden their home, some of them quite distinctive, and the place becomes particularly active during the migratory seasons of spring and fall.

One autumn, that long-ago and rather horrible autumn of 1995 when I was fighting the New York State Department of Health, an owl about twelve inches high perched on a tree right outside a window about two feet away from my office manager's desk.

For two days, the owl visited, sleeping all day, its head buried in a wing. Occasionally, it would awaken and look inquisitively at me or at the members of my staff.

At night, it would disappear, presumably to hunt—perhaps in Bryant Park, where mice live, perhaps further north in Central Park, certainly a suitable forage site. In the morning, it would be back by the time the office opened. It seemed unperturbed by the activity inside, as if it felt completely safe, despite its proximity to us. The owl had stopped on its journey south for the winter, an unexpected gift in the midst of Manhattan. After two days, it was gone. It never returned.

Today, years later, as I approach the window of my workroom I start thinking about the owl, with its searching eyes and tilted head. I immediately feel a sense of relaxation in my gut and, as if by magic, all concerns about the day, all thoughts about cancer, editors, agents, and uncompleted books in need of finishing, all that goes away. I begin smiling, feeling a sense of pleasure, not of urgency. I become a little saddened thinking of the owl and how it helped me forget, at least for a moment or two, my legal battle for survival.

The thought of the owl, as simple a thought as it is, has itself enormous repercussions. Any thought, of whatever type, pleasant or unpleasant, happens in the cerebral cortex. That's what the cortex does: it allows us to think, to visualize, to remember. When we think pleasant and relaxing thoughts such as that of my owl, within milliseconds the cortex sends inhibitory signals to the sympathetic centers in the posterior hypothalamus and stimulating impulses to the parasympathetic areas of the anterior hypothalamus. The sympathetic nerves turn off, the parasympathetic system turns on, and the excitatory impulses from the posterior hypothalamus to the cortex stop. Anxious thoughts and feelings come to a halt.

As I walk toward the window, it's as if I have all the time in the world. I decide that I am going to forget about the book for a moment and all that needs to be done, and instead stand and look outside, into the courtyard. With the sympathetic system winding down, there just is no rush. I look out the window and gaze at the leaves of the trees, all very quiet in the still late afternoon light. The noise from the world—the questions from my staff, the extraordinary and understandable and sometimes desperate needs of very sick patients, the sound of the phone, the concerns about patients, clinical trials, books, all that is hushed.

When I think about the owl, the hypothalamus is receiving instructions from above, from the cortex, but it is also the target of signals from below. Even before I have stopped moving, the somatic motor nerves to the muscles adjust, the contracted muscles in my legs begin relaxing, and the relaxed muscles flex slightly. The proprioceptors, the microscopic organelles in the muscle fibers, immediately inform the hypothalamus that motion is coming to a halt. Overall, as the parasympathetic nerves take over, there is a generalized relaxation in all muscle groups, including those in my gut. The pit in the bottom of my stomach is gone; my shoulders and arms feel droopy, not at all tense. This further inhibits the posterior and further excites the anterior hypothalamus.

In a sense, the proprioceptive impulses from the muscles below combine with the input from the cerebral cortex above, to bring the sympathetic system to a near standstill, and the parasympathetic system, before so quiet, has now shifted into action. Of course, this situation, like any situation in our lives, is complex; the sympathetic system doesn't turn off entirely. Remember, I am still standing, though no longer walking, and if it did turn off completely, I would drop to the floor in a faint. But the pulse does slow, cardiac contractility and blood pressure do go down somewhat, and blood does return somewhat to my gut and to my face. My blood sugar levels I know are declining from their sympathetic high.

The anterior hypothalamus, like the posterior, sends signals to the cortex, but they are relaxing signals that reinforce the quiet brought on by the thoughts of the owl. A deep calm comes over me, a calm with no demands, no threats, no deadlines: a quiet, parasympathetic calm that began with the thought of an owl and that increased when I stopped moving. Movement is always a sympathetic action, always. Great yogis and relaxation therapists know the importance of muscle relaxation and stillness as well as quiet thoughts to reduce the effects of stress on the body. Their thinking is very correct.

My thoughts begin to drift, in a less organized pattern, without urgency, without anxiety. I continue thinking about the owl and owls I have seen at other places. I think of the family farm in Vermont, and how wonderful it must look now, in late spring, with all the greenery blossoming, coming back from the dreariness of the North Country winter. I think about the brook that crosses the land, the 180-degree view from the highpoint of the farm. Minutes pass, and I realize I am smiling.

When the sympathetic system fires, the cortex is ready for action, quick and practical action, aggressive if need be. When the parasympathetic system turns on, the cortex lapses into quiet, dreamlike states. Such thoughts may not seem, at least on the surface, productive, but they are the origins of creativity in every field, be it music, literature, science, or architecture. Creativity comes out of the parasympathetic side, out of thoughts of owls, out of Proust's sudden recollection of a madeleine pastry from childhood, out of Hemingway musing about his long-ago life in Paris. Sympathetic thinking tends to be very linear—get the prey, defend against the enemy, run from the fire. Parasympathetic thoughts, parasympathetic driftings, are less pragmatic but often multidimensional, allowing us to think in new and unexpected ways, allowing us to see situations and problems—and potential solutions—differently.

After several minutes of mental meanderings through the fields of Vermont, I feel calm enough to resume work. I know that I will work best if my sympathetic system is turned on somewhat, but not too much, so that I have the drive to work, the motivation to take on this enormous project, and the energy in my brain to do what needs to be done. Too much sympathetic activity produces only anger, impatience, annoyance, a drive for survival, certainly not a creative state. The sympathetic system has no time or use for memories of owls or the landscape of Vermont; such musings have no practical use to the sympathetic mind. But the parasympathetic system knows better: it is not impatient; it brings out memories from the deepest recesses of the brain, to give a context and color to thought, to give meaning to our lives.

To work effectively, with the writing, I know I want my sympathetic and parasympathetic systems to be in balance. Certainly, I require the calm that patiently brings up my thoughts, allowing them to come together in a creative, nonlinear way, but to get the job done I also need motivation, drive, ambition, and quick thinking. Without some sympathetic drive, disaster overtakes creativity. Many psychiatrists and academic scholars have remarked how often very successful artists, be they writers, poets, composers, or painters, are infused with bouts of severe, unrelenting depression. Many succumb to alcoholism, a form of self-medicating behavior that helps relieve, though only temporarily, the endless melancholy of severe depression. I remember once listing the number of Nobel Prize-winning authors who suffered from alcohol abuse, and how astonished I was at the number—Hemingway, Steinbeck, O'Neill, and Sinclair Lewis, to name just a few.

Such depression follows when the parasympathetic system is on too strong. Indeed, creativity flows through the parasympathetic nerves, but if the parasympathetic system becomes too powerful, too dominant, and the sympathetic system too weak, too passive, despair can become an unending torment, affecting productivity, marriages, relationships, even the ability to get out of bed in the morning. I remember reading about Ernest Hemingway's final months in the excellent and exhaustive biography by the Princeton scholar Carlos Baker. Hemingway, by this time a lauded hero of literature, had spiraled into an interminable depression. Though afflicted with melancholy throughout his life, in his final days, Ernest's depression was so great he could no longer write, so painful was it for him to organize his thoughts into coherent sentences. Though creativity requires a parasympathetic bent, without discipline, organization, and drive—all sympathetic qualities—nothing is going to happen.

During that bleak period in Hemingway's career, then-President-Elect John F. Kennedy had requested the author write some words, just a brief paragraph or two, nothing more complicated, that he might read during the inauguration to be held in Washington in January of 1961. Ernest was so depressed that despite repeated attempts, he could never finish a single paragraph that satisfied him. He was brought to tears, convinced his creative life was over. Some months later, he ended his life with a shotgun blast to the head. Poor Mr. Hemingway was too parasympathetic, though all the psychiatrists he had consulted at the Mayo Clinic knew nothing of this. Tragically, depression, as the press has so often pointed out, haunts the great Hemingway family: his father, a doctor, committed suicide; Ernest's sister committed suicide; his granddaughter, once the toast of the New York social scene, committed suicide not too long ago.

In that five-minute period, from the time I left my desk until the time I ended up standing by the window of my workroom thinking about owls, certainly a lot had happened. What amazes me, as I think about it, is just how smart our nervous system is. My brain deliberately put the thought of an owl in the forefront of my thoughts, ahead of everything else, to slow down my sympathetic system, knowing that in a state of sympathetic overdrive I will be too anxious, annoyed, and impatient for the patient job writing must be. It knew what I wanted to do; it knew what I needed to do to get there. The owl was put into my consciousness to make me dreamy, thoughtful, calmer, to make me more parasympathetic.

My brain then used the response to slowed motion and muscle relaxation to reinforce the effect. By the time I have stood at the window for two minutes, and no longer, I am quieted enough to face the daunting task of putting word to paper (or in this case, to computer). The process had worked perfectly, without any attempt on my part. My autonomic system was essentially in balance. In Hemingway's case, his sympathetic system, so exhausted from years of stress, alcohol, travel, and work, simply could not turn on at all. The final paragraph could never be written.

In every second, indeed in every millisecond of our lives, the autonomic system allows our bodies, with their 100 trillion cells, with their organ systems and highly developed brains, to adjust instantly to the environment around us and to the very thoughts within us. The responses are near instantaneous, the adjustments in our physiology and biochemistry remarkable, all allowing us to live the complicated lives we lead. There is no aspect of our days, from standing up to writing a book to remembering the unhappiness of a legal battle or the pleasantness of a visiting owl, that does not directly involve the autonomic nervous system and its two opposing branches. This system makes our lives literally possible, in a fundamental physiological way, but even more profoundly, this collection of nerves defines much of who we are: our thoughts, our personalities, the way we react to everything around us from the sound of a phone to sunlight in a city garden. This system regulates our moods and determines, in many ways, our dreams, hopes, emotions, successes, and failures—all the things we are.

Overview of the Nervous System

How does all this happen? How does our nervous system know what to do and when to do it, usually correctly, usually in the right way and at the right time? How can we change our position, for example from sitting to standing, while at the same time our blood pressure remains constant, ensuring no loss of blood supply to the brain? How can our moods shift from sadness to joy, and back again, at times with no more effort than a fleeting thought and a distant memory?

All nervous system action happens ultimately at the level of the neuron, the fundamental nerve cell. The brain, the spinal cord, and their appendages, such as the cranial and spinal nerves that travel to all regions of the body, as complicated as they are, consist of just two different types of cells: the neurons and the glial cells. This latter group consists of supportive cells dispersed through the nervous system that serve the same function as connective tissue cells in our other organs. In each of us, the neurons number about 100 billion, the glial cells about nine times as many. The numbers are truly staggering.

Neurons come in several different types and a variety of sizes and shapes, but all have a unique microscopic appearance that differs from that of any other cell in the body. Nerve cells have a soma, or cell body, a nodular structure that contains the main metabolic machinery of the cell. Here lies the cell nucleus with its DNA, the central computer of the cell. Here, in the soma, is the main collection of cytoplasm with its endoplasmic reticulum and Golgi complex, the subcellular structures responsible for making proteins, fats, and the neurotransmitters essential for nerve cell action.

In most nerve cells—though not in all—sprouting at one end of the soma are the dendrites, cell extensions that often appear under the microscope as the dividing branches of an old oak tree in winter. In fact, so close is the botanical resemblance that histologists refer to the dendrites as arborizing. These cytoplasmic extensions function essentially as the antennae of the cell, receiving incoming information, in the form of neurotransmitters, from other nerve cells.

At the end opposite from the arborizing dendrites, we find the long, tube-like axon, essentially an extension of the cell cytoplasm. Most neurons have a single axon that travels from the soma to the target cell of the nerve, whatever that target may be, such as another nerve cell, a muscle cell, or the cell of some gland. The axon can vary in length from microns to a meter (more than three feet) or more, depending on the specific neuron type and its function. Tiny vesicles filled with neurotransmitters manufactured in the soma travel down the axon by a process of cytoplasmic streaming, equivalent to small pebbles being carried by a cascading Rocky Mountain stream in spring.

At the axon tip, the point furthest from the soma, these vesicles accumulate; when the appropriate signal comes down the axon, the vesicles attach to the axon membrane, and then release their contents into the space between the neuron and its target cell. This microscopic region between the axon of a neuron and the dendrites of another nerve cell, or between the axon and a muscle or gland cell, is called the synapse. Across this microscopic region, nerve signals in the form of neurotransmitter molecules move from the neuron to its target cell. This is how, in the nervous system, information travels.

I think much of the confusion medical students experience when trying to master neuroanatomy results because they become so enmeshed in the elaborate details of structure that they forget that nerve activity overall is really quite straightforward. Though our billions of nerve cells are arranged in complex patterns, they really serve three basic functions. Some nerves, the sensory nerves, bring information to the spinal cord and brain: there, in the central nervous system, other neurons process and interpret the information and then make decisions based on what's coming in. The motor nerves, the nerves of action, then carry out the directives of the brain and spinal cord.

Sensory information can originate in all regions of the body: from the skin, the muscles, the internal organs, and the specialized organs such as the eye, the ears, the nose, and the tongue. Information about the pain, pressure, and temperature originates in the sensory receptors of the skin. The microscopic muscle spindles, located in all the large, striated muscles of our limbs and trunk, send information about position to the brain, to assist with decisions about movement, balance, and coordination.

Sensory nerves in the gut relay the status of the stomach and intestines, in terms of the presence or absence of food. All this information comes into the central nervous system, the spinal cord and the brain, continuously, whether we are awake or asleep. Other sensory nerves, the nerves of the special senses, transmit the unique information from the head: these include the optic nerve for vision, the auditory nerve for sound, the olfactory nerve for smell, and the glossopharyngeal nerve for taste. This information comes into the brain directly, from the cranial nerves of the head.

The motor nerves carry signals for action from the central nervous system to the tissues, organs, and glands of the body. Motor neurons that specifically control the skeletal and striated muscles are called the somatic, or voluntary motor nerves, because they allow for willed movements, such as walking, writing with a pen, or throwing a baseball. Somatic motor nerves connect only to the striated muscles of the body, and not to any of the internal organs or glands.

In addition, another set of motor nerves causes contraction (or again, relaxation) of cardiac and smooth muscle. Cardiac muscle is the very specialized muscle found in the heart, whereas smooth muscle consists of individual muscle cells, unlike the complicated muscle fibers of skeletal muscle that line all blood vessels, the gastrointestinal tract from esophagus to rectum, and other internal organs such as the gallbladder and urinary bladder. Contraction or relaxation of smooth muscle in the circulatory system allows for precise control of blood pressure and shunting of blood where it is needed, such as to the skeletal muscles and heart during activity or to the gastrointestinal tract during a meal.

Contraction of the smooth muscle that lines the stomach and small and large intestines provokes peristalsis, the powerful muscular movement that churns food in the gut to speed up the digestive process and propels waste toward the rectum for excretion. When the smooth muscle of the gallbladder contracts, bile flows into the small intestine to enhance digestion of fat, and in the pancreas, contraction of the muscle cells lining the ducts pumps digestive enzymes and bicarbonate toward the duodenum.

Contraction or relaxation of the smooth muscle in the eye permits accommodation to different intensities of ambient light as well as focusing for distant and near objects. Contraction of smooth muscle in the bladder allows for urination.

Additional motor nerve connections to the various exocrine and endocrine glands, such as the pancreas, the microscopic glands lining the stomach and intestinal tract, the adrenals, and the sexual glands, directly control secretion of a host of enzymes and hormones. In these cases, the nerve endings stimulate the secreting cells to start releasing their product, be it a hormone or an enzyme. Motor nerves also directly or indirectly control the spleen and thymus and, through their neurotransmitters, the individual cell types of the immune system.

These nerves that regulate cardiac and smooth muscle, glands, and immune function are, of course, our old friends of the autonomic nervous system, which operate without the need for will or conscious control. The autonomic nervous system is a motor system, a system that makes things happen. It reacts to signals from the brain, but it is not a sensory system, bringing information toward the brain. As we shall see, the somatic motor nerves that control the large muscles of the limbs and trunk are different in terms of microscopic structure and overall anatomy from the autonomic nerves that control the cardiac muscle, smooth muscle, and glands.

To review, it is useful to keep thinking simply: the sensory nerves bring information from all corners of the body, from the skin, muscles, internal organs, etc., into the spinal cord and brain, collectively grouped as the central nervous system. In the brain and spinal cord, another set of neurons interprets the incoming signals, decides on a course of action, and then sends signals outward to bring about the desired result. The two classes of motor nerves direct the tissues, organs, and glands of the body to carry out the wishes of the brain and spinal cord. The somatic motor nerves regulate the striated muscle groups of our limbs and trunk, for movement, balance, and fine coordination, and the autonomic nerves control cardiac muscle, smooth muscle on the internal organs, and the exocrine and endocrine glands. Stimulation of smooth muscle and glands allows for the physiological functions of circulation, digestion, respiration, and endocrine secretion, functions that permit us to survive in whatever environment we may find ourselves in.

Though neuroanatomists traditionally divide the motor system into the somatic and the autonomic collection of nerves, and though indeed these two systems are distinct anatomically, there is a considerable amount of interaction between these two. They do not exist in isolation. As we have seen, when the striated muscles of the limbs contract during walking, excitatory signals travel to the posterior hypothalamus. The sympathetic nerves start firing, while at the same time the parasympathetic system tones down; on the other hand, a generalized relaxation of skeletal muscles groups stimulates the anterior hypothalamus and the parasympathetic nerves, while inhibiting the sympathetic. In this way, the somatic muscle system can influence autonomic activity.

But the reverse is also true. The autonomic nervous system can affect the somatic motor nerves and the striated muscles. For example, certain mental activities—such as worrying about a book that needs to be written—will, through connections from the cortex, immediately turn on the sympathetic centers in the posterior hypothalamus. Heart rate increases and blood shunts to the brain and the skeletal muscles, but in addition, this mental calisthenic will activate the motor centers in the cerebral cortex, and muscles will start tensing.

So the somatic and autonomic systems, it is important always to keep in mind, are closely interrelated. It is not poetic license when a patient says, "My gut feels tight when I get stressed out," because quite literally, under emotional stress, sympathetic activity signals the motor centers in the brain to contract skeletal muscles in general, but particularly certain muscles in the abdominal wall. It is not mythic to say that a pleasant thought relaxes the gut; it really does happen. The relationships are subtle but, to me, quite amazing.

But I jump ahead of myself. I want to return to the neuron, the single cell that is the foundation of all nervous system tissue, and the foundation of all nervous system activity. How does a neuron do what it does, transmit "information," to use my own term?

Nerve cells are unique in many different ways, but it is their ability to transmit electrical impulses that in my mind truly distinguishes them from other cells and tissues of the body. Neurons can do what they do because they can transmit electrical impulses, in some respects, as can an electrical wire. Other cells, such as cardiac muscle cells, can conduct impulses to some extent, but no other tissue is designed to transmit electrical energy as efficiently, and extraordinarily rapidly, as a nerve cell. Certain nerve cells can transmit an impulse that travels the distance of a football field, a hundred yards, in a second. That is very fast for a microscopic cell.

For this discussion of electrical transmission of neurons, to make things simple, I would like to take a somatic neuron of the voluntary motor system, say, a nerve connecting to the biceps of the arm. Such a nerve, like all somatic motor nerves, has its soma in the spinal cord, while its axon exits the cord, traveling along what we call spinal nerves, until it reaches its point of contact in the muscle fibers of the arm. The motor cell bodies that innervate the biceps specifically lie in the cervical spine at the levels of the fifth and sixth cervical vertebrae and travel through the brachial plexus of nerves in the armpit until they reach the biceps.

The great majority of nerves, like this motor nerve lying quietly with its cell body in the anterior, or front, portion of the cervical spinal cord, react to signals from other nerves. In this case, these nerves can be sensory nerves that are sending information about position from the biceps itself. Sensory nerves differ from somatic motor cells in a basic anatomical way; somatic motor cells that connect to striated muscle always have their cell bodies, or soma, in the anterior portion, known as the anterior horn, of the spinal cord.

Sensory nerves that carry information toward the central nervous system, however, have their cell bodies adjacent to but distinctly outside the spinal cord. These cell bodies are located in what we call the dorsal roots of the spinal cord, small nodules positioned next to the spinal cord along its entire length down the back. These spinal sensory nerves have no dendrites, but instead have an axon that bifurcates shortly after exiting from the soma. Each half of the split axon goes in the opposite direction, one ending in the periphery of the body, be it in the skin, the muscle, or an internal organ. The other half of the axon goes toward the spine, entering the posterior horn of the spinal cord. In sensory nerves, information always begins at the periphery and moves toward the spinal cord.

In the cord, the sensory axon can connect directly with the dendrites and cell bodies of somatic motor nerves. Such direct connections between sensory nerves and motor nerves allow for simple reflexes, such as the patellar reflex, in which the leg extends when the kneecap is hit with a rubber hammer. These reflexes involve only two nerves, a sensory and a motor nerve, and do not require input from the higher centers in the brain. Such a system allows for a rapid protective response, without the need for discussion from the motor cortex or other areas of the thinking brain.

For example, if your finger should touch a hot pan, within a millisecond heat and pain receptors in the finger will send information directly to the motor nerves of the biceps, causing contraction and near instantaneous withdrawal of the arm. We don't have to think, and ponder, and reminisce about prior experiences and the deeper spiritual meaning of the hurt finger. We just get our hand out of there. It's a useful system that bypasses more complicated and time-consuming activities in the brain itself.

However, our motor nerve sitting in the spinal canal at the C5 level does receive axon connections from nerves with their cell bodies higher up, in the lower portions of the brain and in the motor centers of the cerebral cortex. If we decide we want to lift up our suitcase or write a letter (with either pen or computer), our higher centers send out the appropriate response through the somatic motor neuron at C5 and the biceps start to contract—not as a reflex, but as a willed effort.

Like most if not all nerve cells, our somatic motor neuron responds to chemical messages in the form of neurotransmitters. In this particular case, the motor nerve reacts to the transmitter acetylcholine, released by either the sensory nerve as part of a reflex, or from one of the nerves originating in the higher areas of the brain. The transmitter makes its way through the narrow space, the synapse, between the incoming axon (from either the sensory or a higher neuron) and binds to any of the literally thousands of protein receptors for acetylcholine on the membranes of the dendrites of our biceps motor neuron. The soma, the cell body of our motor nerve, and even the axon also contain receptor proteins for acetylcholine, but it is estimated that 85 percent or more of the receptors are on the arborized dendrites. When the transmitter attaches to the protein receptors, in both the dendrites and the axon, ion channels, small pores located on the soma and axon, start opening, allowing sodium ions with a positive charge to rush into the nerve cell. This is a very important phenomenon, essential to any understanding of how our nervous system works.

When at rest, when not firing, nerve cells have in their interior an electrical charge, specifically a negative electrical charge that has been measured at about –65 millivolts. Negatively charged proteins along with negative ions such as phosphate tend to keep this charge fairly constant. In addition, positive ions such as sodium, which would tend to be attracted to the negative charge inside the cell, are extruded continuously to the outside of the cell through what we call the sodium pump, a microscopic membrane engine that literally pumps out sodium into the extracellular fluid, the fluid that bathes all our cells. As a result of this action, sodium accumulates in high concentration in the extracellular fluids along with the negatively charged chloride ion.

As long as the charge inside the neuron stays negative at –65 millivolts, the cell remains quiet, doing very little of anything. However, when certain neurotransmitters such as acetylcholine open up sodium channels, the positively charged sodium ions rush in, attracted to the negative internal charge. In electrochemistry, remember that opposites attract. As the sodium floods the inside of the soma and axon, the charge becomes less negative and more positive; when it finally reaches approximately –45 millivolts, the cell technically depolarizes, a term that simply means an electrical current passes rapidly through the soma and down the axon. This current is called an action potential.

Although an electrician knows that an electrical current can pass through a wire in either direction, in the case of a neuron, electrical currents move in one direction only. In motor neurons, the action potential always travels from the dendrite and soma region down the axon toward the axon tip, but never from an axon toward the soma and dendrites. In the case of a sensory neuron with a split axon going in two directions, the impulse travels from the peripheral sensory area toward the soma initially, then onward to the spine. This one-way movement of electricity in nerves is an important adaptation, because it allows precise control over the direction information flows.

As the current instantaneously passes down the axon of a motor neuron, at its tip, another series of events takes place. A second group of ion channels, small pores in the axon tip membrane, open up, allowing positively charged calcium ions to enter the cell from the extracellular fluids. Calcium ions, which like sodium have a strong positive charge, tend also to accumulate outside of the cells, in the extracellular bath. However, when the calcium channels open up, calcium ions rush into the axon tip.

The tip of any nerve axon is, remember, filled with tiny vesicles that themselves serve as reservoirs for neurotransmitters. In the case of somatic motor neurons like the one we are discussing, with its axon connecting to a biceps muscle fiber, acetylcholine is the main transmitter. A single vesicle in the axon of a motor nerve can contain up to ten thousand molecules of acetylcholine. When the calcium ions rush in, through a complicated and still undeciphered mechanism, the vesicles merge with the axon membrane, before discharging their contents outside of the cell, in the synapse.

The acetylcholine quickly travels the distance from the motor nerve axon tip across the synapse to a receptor on the muscle fiber membrane. As the acetylcholine molecule binds with its receptor on the muscle fiber itself, like a key in a lock, contraction of the muscle fiber begins. This process in muscle involves the release of calcium from internal storage sites, which in turn results in the muscle cells shortening.

After depolarization, the creation of the action potential electrical current, the nerve cell then enters a period of rest. The sodium pump rapidly causes efflux of the positively charged sodium ions out of the cell into the extracellular fluid, the negative charge inside the cell is restored to –65 millivolts, and all is quiet. Of course, if there is much action going on, and signals keep coming in to our motor nerve at C5, it will then fire again, repeatedly, keeping the biceps contracted. If the signals do not stop coming in, eventually, the system breaks down: first, at some point the motor nerve is going to run out of neurotransmitters unless it gets a rest, and second, at some point, as wastes from the contraction process start building up, and the muscle cells start running out of calcium, contraction will end. The muscle technically becomes fatigued. Other than at certain extremes, the process is indeed very efficient.

What I have described here is an excitatory response, the activation of a somatic motor nerve and the subsequent contraction of a muscle. Nerve signals can also inhibit; certain neurotransmitters such as gamma-aminobutyric acid (GABA) or the amino acid glycine, which in the central nervous system doubles as a transmitter, block action potentials and nerve transmission. Although the details aren't critical for our purposes, briefly, such a response occurs when a nerve releases an inhibitory molecule such as GABA into the synaptic connection with another nerve, say our motor neuron at the C5 level. In such a circumstance, GABA, like any other transmitter, will bind to receptors on the membranes along the dendrites and cell body, but this time, chloride channels open up, allowing the negatively charged chloride ions to come swarming into the cell. Although the negative charge within the neuron would normally repulse the negative chloride ions, the pump is so strong it overrides this uphill electrical gradient and the chloride comes in, pushing the charge within the cell in a more negative direction.

Action potential, the electrical current within a neuron, occurs only when the internal charge becomes less negative and more positive, so the increasing negativity leaves the cell quieter and more resistant to response. Inhibitory reactions are as critically important as an excitatory response. Imagine what would happen if we had no mechanism to block nerves; the amount of sensory input in a second could overwhelm the nervous system and lead to hyperstimulated states, even grand mal convulsions and brain collapse. A seizure can result if the inhibitory systems aren't working the way they should. It isn't enough to be able to react; reactions need to be controlled, and very carefully.

Although of course I have simplified the process for the sake of this particular discussion, it is fair to say that information comes into the central nervous system, where information is processed and then acted upon, all through action potentials and the subsequent release of stimulatory—or inhibitory—neurotransmitters. As simple as it may seem, there is no other way anything happens in the nervous system, including the brain. It doesn't matter whether the process is the memory from a distant past, the solving of a problem in differential calculus, or moving one's hand off a hot stove. It's a question of electrical currents and the release of neurotransmitters. However complex our brains may seem, their physiology breaks down ultimately to nerve currents and the transmitters that they cause to be released.

Nervous System Anatomy

I remember so well the spring of my first year of medical school. I was overwhelmed, confronted with the mass of basic science information that needed mastering. It wasn't a good time for me. It was a period of great confusion, restlessness, self-doubt, and considerable despair—quite a different state of mind than a year earlier, when I was preparing to begin medical school. When I had two years earlier decided to switch careers, leaving my budding career as a novel writer and turning down a lucrative book contract—everything as a writer I had worked toward—to go back to school and pursue premedical studies at Columbia, I knew I was on the right road.

From day one, as I faced the rigors of genetics and organic chemistry, I didn't look back. I didn't regret putting my book projects on a shelf and turning down the financial offer. I didn't regret living at my parents' house, a prodigal son returning home at age twenty-nine to become a doctor and research scientist. I didn't mind the long commute from Flushing, in not very romantic Queens, to the Columbia campus on the Upper West Side. The things most premedical students trudge through and learn to dislike, the heavy science course load, I really enjoyed. I enjoyed studying; I enjoyed this new world of cell biology and biochemistry, even organic chemistry, which no one is supposed to like.

I had ended up at Columbia because I read too much. I had always been a voracious reader, at times, during my journalism and fiction-writing years, reading a book every day or two, in all fields, from Hemingway and Capote to wildlife ecology and eventually medicine and biochemistry. I became interested in nutrition, through my endless reading, and particularly nutritional effects on mental illness. I even published several articles on such topics that generated, at least in some circles, considerable discussion and interest. I remember working endlessly on my novel by day, and reading at night the works of scientists such as Hoffer and Osmond, who in the early 1950s first proposed high-dose vitamin treatment of schizophrenia.

My reading led me in new and somewhat unexpected directions. From my belief that poetry and art explained far more of life and were far more important than the calculated reductions of cold-hearted scientists, I had done a complete turnaround and come to think that biochemistry was art, and that biochemistry explained the human condition with more wonder than poetry ever could. The day I decided to go back to Columbia in late August of 1977 was the same day I turned down the book offer and put the novel in a closet, and it was the last day I ever read a page of fiction. I was determined to forge a new career as a research scientist, unraveling the biochemical basis of the mind and, in turn, of human disease.

I did extremely well at Columbia and was accepted to every major medical school to which I applied, from Stanford to Johns Hopkins. Though normally medical schools, like undergraduate colleges, send out their acceptances in the spring, by November of 1979, the year I applied, I had been accepted everywhere I could have wanted to go. I remember, in October, when my acceptance from Johns Hopkins came in, the sense of relief, victory, and accomplishment I felt. I had succeeded, overcoming the doubts of friends, the doubts of writer colleagues, and, most importantly, my own doubts about myself.

I seriously considered going to Hopkins, because of its strong program in neuroscience. Solomon Snyder, the dean of neuropharmacology, had his lab at Hopkins, peopled with many of the best minds in the neuroscience field. Yale too—I had been accepted there some weeks later—had a great program in neuroscience and had a fair number of older students like myself. I thought I might feel at home there. Then there was Columbia, a superb research center in New York, though not in the most convenient location, with wonderful resources.

As the cover profile of me in *The New Yorker* magazine in February 2001 reported, I ultimately decided to go to Cornell, which may have lacked the "prestige" of Yale, Hopkins, or Stanford, but which had Sloan Kettering and the Rockefeller Institute, both preeminent research institutions. Plus, it was in New York, on the East Side of Manhattan where I had lived for years during my writing days. It was in my old neighborhood. Most importantly, Cornell had Dr. Robert Good, the president of the Sloan Kettering Research Institute, one of the great scientists of his generation, a giant in medicine, free thinking, freewheeling, loved and ridiculed, a man who was on the cover of *Time* one year and attacked in the press a year later when one of his research fellows, in the famous case that haunted him the rest of his career, faked results in an animal transplantation experiment.

I knew about Dr. Good from my journalism days. He seemed to be a giant in a field of giants, the man who had successfully completed the first bone marrow transplant in 1968, while he worked at the University of Minnesota. He had published in physiology, neuroscience, and nutrition, as well as in his home turf of immunology. He had first reported the existence of B and T cells, two main cell lines of the immune defense system that are followed in the popular press on what seems to be a weekly basis. Dr. Good had helped unravel the importance of the thymus, a central regulatory organ of immunity that previously had been thought to be vestigial, with no function of any substance.

I thought Dr. Good, if I went to Cornell and got to know him, would understand someone like myself, who did things differently, often in reverse, my mind never seeming to understand the right and simple way of doing things. He probably would understand someone who gave up novel writing for the pleasure of studying organic chemistry at age twenty-nine. He would understand, I thought, someone who was interested in nutrition, and the brain, and how nutrition and the brain affected everything, even cancer—Dr. Good's own personal latest challenge. With Dr. Good in mind, it took, as Michael Specter wrote in *The New Yorker*, about "five minutes" (48) to make up my mind about medical school. It would be Cornell.

Yet here I was in the spring of the first year at Cornell, restless, bored, and depressed. I had a nasty flu that lingered for weeks, almost like an Epstein-Barr infection, and left me tired and unable to concentrate with my usual precise focus. In retrospect, I am sure the stress had broken down my resistance, but sick or not, the demands of medical school continued. I felt lousy and restless, in a profound way questioning the choices

I had made and finding science—as I had originally found it as an undergraduate—boring, overwhelming, and tedious.

The joy I had felt at Columbia, the joy I had experienced studying cell biology on a Saturday afternoon in my bedroom in Queens, preferring lessons about cell membranes instead of the odes of Yeats or Byron, seemed strangely gone. At Cornell, in the spring of 1980, neuroanatomy was the last tedious straw, a straw the size of a log on my shoulders, with detail beyond, it seemed, reason or understanding, without meaning or practical usefulness that I could see. I couldn't even understand why I was at Cornell, or why I had ever thought about going to medical school.

It wasn't until I met Dr. William Donald Kelley, with his theories about nutrition and autonomic nervous system balance, that neuroanatomy and neuroscience suddenly came alive and my enthusiasm for science and medicine returned. If I owe Dr. Kelley nothing more than the return of my enthusiasm, I owe him a lot. I remember so well, my third year of medical school, the main clinical experience when the basic science years are finally done, spending every free moment—including Saturday afternoons—reading neuroscience and physiology and restudying the anatomy I had learned so badly the first time around.

I guess it has always been my curse to do things in my own way, which so often seems different from the way the rest of the world does things. While my colleagues in medical school were so pleased to be in the clinical sciences and done forever with things such as neuroscience, I was back at the textbooks, finally understanding neuroanatomy, and finally appreciating the extraordinary workings of the nervous system. I hadn't been wrong, as a somewhat naïve applicant to medical school in 1979; there was poetry in the biochemistry and anatomy and physiology of the brain. I had just gotten lost.

The second time around, it didn't seem that complicated. Although the minute details of the brain, the spinal cord, and the nerves that reach into every corner of our bodies at first glance seem, as they did to me years ago, a little bit too much, it helps to always keep in mind that the nervous system, even in its details, involves bringing information into the brain, interpreting the information, and sending out messages and commands for an appropriate response.

Think about something as commonplace as touch. It's an important ability, to sense something in our environment; it helps us locate ourselves, warns of objects in our path, and tells us the nature of objects we can use for our benefit or avoid if harmful. Even such a seemingly simple process as touch sensations involves a variety of different types of nerves, and in some cases even microscopic little organelles such as Meissner's corpuscles, which are distributed in high concentration on the fingertips and lips. These sensory capsules each consist of a single nerve and help interpret the location of subtle, delicate touch. Kissing, for example, gets some of its beneficial effect from Meissner's corpuscles.

Merkel's disc, also found in the skin, is another type of sensory nerve ending in the finger tips, lips, and elsewhere that helps monitor touch on the skin over time. Meissner's corpuscles tell us where we are being touched, while Merkel's disc tells us for how long we are being touched. Ruffini's end organs, yet another type of sensory nerve receptor, specifically relay information about prolonged deep touch, into the skin and underlying connective tissues. If a fifty-pound bag of potatoes should decide to take up abode on your abdomen, the Ruffini end organs will let the brain know there is a major pressure factor at work on the body—and where this factor is, even without the need for sight. Temperature and pain receptors in the skin are equally as complex, equally as sophisticated.

Another group of sensory nerves that connect to the muscle spindles monitors the state of contraction or relaxation of every muscle fiber group in every striated muscle in the body and sends back to the central nervous system continuous information every second, to help the brain coordinate even the slightest of movements.

It might be helpful if, for a moment, we follow the trail of a sensory impulse of the sensory nervous system. For the sake of discussion, let's say an action potential originating in the muscle spindle of one of the fibers of the biceps muscle, a major flexor of the arm I mentioned earlier when describing a motor nerve. The biceps, part of the striated voluntary muscle system, are located on the inside of arm, in the group of muscles that when contracting draw the fist toward the shoulder, in what we call a flexion motion. As the biceps contracts, a set of opposing muscles on the elbow side of the upper arm, including the triceps, relaxes, allowing the arm to curl up on itself.

Let's say the biceps has contracted—and the extensors have relaxed—on signals from the decision-making centers in the brain to help us pull a suitcase down from the overhead bin of an airplane. As the muscle shortens, which is what happens with contraction, the spindle itself shortens, and this activates certain sensory nerves with their receptors in the spindle. This leads to an action potential in the sensory nerve signaling biceps contraction—remember, nerves transmit information only when action potentials occur—which travels down the long axon of the sensory nerve toward the cell body, located in the dorsal root ganglion in this case, which would be located adjacent to the opening between the fifth and sixth cervical vertebral bodies. Remember that most sensory nerves, at least below the head itself, have their cell bodies not in the spinal cord but in the dorsal roots.

I would like, for a moment, to consider the spine and the spinal cord, and what these words actually mean. I realize most of us have a strong familiarity with these terms, because we all know in a general sense what the spine is, particularly nowadays when back pain and back injuries are so common. When I use the word *spine*, I use it specifically to include the bony vertebral bodies that cover and protect the actual spinal cord collection of nerve cell bodies and axons that run toward and away from the brain, sitting at the top. The spinal cord nerve mass is a thick cord-like structure that runs through the seven cervical vertebral bones of the neck, the twelve thoracic bones of the upper and mid-back, the five lumbar bones of the lower back, and the five fused bones of the sacrum.

This nerve cord has a very precise and specific anatomy. Sensory nerves send their axons through the spaces between vertebral bodies, into the spinal cord itself. Each sensory nerve enters the spine not in a random way, but at a precise level of the spine. In the case of a sensory nerve transmitting electrical impulses from the biceps, the axon leaves the dorsal root ganglion located adjacent to the opening between the C5 and C6 vertebral bodies, to make its way into the dorsal, or back, portion of the spinal cord, where sensory axons usually terminate on the dendrites of another set of neurons. This is an oversimplification; certain sensory nerves cross over to the other side of the cord, while others make their way to the anterior, front "horn," but for our purposes, it is enough to say the sensory axons synapse onto other intermediate nerves in the dorsal horn.

Impulses from the first nerve, carrying position information in from the biceps, release neurotransmitters, such as acetylcholine, which then activate entire groups of what are called interneurons—one target of the primary sensory nerve cell. These are short nerves that travel only within the spinal cord itself. Some interneurons extend only within the same spinal levels and cross to the front of the cord, to synapse onto motor neurons with cell bodies located in the anterior horn. These interneurons allow for the classic spinal reflex mentioned earlier, when the leg extends when the doctor hits the kneecap with a rubber hammer, or when the arm flexes, in response to a tap in the crease between the upper arm and the forearm. The same response is at work in the real world outside the doctor's office, for example, when your finger touches a hot stove by mistake; before the thought of what has happened has reached the brain, the biceps are flexing, bringing the arm away from the source of danger. Such reflexes involve a circuit of impulses, from the incoming sensory nerve, to the outgoing motor nerve that leads to the appropriate contraction.

Even a simple reflex such as this, moving the arm away from a hot pan or lowering a suitcase from the overhead bin on an airplane, is a little more complicated than flexion of the biceps. The extensor muscles of the arm, such as the triceps, extend the arm out straight when they contract. These are located on the elbow side of the upper arm, and they work in opposition to the flexors. When the flexor muscles contract, the extensors must relax—otherwise, there will be a profound stalemate and the arm won't move at all. As one group of interneurons tells the flexors to flex, bringing the lower arm toward the body, another group of neurons inhibits the extensors, allowing them to relax—all within microseconds, and all without any need for higher brain input.

This reflex occurs at the spinal level, in this case, primarily at the level of C5–C6. I say primarily, because another set of interneurons also travels up and down the spinal cord, to allow the reflex to spread to additional muscle groups if needed. As you can see, although we tend to think of the spinal cord as a simple place compared with the brain, and more of a place for impulses to pass through on the way to the sophisticated centers higher up, even simple reflexes involve precise coordination at the spinal level.

As all this activity is going on, the incoming sensory nerve axon from the biceps also connects directly to a second set of sensory nerves, which when activated transmit an action potential along their own axons on the cord to the base of the brain, neatly protected within the skull. For any complex movement, such as pulling a suitcase down from an overhead bin, there is far more involved than just simple reflex response. Reflexes at the spinal level are clearly involved, but this is also a pondered movement, involving thought and willed action—all events occurring at the highest levels of the brain in the cerebral cortex. While the spinal cord makes things happen quickly, spinal reflexes tend to be very gross movements, very imprecise; lifting or pulling down a suitcase is a complicated gesture, requiring fine and precise movements, in sequence, not the sudden uncontrolled contraction of the arm. Such fine coordination requires input from the brain.

In the brain, as in the spinal cord, incoming information from sensory nerves keeps going upward and forward, from the lower parts of the brain to the highest levels in the cerebral cortex. It is interesting to me that as the incoming impulses move geographically literally from the lower to the higher sections of the brain, they are also moving from the regions controlling basic functions, such as respiration, to those centers in the cortex responsible for our most sophisticated thinking processes. Anatomically, the lowest part of the brain, at the top of the spinal cord and at the base of the brain, is the brainstem; this itself, consists, in order from lower to higher, of three distinctive components: the medulla, pons, and midbrain. These three regions are really thickened, more elaborate extensions of the spinal cord, but with quite sophisticated functions. They can serve as a simple relay station for sensory impulses going to still higher areas in the brain, such as the hypothalamus, the thalamus, and, eventually, the cerebral cortex.

Alone, the brainstem is far more than merely a passage to higher planes; it is an elaborate computer that helps regulate many basic sympathetic and parasympathetic system motor activities necessary for life, such as gastrointestinal function, respiration, and heart function. At the brainstem level, these activities can operate without the need for conscious or more complex, higher input. Though the higher centers, as we shall see, profoundly influence brainstem autonomic centers, they can operate independently. For example, animal experiments from decades ago showed that even if connections to the higher centers of the brain are severed surgically, the brainstem will still continue its work, the autonomic centers remain functional, and respiration, cardiovascular activity, and even digestion continue on, to allow for life.

In addition to such basic autonomic regulation, the brainstem also serves as the center for maintaining position against gravity, an activity alluded to earlier. We may take for granted how easy it is for us to stand tall, but it's a fairly delicate maneuver. One misplaced impulse, and you aren't going to be standing.

To keep us straight, the reticular formation within the medulla, the first part of the brainstem, sorts out incoming information from proprioceptors of the muscles of the legs and trunk, as well as impulses arriving from the vestibular nerve, the nerve in the ear that senses our position in space. As these incoming impulses come together in the medulla, our position in the environment is accurately and instantly sensed. Appropriate motor signals then go down the spinal cord, to the muscles along the spine and to the extensor muscles of the leg, which, when contracting, allow us to stand against the enormous and constant force of gravity. Interestingly, in the same area of the medulla lie a series of inhibitory nuclei that send motor signals to prevent the antigravity muscles of the neck and the extensors of the leg from becoming too tense.

As we stand in the airplane aisle, all this signaling in the medulla happens, from millisecond to millisecond, without any conscious thought or input. It's nice to be able to stand without having to think about standing. Meanwhile, as the sensory signal from the biceps passes through the brainstem, it connects to local neurons to let them know what is going on in the arm. The action potential from this specific area quickly gets shunted to the autonomic centers in the brainstem that control blood circulation, to let them know contraction is in progress and an increased blood supply is still needed. So, in a fraction of a second, nerve signals from the proprioceptors of the muscle tell the brainstem in a very precise way what needs to be done, almost instantly.

As all this is happening, the impulse from the biceps moves on to the next higher level, to neurons with their cell bodies housed in the hypothalamus. This is an extraordinarily complex suborgan within the brain that interprets incoming information from the lower sensory nerves in a far more sophisticated way than the brainstem does.

From the earliest days of the last century, the hypothalamus was correctly thought to be a center, if not the main center, for maintaining homeostasis, that is, biochemical and physiological balance within the body, from second to second in a changing environment. It sorts out our complex state of biochemical and physiological affairs and dictates responses to allow the best possible course of action. Although, like the brainstem, it does respond to signals from the higher cortical centers, the hypothalamus can do much on its own, based on its own analysis of its sensory input. This small collection of neurons can do this through its direct control of most endocrine function, of our friend the autonomic nervous system, and of most drives such as hunger and sex. Much of the subtle shades of human emotion are controlled in the hypothalamus.

It would appear, from what I have said here, that the brainstem has many of the same qualities as the hypothalamus, in that it too can regulate autonomic function on its own, without input from anywhere above—including input from the hypothalamus itself. But the brainstem works on a gross level, to keep things going, whereas the hypothalamus adds enormous precision and flexibility to our reactions. I like to think of the brainstem as the autopilot control of the body; the autopilot of a car, say a nice Lexus (no, I don't own a car at all, let alone a Lexus, but I have been in one, twice), allows us to chug along rather automatically, without much thought needed, but without much subtlety. The car can't turn and it can't speed up or slow down, but it keeps the car going. The hypothalamus is the car with a driver, off autopilot, who controls every movement, who can make the car speed up, slow down, stop, turn right, turn left, or even turn around (hopefully, not on a six-lane interstate).

I would like to stop for a moment in our journey through the nervous system and think about the hypothalamus, because, as we shall see, it is so central to any understanding of the autonomic nervous system. The hypothalamus is really quite small, the size of a small nut, and in volume only 1 percent of total brain mass, not very impressive certainly in terms of size. It lies right above the midbrain, at the top of the brainstem, and at times is considered the most "northerly" part of the brainstem itself. To look at it from another perspective, the hypothalamus is the lowest region of the high brain centers of the cortex. I think of it as the transition point between the lower brainstem regions in the medulla, pons, and midbrain, which don't think, and the higher centers in the cerebral cortex, the ultimate center for higher intellectual processing and skills.

The hypothalamus is important neurologically, but it is also the connection between the nervous system and the hormone-producing endocrine glands. Attached to the lower side of the hypothalamus by a "stalk" is the pituitary, known to generations of medical students as the master gland of the body, the gland that controls the major glands such as the thyroid, the adrenal glands and the gonads, the ovaries in women, and the testes in men. If the pituitary is the master gland of the body, the hypothalamus is its primary nervous system commander.

Over the past fifty years, neuroscientists have learned that each region of the hypothalamus has a specific function and these regions have been carefully mapped out in great detail. A particular section within the hypothalamus that serves a specific function is referred to as an "area" or "nucleus." Here the term *nucleus* does not mean, as we learn in high school biology, the center of an individual cell, but rather a collection of nerve cell bodies that control a particular activity, say bladder contraction or hunger. Traditionally, neuroscientists divide the hypothalamus itself into the anterior, or frontal section, and the posterior, or back half. These have very different and often, as we shall see, opposing functions.

The anterior hypothalamus, for example, specifically two regions within the anterior hypothalamus called the paraventricular and supraoptic nuclei, controls the release of the posterior pituitary hormones oxytocin and vasopressin, both involved with salt and water balance in the body.

Critically for our discussion, the anterior hypothalamus, more than any other brain region, is the control center for the parasympathetic nervous system. When the anterior hypothalamus becomes active—in response, of course, to certain sensory information coming in from either the higher cortical centers or the lower brain centers and peripheral sensory receptors—the parasympathetic system becomes active. Parasympathetic function is very precisely organized within the anterior hypothalamus, with different areas, or "nuclei," controlling specific parasympathetic nerve functions. For example, the "medial pre-optic area" of the hypothalamus, when active, will stimulate parasympathetic nerves that contract the bladder when it is full, slow the heart rate, and lower blood pressure, such as occurs when we are resting. The "posterior pre-optic area," when stimulated, turns on the parasympathetic nerves that lower body temperature through sweating and dilation of the blood vessels in the skin, both of which help release heat.

The posterior hypothalamus controls the anterior pituitary, which, when active, releases peptides that in turn regulate the thyroid, adrenals, and gonads. When the thyroid turns on and releases thyroid hormone into the blood system, metabolism speeds up and temperature rises—a useful sequence of events if the environment is cold and the body is in need of warming. The adrenal cortex releases a host of hormones that help convert stored energy in the form of fats and glycogen into available energy in the form of fatty acids and blood glucose—important during times of physical or emotional stress, when metabolic needs can increase dramatically. The adrenal cortex hormones also help keep blood sugar and blood pressure levels from getting too low.

Importantly, the posterior hypothalamus is the central monitor for most sympathetic activity. When the posterior hypothalamus is active, the sympathetic system becomes active. For example, should we suffer unfortunately a severe hemorrhage after an accident, or a state of dehydration with severely low blood pressure, warning signals are transmitted to the posterior hypothalamus indicating there's a problem. The posterior hypothalamus jumps into action, and in turn the sympathetic system turns on full blast. Heart rate goes up, the heart beats harder, cardiac output increases, and blood pressure goes up. The arteries that carry blood to the skin and intestinal tract constrict, so the preciously low blood supply can be efficiently diverted to the more essential regions of the body such as the heart and brain.

A specific posterior hypothalamus area, the perifornical area, when active, stimulates hunger, produces anger, and raises the blood pressure. Scientists know this because in laboratory experiments from decades ago, if they sent an electrical current into this specific nucleus in a laboratory animal, the animal got angry and its blood pressure went up, even if there was no evident reason to be mad. The fact that rage and high blood pressure are both under the control of the same area explains why anger generally raises blood pressure; they cannot but go together. Of course, rage has a value, as a protective response to a perceived threat or to frighten an enemy off, and in danger, it helps to have not only rage, but also blood pumping more strongly to the brain to allow rapid thinking and decision making, to the heart itself, and to the muscles to allow for increased physical strength. Though high blood pressure is of course a serious epidemic problem, it makes biologic sense to have anger and hypertension related. We have a problem when anger becomes constant, uncontrolled, or inappropriate; then, high blood pressure, with all its devious effects, becomes a disease.

It's interesting to me that the centers for hunger, in the perifornical area, and thirst, in the lateral hypothalamus, are also in the posterior hypothalamus. When we need calories, nutrients, or water, these nuclei turn on, and the sympathetic system turns on. It makes sense that if we're hungry or thirsty, the sympathetic system would fire. To find food, or water, we need to move, maybe tackle a bear or cow, or jaunt through a steep ravine (to the stream below). Such tackling and jaunting are both definitely sympathetic phenomena. The restfulness and calm of the parasympathetic nervous system would be of little use in tackling bears or sliding down ravines.

Hypothalamic control of autonomic function is really, at least to me, quite an extraordinary thing: when an animal, or a human, is out seeking something to eat and something to drink, the sympathetic system will be quite active, and the parasympathetic nerves will be nicely inhibited. This makes sense, as I have now discussed, but once food is in the gut, the reverse holds; the parasympathetic nerves take over, and the sympathetic system tones down. This allows digestion to take place, a purely parasympathetic activity. We need our sympathetic system to find and subdue our food—even in the hectic lines of my Whole Foods supermarket—but we need our parasympathetic nerves to get the food digested. This parasympathetic switch explains why we—and lions and tigers and bears—get tired after a large and sometimes even after a small meal: our sympathetic system is down for the count.

Just a few paragraphs earlier, I remarked that brainstem nuclei regulate at least at one level, digestive function, respiration, and cardiac function, and can do so independent of higher influence. However, the brainstem is itself influenced by the hypothalamus directly, through neuron connections between the two regions.

I have already made the point, hopefully clearly, several times that the sympathetic and parasympathetic nervous systems have opposing functions throughout the body. This concept first came up when I discussed the pioneering work of Francis Pottenger. Not only do these two systems of nerves have opposing functions; they are reciprocally inhibiting, to use the correct neuroscience term. This means that the sympathetic and parasympathetic systems not only have opposite effects on the gut, the lungs, or the heart, but actually inhibit each other. When the sympathetic system fires, it turns off the parasympathetic system. And, vice versa, when the parasympathetic system fires, it turns off the sympathetic system, if not completely, at least fairly significantly.

All this reciprocal inhibition happens in the hypothalamus; here, as we have seen, nerve impulses come in from below, from the sensory nerves in the periphery. In addition, there are sensory and motor nerves that run back and forth between the anterior and posterior hypothalamus. These nerves carefully and closely monitor the other half and tell each half what the other half is doing. There are no secrets in the hypothalamus.

Let's say we're dehydrated after a long hike in mid-July in Arizona, and our blood volume is down. As we know, the posterior hypothalamus senses the problem and tells the sympathetic system to turn on at once, to conserve blood and send it where it will be needed most. In addition, motor neurons with their cell bodies in the posterior hypothalamus travel across town to the anterior half and turn off the parasympathetic centers. This is a good thing, because if we're dehydrated and the parasympathetic stays active, it will fight to keep the blood pressure down, not exactly what we need. This reciprocal inhibition is quite useful in a situation like this. With the blood pressure dropping because of dehydration, the sympathetic system will divert blood to the organs that need to be kept going if we are going to live, the brain and the heart, and at the same time prevent the parasympathetic system from sending blood to the skin and gastrointestinal organs. The system reinforces itself, precisely.

I have been talking about the anterior hypothalamus, or the posterior hypothalamus, turning on or turning off, and as a result, the parasympathetic or sympathetic turning on or off, as if this were an all-or-nothing scenario, like a light switch going on and off, but this isn't really the case. The sympathetic system can turn on a little bit, or somewhat or a lot, and the parasympathetic system can be at the same time inhibited a little, somewhat, or a lot. The reverse is true; the parasympathetic nerves can turn on barely or completely, and the sympathetic system can be suppressed barely or completely—with all gradations in between quite possible. This is the marvel of the hypothalamus, the driver of the autonomic system; it allows precise movements, shifts, and changes in autonomic activity, depending on the minutest information coming in via the sensory nerves.

If we are a little dehydrated, after a mild hike not in July but in September and not in Arizona but in Maine, then the sensory input will indicate mild dehydration. Sensory nerves can be that specific, and the hypothalamus can react, specifically. The sympathetic areas of the anterior hypothalamus, including those areas needed to raise the heart rate, cardiac output, and blood pressure, will turn on, and they will turn on only slightly. In reverse, the parasympathetic centers in the anterior hypothalamus, including those that would tend to slow the heart rate, reduce cardiac output, and cause vasodilation and lowered blood pressure, will be suppressed, but only slightly. The hypothalamus—and not the brainstem—allows for such precision.

If the signals are strong enough, such as severe blood loss after a car accident or eating a big meal, an entire hypothalamus half, either the posterior or the anterior hypothalamus depending on the nature of the input, can turn on completely or, conversely, be inhibited completely. In a case of dangerous dehydration, the hypothalamus will be barraged with a strong assault of worrisome sensory indicators that low blood pressure is starting to cause serious problems, and that not enough blood is going anywhere, including to the brain and to the heart. The entire posterior hypothalamus will become strongly active, turning on the entire sympathetic system fully. At the same time, all the nuclei in the anterior hypothalamus will be strongly inhibited.

In our particular example, we had been following the path of a sensory impulse from the biceps, sending the message that the muscle has been contracting. Muscle contractions always turn on the sympathetic system, and muscle relaxation always turns on the parasympathetic nerves. Of course, the degree of turning on or turning off of the sympathetic and parasympathetic systems depends on the degree of muscle contraction. There's an obvious difference between our simple example of a limited biceps contraction and the widespread muscle activity that goes on when you run fast up a steep incline, where scores of muscles are contracting, and quite powerfully, at once.

Limited muscle activity, such as the contraction of the biceps as we lower a suitcase from an overhead bin, is hardly a momentous activity; it involves a limited number of muscles contracting briefly. The posterior hypothalamus turns on slightly, and the sympathetic system turns on slightly. The parasympathetic centers in the anterior hypothalamus turn off, again, slightly.

What amazes me is that the response will tend to be localized, affecting primarily the sympathetic and parasympathetic nerves that feed into the arm. The hypothalamus is capable of such sophistication that not only can it turn on (or off) the entire sympathetic or parasympathetic systems as a unit, but it can turn on either system in one area of the body only if that is what is needed—in this case, the nerves to the right arm. The hypothalamus is a driver indeed, with great skill.

As you can see, a lot happens at the level of the hypothalamus. But there's more that needs to be done. The hypothalamus is somehow able almost instantly to sort out the enormous mass of incoming information, including the action potential from the biceps, and decide which impulses can be dealt with locally, just in the hypothalamus, and which need to be sent upstairs, toward the higher centers. In this case, the simple sensory impulse from the biceps sets up a cascade of events in the hypothalamus itself, turning on the posterior hypothalamus and the sympathetic system (again, a little bit and in a largely limited area) and turning off the anterior hypothalamus and, with it, the parasympathetic system (but a little bit, and mostly in the biceps). The hypothalamus knows that the biceps are in motion, performing a series of movements with a conscious end, and conscious ends are the business of the cortex. So what might seem to be a simple signal from the biceps will be sent to the next level in the brain hierarchy, the thalamus, which sits just above the hypothalamus (*hypo* means "below," aptly put in this case).

Although the hypothalamus does many things, in one respect I like to think of it as a sensory filter that sorts out what needs to be sent above and beyond, to the thalamus, and what can be dealt with locally. If the hypothalamus decides which impulses are being sent on, the thalamus decides where in the higher centers the information needs to go. The thalamus is like a sophisticated mail sorter for incoming sensory mail. It can send the sensory input in a number of different directions, but in the case of contraction impulses coming from the biceps, the target is fairly straightforward: the portion of the sensory cortex that receives input from the arm.

The thalamus does have projections, which is another term for nerve connections, back down to the hypothalamus, so the hypothalamus knows in a sense what the thalamus has decided to do with the incoming impulses. For example, should a signal from the hypothalamus indicate that the sympathetic system need not be particularly active, the thalamus will send inhibitory neurons back to the posterior hypothalamus for reinforcement. It can also, as needed, send activating impulses back to either half of the hypothalamus.

I have used the term *cortex* repeatedly, and now some further clarification seems warranted. If one were to think of the brain, perhaps somewhat unceremoniously, as a cantaloupe or honeydew melon, the cerebral cortex would be the thick skin, or rind. That I think is a good image to keep in mind, though it hardly does justice to the enormous importance of the cortex to our higher human intellectual function. The cortex really is the center of cognition, but it also is used for interpreting incoming sensory function and directing sophisticated motor activity. As I have shown, a simple withdrawal reflex, such as happens when you remove your hand from a hot pan, can occur at the level of the spine only, without the need for input from higher up. However, the cortex allows for precise, elaborate movements, based on a conscious thought, such as deciding to open the overhead bin and pull down the suitcase. This kind of conscious decision making occurs only at the level of the cortex.

The cortex can use input from a variety of sources to orchestrate very detailed muscle movements. In this case, we consciously know the airplane has landed, we are getting our luggage down from the overhead bin, and we need to get moving off the plane. A great deal of information comes into the cortex, to help it make the decisions that need to be made. Here, information from our eyes has been coming into the cortex, allowing it to assess accurately the location of the bin handle; which suitcase, based on memory and prior knowledge, is ours; the distances that need to be traversed to reach the suitcase; and the pattern of extension and flexion needed to bring the suitcase down. The cortex alone can make sure this movement happens smoothly, and that it happens at all. The lower areas in the spine up to the thalamus cannot get a suitcase down from a bin.

The cerebral cortex is divided into the right and half lobes, with each half reasonably a mirror image of the other. The mirroring isn't exact, and the differences between the right and left hemispheres of the brain have been the subject of considerable scientific investigation and much popular culture mythology. Roger Sperry, the eminent Cal Tech neuroscientist, won the Nobel Prize in 1981 for his many years of study of the differences between the right and left halves of the cerebrum. The left hemisphere has been tradition- ally portrayed, with some justification, as the analytical brain; the right brain, again with some justification, the "emotional" poetic brain. We shall refer to such concepts later.

In terms of some basic anatomy, each cerebral hemisphere is itself divided into lobes, geographical sections that are associated with very specific functions. These lobes are separated from one another by actual grooves in the brain, called fissures, or sulci. The frontal lobe, the area of the brain behind the forehead, is really the center of our highest intellectual ability. Here we can make conscious decisions, think, daydream, do math problems, write symphonies, or write books.

I do not mean to imply that the cortex alone in the brain is involved with such cognitive activities; as in any other part of the brain, input comes in from a variety of directions, and other sections of the brain can influence thought, consciousness, and emotion. But thinking along with conscious decision making is a primary activity of the frontal lobe. This part of the brain is also the center for striated motor control, that is, regulation of what are known as the voluntary muscle acts, such as pulling a suitcase down from an overhead bin, an activity we think about. Centers for such activity lie in the back part of the frontal lobe, in what is called the motor strip, which runs longitudinally, or up and down. Each point along the motor strip is responsible for a specific muscle group, such as the flexors in the arm or the extensors of the leg.

The central sulcus, a perpendicular fissure located about midway along the brain, going from front to back, separates the frontal lobe from the parietal lobe. The parietal lobes are of particular interest to us right now, with our example of incoming sensory information from the biceps, because the parietal lobe is the center for receiving and interpreting incoming sensory information from receptors all over the body. Incoming impulses to the sensory cortex are specifically localized. There is, for example, an area of the parietal lobe that receives information only from the arm. There is another area for the legs, and a fairly big area for the lips, which are a very active area with sensory input—another reason for the particular attraction and excitement of kissing.

The sensory cortex interprets all this incoming data and then decides what needs to be done. In this case, the motor cortex, lying on the other side of the central sulcus in the back part of the frontal lobe, must be told which muscles of the right arm need to keep contracting and which need to be relaxing so our arm doesn't suddenly freeze in midair, with a heavy suitcase on its end. Fortunately, the sensory cortex has multiple neuron connections that travel directly to the motor strip, so it can send its directions with near-instantaneous speed. It quickly and continuously, as long as needed, tells the motor cortex specifically which muscles need to be contracting and relaxing to allow a specific movement, no matter now slight, to occur.

Continuing our brief anatomy lesson, the occipital cortex, located at the back of the brain, specifically receives information related to vision. The temporal lobes, one in each cerebral hemisphere, are responsible for hearing and for speech: strokes in this part of brain produce aphasia and dysphasia, difficulty getting the right words out. In addition, the temporal lobes house the complex limbic system, with its hippocampus; simply described, this region is essential for storing certain memories, particularly those related to emotion.

So, let's return to our incoming biceps reflex, arriving in the sensory strip of the parietal cortex. The suitcase is in your arms, and you are about to let it drop to your right side. The sensory cortex is receiving a considerable amount of information at this point, including conscious input about your position on the airplane, whether the doors of the plane are open or not, whether the passengers have started moving down the aisle, and where the suitcase is in its journey from bin to your side. All of it is sorted according to memories coming in from places such as the limbic system that remember other airplane trips and other "deplaning" operations, and how it works and what you need to do. You might also be thinking about why you are even on the plane.

The sensory strip in the parietal lobe is also receiving those impulses that move through without conscious awareness, such as the action potential that began in the proprioceptors of the biceps, which tells all about its state of contraction or relaxation. You thought getting off a plane was a simple maneuver, but there is much information coming in. Fortunately, the cortex can, without any difficult thinking, figure out what you want to do and how to do it. It quickly makes a decision: the biceps can relax, but the extensors such as the triceps now need to contract in order for you to hold the suitcase at your side.

This might seem like a simple conclusion to reach, but even for this little movement, a lot needs to be done. Inhibitory signals, to use the technical term, travel from the sensory cortex to the biceps region of the motor strip to turn off contraction, and excitatory impulses go from the sensory cortex to the area of the motor strip controlling the triceps. All the while, all kinds of sensory information keep coming in to the parietal lobe about the weight of the suitcase, how it is moving through space, and what the next series of moves needs to be. Further, you are considering all the options, assuming the line of passengers starts or doesn't start moving, determining how close you are to the passenger in front or back and what each is like (man, woman, attractive, not attractive, etc.), and thinking about how your meeting is going to go and which—in my particular case—patients I am most concerned about, thousands of miles from my office in New York.

All this, coming in to the sensory cortex, which sorts it all out, decides what is most important right now and tells the motor cortex what to do. I have to get off the plane; the sensory cortex knows that's the immediate issue, and I can think about patients all I want, but the biceps is going to relax and the triceps is going to contract and extend the arm, at my side, so I can carry the suitcase off the airplane.

The signals for biceps relaxation and triceps contraction for the right arm begin to move downward through the brain, through those areas of the brain that control our actions. We are now out of the realm of the sensory nervous system and into the realm of the motor, out of the system of incoming information and into the system of action.

Most of the outgoing impulses from the motor strip in the frontal cortex move down a major nerve pathway, known as the corticospinal tract. Some of the neurons responsible for the very fine, precise movements of our fingers and hands travel from the motor cortex and barrel through the various lower areas of the brain such as the thalamus, hypothalamus, and brainstem, without sending off any side branches, like an express train bypassing an intermediate stop between two cities. These express motor neurons end their run not in the brain, but in the anterior horn of the spinal cord at the level of the cervical spine. Here, they connect to another set of motor neurons that exit the spine, then journey down the arm to the hands and fingers.

Many more neurons originating in the motor strip don't make such a direct and quick trip but instead, as they meander down through the brain, make local stops, sending off branches to two areas of the brain known as the basal ganglia and the cerebellum. We find the basal ganglia in the middle section of the brain, surrounding both the thalamus and hypothalamus, like the white of a hard-boiled egg around the yolk. The basal ganglia form quite an interesting area; they receive impulses from the motor cortex and from the sensory strip of the parietal cortex, but from nowhere else, or at least from nowhere else directly. Then, they send signals not to lower areas in the brain or spinal cord, but only back to the motor cortex, in a type of closed circuit. The basal ganglia have no connections to the brainstem, to the hypothalamus, thalamus, or limbic system, no direct connections to the visual occipital cortex or the hearing centers in the temporal lobe. They receive connections from the motor and sensory strip and send impulses back to the motor cortex, and that's it.

They might seem limited, with the territory in the brain they affect, but without the basal ganglia, we couldn't lead the lives we lead. This small area gives us the power to perform complicated willed movements smoothly, effortlessly, quickly, in the right order, in the right sequence, without much thought once we have decided what it is we want to do. Dr. Guyton (1956, 657) listed in his text such movements as "cutting paper with scissors, hammering nails, shooting a basketball through a hoop, passing a football, throwing a baseball, the movements of shoveling dirt."

These are complicated activities we must first decide to do—we decide to ride a bicycle or shoot a basket—but once willed, they usually proceed without much conscious input needed. Once we're on a bicycle or hammering nails, we don't have to think each motion through. A professional basketball player doesn't think out each move during a jump shot; he or she just jumps, usually with precision. Once we have told the cortex what we want done, the basal ganglia tell the cortex how to do it. It's a good system, and it generally works remarkably well. I like to think of our basal ganglia as the difference between the movements of a professional baseball pitcher and the rather unrefined motion of an earthworm.

Earlier, before I mentioned the term *basal ganglia*, I did discuss the enormous amount of sensory input that goes into the simple movement of pulling down a suitcase from the overhead bin. All this input—from our special sense organs such as our eyes and ears, from the proprioceptors in the muscles, from the memory storage vaults in the hippocampus—comes together in the sensory cortex and then is funneled to the basal ganglia. From there, signals travel back to the precise motor cortex areas needed for the smooth sequence of movements—all without conscious input. Parkinson's disease occurs when nerves that send inhibitory impulses into the basal ganglia are destroyed. In such a condition, the basal ganglia go out of control, and the patient can suffer a variety of awkward, uncontrolled movements, including a tremor even at rest and very rigid, tense muscles. Such patients may be unable to initiate certain movements, such as walking, but once they are walking, it may be difficult to stop!

Next, we move on to the cerebellum, which I always picture as looking like a small cauliflower, sitting piggy back on top of the medulla and pons, the first two segments of the brainstem. It is often referred to, as Dr. Guyton (1956, 647) said, as a silent area within the nervous system because incoming impulses do not lead to any conscious sensation, nor, when any part or portion of the cerebellum becomes excited, does any specific muscle contract. However, without the cerebellum, just as without the basal ganglia, we wouldn't be human, or at least, we wouldn't be capable of much distinctly human activity, as Guyton (1956, 647) reported, "such as running, typing, playing the piano, and even talking." The cerebellum helps with the timing of rapid muscular activities and makes sure a series of fast movements, such as playing Bach well, occur in the right order, again, effortlessly. Should the cerebellum be damaged, such fast, precise activity, even though the muscles themselves may be perfectly normal, will not occur.

The cerebellum receives information from millisecond to millisecond directly from the motor cortex on the status of every striated muscle in the body, from the face to the big toes. In addition, an enormous amount of sensory information comes in from all over the body, arriving via connections coming up from lower down in the spinal cord and coming down from the sensory areas of the cortex. That is a lot of information coming in from several areas. But it's not arriving just for effect: above and beyond this mass of incoming data, the cortex lets the cerebellum know in advance each movement it wants done, and in what sequence.

Once given its orders, the cerebellum takes what would seem to be an overload of motor and sensory information, including impulses from the spindles of the various muscles, and compares what is actually going on in the muscles with what the higher-thinking cortex wants to be happening. As Guyton (1956) wrote, "If the two do not compare favorably, then instantaneous appropriate corrective signals are transmitted back into the motor system to increase or decrease the levels of activation of the specific muscles." All this goes on, remember, without much conscious input.

The cerebellum, with far more precision than the most advanced computer, plans each movement, each complicated series of muscle contractions and relaxations, a fraction of a second in advance, thus allowing for a continuous, smooth series of movements. Imagine if a classical pianist had to consciously plan each finger action in advance; piano playing, and life as we know it, would be impossible.

With our simple movement of bringing a suitcase from the overhead bin to our side, both the basal ganglia and the cerebellum are very much involved. The basal ganglia allow us to plan and initiate the motion, and the cerebellum allows the fairly rapid activity to occur in proper sequence: first the flexors flex and the extensors relax; then the flexors relax and the extensors extend and bring the suitcase to rest, held at our side, our right arm extended fully. All this happens very quickly.

Even a commonplace motion like bringing a suitcase to our side ultimately depends on the motor neurons that feed into the flexor muscles of the right arm, with their cell bodies, remember, in the anterior horn at the level of C5–C6, their axons exiting between the C5 and C6 vertebral bodies. These axons end at the synapse between the nerve ending and the acetylcholine receptor in the muscle itself. In this case, as the flexed arm has reached its maximum point of contraction, the brain now wants the flexor biceps to relax and extend while the extensors are now contracting, bringing the arm into a straight, downward position. The excitatory neurons in the biceps then will be inhibited and stop releasing acetylcholine, as the neurons to the extensors become themselves excited and begin releasing acetylcholine. The biceps relaxes, the triceps contracts, and the arm comes to the side, with the fingers of our right hand holding to the suitcase handle tightly.

Now that we've covered, though somewhat briefly, the physiology and anatomy of the somatic nervous system, there is one point I need to make. I have used the words *nerve* and *nerves* repeatedly, knowing that we all have a fair understanding of what the terms mean in a general sense. I would like to be more specific. A nerve cell is an individual microscopic neuron, whatever its function; sometimes, the word *nerve* is used to mean an individual cell, say a sensory cell carrying information toward the central nervous system, or a motor neuron causing something to happen in a striated muscle. Most of our activities, such as pulling down a suitcase from an overhead bin, involve many muscles and hundreds of thousands of individual "nerve cells," including sensory nerves, neurons in the central nervous system, and motor nerve cells.

A single excited sensory "nerve cell" carrying its action potential toward the central nervous system is not going to cause much of anything to happen. And an action potential moving down a single motor neuron ending in the biceps is, by itself, too weak to cause any movement in the muscle as a whole, with its thousands upon thousands of muscle fibers that need to be stimulated in synchrony all at once for anything significant to happen. To perceive even the slightest of sensations, such as pressure on a finger, or contraction of the biceps, literally thousands upon thousands of individual sensory neurons must be activated, and for a muscle to contract, literally thousands of individual motor neurons must go into action.

The axons of individual sensory and motor neurons do not make their own way to or from the spinal cord through the complicated anatomy of the body. Instead, sensory and motor axons carrying impulses toward or away from the spinal cord move as groups of tens of thousands of axons together in what are called spinal nerves, collections of axons and supporting connective tissue all encased in a tough fibrous coating. Spinal nerves are quite large and easily visible during surgery or during dissection of a cadaver. It's useful to think of a spinal nerve as an underground electrical or telephone cable in the city, carrying thousands of individual wires, the equivalent of axons, to a particular neighborhood, with perhaps thousands of individual apartments and homes.

Spinal nerves exit from the spinal cord between the vertebral bodies along the length of the spinal cord, with the exception of the first cervical nerve, which exits in the space between the first cervical vertebra and the skull. Spinal nerves innervate all areas of the body below the skull and certain areas of the head and neck, and each spinal nerve innervates a specific limited part of the body. In the case of the somatic nervous system, the area of distribution for a particular spinal nerve is referred to as the segmental distribution for the nerve. Remember, when we talk about the somatic nervous system, we're talking about sensory input from peripheral receptors that eventually activates—or inhibits—motor nerves that target striated, "voluntary" muscle only.

At any given level of the spinal cord, the spinal nerves come in pairs, one exiting on the right side of the cord and serving a particular area on the right side of the body, its pair nerve exiting on the left side of the spinal cord and serving the mirror image area on the left side of the body. There are thirty-one pairs in total, running the length of the spinal cord: eight cervical spinal nerves, responsible for the sensory and muscle areas of the head, arms, and neck; twelve thoracic nerves, which innervate the skin and muscle regions of the chest; the five lumbar spinal nerves that extend to the skin and muscles of most of the legs; the five sacral nerves that control the skin and muscles of the groin and upper thigh; and the single coccygeal nerve, which controls a small area in the lower back.

In addition to the thirty-one pairs of spinal nerves, there are twelve paired cranial nerves. These differ from the spinal nerves in several basic ways. First, the cell bodies for the sensory cranial nerves do not lie adjacent to the spinal cord, as do the cell bodies of the spinal sensory nerves, but rather in the brain itself. Similarly, the cell bodies for the motor cranial nerves do not lie in the spinal cord, as do the cell bodies of the spinal motor nerves. Instead, like the sensory cell bodies, they lie in the brain substance. Each cranial nerve also exits the skull directly, to travel toward its target organ, with no connections to the spinal cord of any type; these nerves originate in the brain and transit through the skull—hence the designation *cranial nerve*.

The twelve cranial nerves are really quite a heterogeneous grouping with a variety of different functions. Some are purely sensory, some are purely motor, some relay special sensory information about vision and hearing, and others are largely autonomic. But in structure, they are, like the spinal nerves, large visible nerves, consisting of axons and connective tissue and surrounded by a tough fibrous coat.

I will now refer to cranial nerves, so I feel it useful to list them and briefly explain their function:
- Olfactory nerve: Carries the impulses related to smell
- Optic: The special sensory nerve for vision
- Oculomotor: A parasympathetic motor nerve that causes the pupils of the eye to constrict
- Trochlear: Controls the tracheal muscle of the eye orbit, which helps with eye movement and focusing
- Trigeminal: A largely sensory nerve of the skin and muscles of the face, and of the teeth
- Abducens: Controls the abducens muscle of the eye orbit, important for visual tracking
- Facial: A motor nerve of the facial muscles, important for expression and speech
- Acoustic: The nerve for hearing and balance
- Glossopharyngeal: Responsible for taste

- Vagus: The large wanderer of the parasympathetic system that innervates the organs of the chest, including the lungs and the heart, and all the digestive organs above the level of the descending colon
- Accessory: The motor nerve of the trapezius muscle of the back
- Hypoglossus: A motor nerve of the tongue

We have now followed, in some detail, the journey of a sensory impulse from its peripheral receptor in a specific somatic muscle, the biceps, right up the spinal cord to the highest levels of the thinking brain, the cerebral cortex, where decisions about action take place. We have then followed the motor impulse down from the cortex, through the basal ganglia and cerebellum, down the anterior horn of the spinal cord to the muscle receptor on the biceps itself. Now, having discussed the somatic sensory and motor system, we are ready to approach the autonomic nervous system again, the system so crucial to an understanding of how we treat cancer, and all other disease.

The Autonomic Nervous System

Neurophysiologists, for more than a hundred years, have distinguished the somatic voluntary nervous system from the autonomic nervous system. Such distinctions give some order to a complex topic and allow the mind to create comfortable categories. As we have seen, the somatic nervous system is the collection of motor neurons that innervate and regulate all the striated, or as scientists also call them, voluntary, muscles of the body. The term *voluntary* refers, of course, to the fact that these are the nerves and muscles that allow us to carry out a nearly infinite number of willed, intentional movements, movements that require some level of thought at the levels of the cerebral cortex. However, it is useful to keep in mind that these same muscles also allow reflex responses, such as removing your hand from a hot pan, that occur initially only at the spinal level, without the need for higher cortical input. Though reflexes aren't usually "voluntary," any activity in these muscles still comes under the domain of the somatic nerves.

The autonomic nervous system (ANS), as we have touched upon before, is that collection of nerves that regulate the automatic activities in our body, such as digestion, blood flow, breathing, the secretion of hormones, and immunity, processes all essential to life. These activities all generally are assumed to be beyond or beneath the need for conscious input. Interestingly, the ANS was first named by the brilliant Cambridge University neuroscientist J. N. Langley in 1898—when our friend Dr. Beard was busily formulating his trophoblastic hypothesis up north in Edinburgh.

The distinction between the somatic nerves and the ANS, however useful as a teaching device, is really quite arbitrary. In my prior description of a somatic muscle movement, the lowering of a suitcase from the bin in an airplane, we saw how a willed movement—we consciously know we have to get off the airplane, and our brain does what is necessary to make it happen quickly and efficiently—does of course involve, and in fact requires, thought processes in the sophisticated cerebral cortex (the rind of the melon in my analogy for the brain). It also involves, and in fact requires, autonomic responses for any muscle activity to occur smoothly, or to occur at all. Though neuroscientists, trying to make a point, differentiate the voluntary motor system from the autonomic, the fact is that most of what goes on even with such a simple maneuver involves autonomic nerves.

The moment we think of an action, even before the action begins, signals from the motor cortex move downward through the basal ganglia and the cerebellum and, almost instantly, to the motor nerves that go right to the appropriate muscles, indicating which muscles should start contracting and exactly how much contraction is needed, which should start relaxing and exactly how much relaxation is needed, and which need to do nothing. Still other neurons from the motor cortex branch off on their journey to the posterior hypothalamus with its sympathetic autonomic centers, to let it know something is about to happen, where it is going to happen, and how it is going to happen. The thought of a movement always turns on the posterior hypothalamic sympathetic centers. Then, almost instantly, while the flexors are starting to contract and the extensors are starting to relax, the posterior hypothalamus alerts the brainstem cardiovascular centers, so that precisely the right blood vessels in the right muscles will start dilating to allow increased blood flow in exactly the right amount—a sympathetic phenomenon. Muscle action requires oxygen and nutrients, and an increased blood supply provides just this.

For a willed, "voluntary" conscious movement to occur, the autonomic system is always involved and must always be involved, working together with the somatic system to allow the movement, however slight or however grandiose, to occur with ease. We may not need to think about autonomic functions, but with any willed activity, the autonomic system is there working with us and for us.

The hypothalamus receives input from below, as well as from above, from the cerebral cortex. As the impulses are coming in from the motor cortex, as we have seen, sensory signals from the various involved muscle spindles in the contracting and relaxing muscles start moving quickly toward the spinal cord, up to the brainstem, to the hypothalamus on their way to the sensory cortex. There, in the posterior hypothalamus, the message that muscles are in the process of actively contracting further stimulates the sympathetic centers. The thought of movement has already alerted the hypothalamic sympathetic nuclei to start waking up, but movement itself, even a slight motion such as scratching your face, turns on the posterior hypothalamic sympathetic centers. Of course, the hypothalamus is very smart, and it tells the sympathetic system just how much it needs to turn on—and turns off the parasympathetic anterior hypothalamic nuclei, at least to some degree.

Then, as part of this wonderful circuit, downward impulses from the hypothalamus relay what is wanted to the autonomic centers in the brainstem, then on to the sympathetic and parasympathetic nerves themselves. As the sympathetic nerves are revving up, blood supply to the skin and to the gut lessens. As I bring the suitcase to my side, I become slightly paler, as blood is diverted from the skin, and digestion diminishes slightly. Pulse rate and the strength of cardiac pumping increase, to increase blood supply to the muscles. For such a brief and simple act, the effects will indeed be mild, consciously unnoticed, but the effects are there without ongoing higher input.

So the hypothalamus responds, in most cases appropriately, to incoming sensory messages from the muscle spindles, but in addition, it also relays these sensory signals from the muscle spindles of the contracting biceps upward and onward, to the thalamus, and ultimately to the sensory cortex. There, the incoming information is sent on to the motor cortex, for the next set of adjustments and instructions. The signals start coming down again—and all within milliseconds.

The distinctions between the voluntary, somatic nervous system and the autonomic nervous system are really very arbitrary. The fact is, they really do work together, must work together, and always work together, whether you are scratching your head, running from an oncoming bus, or digesting a meal. Here, I have shown how a simple willed movement, the pulling of a suitcase down from an overhead bin, involves the somatic motor system and the striated skeletal muscles but also requires very subtle maneuvering, to use that word again, of the autonomic system.

Willed movements do involve and influence the autonomic nervous system in each second of our waking lives, but the reverse is also true: autonomic activities, such as blood flow, digestion, and breathing, always affect the somatic system, the so-called "voluntary" nervous system. Signals from these routine autonomic activities also, through connections in the hypothalamus, influence our voluntary muscles.

I like to think of the hypothalamus, seated as it is in the center of the brain, as the true crossroads of our bodies, connecting the higher centers to autonomic nuclei of the brainstem and connecting these "lower" autonomic areas back up to the cortex. The influence works both ways, as we shall see, profoundly.

Autonomic Nervous System Anatomy

It's helpful to think of anatomy in general, and neuroanatomy specifically, as a wonderful roadmap that tells us, like any decent map, where things are. Think of a trip to a foreign country, say England or Spain; a roadmap is absolutely essential for any productive touring and sightseeing. Initially, a map of a strange new place can be daunting, filled with the names of cities and towns and villages we've never seen before, connected by roads we've never driven and governed by rules we may not know (I still will not drive in England because I will never adjust to the opposite side of the road driving). If we're motivated, we learn where things are quickly, we learn the names of the towns, the cities, the highway names and numbers, and we're the better for it. After a time, and after some travel to these cities and towns and villages and along these roads, they are hardly foreign at all, but second nature to us and as known as our own home territory.

The nervous system is to most of us, to most physicians, a foreign country, with a new geography, with strange names and unknown locations, and with what seem to be complicated connections that are beyond our previous experience. The connections, the nerve highways and the areas they connect, can seem confusing and complicated; however, it's all just part of the map of a new country that takes some getting used to but that can be fairly easily learned and mastered. I think it's important to know at least the basics of nervous system geography. There is much that we can learn about ourselves from poetry, art, music, history, and travel. We are in so many ways ultimately, each of us, what our brains are, and what our brains allow us to be.

To keep our focus, as we begin a somewhat more detailed discussion of autonomic nervous system geography, I think it's important to get back to basics and think about what the nerves actually do. As complicated and fear provoking as neuroanatomy can be even to a medical student, remember that nerves do essentially three things. One set of neurons carries information to the central nervous system, the spine and the brain, from every nook and cranny of our bodies, information about the world around us as well as input from our own internal organs. All these data travel to the spinal cord and brain via the sensory nerves.

There, another set of nerves, those of the central nervous system, interpret and make decisions based on incoming impulses from all over the body. Then, the third set of nerves, the motor nerves, leaves the brain central nervous system (CNS) and travels again to every nook and corner of our bodies, carrying out the specific instructions of the CNS. The motor system, remember, consists of the somatic nerves that control the striated skeletal muscles, and the autonomic nerves, which control our essential "non-conscious" physiology. But, overall, certain nerves carry information in, other nerves interpret it, and other nerves carry out the directions. It's that simple.

Although the various nerves and neurons of the ANS are a motor system, they are of course reacting to impulses carried by sensory nerves that have been evaluated in the CNS. You can't think about the autonomic nervous system and its anatomy, with its sympathetic and parasympathetic branches with all their complicated routings, in isolation, without considering the sensory nerves themselves, which start the whole ball of ANS activity rolling. So, though I have already introduced the idea of sensory nerves, and their travels to and up the spinal cord to the sensory cortex, I would like to think about this system briefly. Though I don't want to overdo the geography analogy, it is useful to think of sensory nerves, wherever they originate, as a true information highway, bringing data back to the CNS.

Sensory nerves come in many sizes and shapes and differ considerably in their appearance and function. Just think of the optic nerve of the eye, which differs so dramatically, in the way it looks under the microscope and in what it does, from the Pacinian corpuscles, the sense organ for pressure of the skin. Indeed there is variation, just as there is great variation in the roadways of any country, say the United States. These include the superhighways of six and eight lanes that traverse counties and states, usually leading to a major metropolitan area, such as my own New York or Washington,

DC. There are also two-lane blacktops winding through the countryside, and dirt roads, like the one that leads to my family's farm in northern Vermont, and the individual streets and lanes of any village, town, or city, again, as in my own New York.

These sensory nerves carry back data from every area of the body, from the big toe to the hair follicles in the scalp, including all areas in between, but wherever they come from, they are always going in one direction, toward the central nervous system, the spinal cord, and the brain. They carry traffic only one way, to the center. And these sensory nerves carry basically just two kinds of informational traffic. Whatever their size, shape, or form, from wherever they originate and however circuitous their path through the body may be, the sensory nerves carry data to the brain about the two great areas of our lives: the external environment, which is the world around us, and the internal environment, which is the environment of our tissues, organs, glands, and blood vessels, from the skin on the surface to the liver, pancreas, and intestines inside. Claude Bernard, the great French physiologist of the nineteenth century, first made this rather important point, however obvious it may seem retrospectively, that input coming into the brain and spinal cord along the sensory nerves really consists of data about the outside universe and the inside universe, the internal milieu, to use the French.

It's useful to think of sensory nerves geographically, beginning from the surface of the skin and moving inward, to the muscles and then to the internal organs. It helps, when thinking about the anatomy of sensory neurons, to consider first those that originate below the head. Wherever they may originate, axons of these neurons carrying impulses back to the spinal cord run mostly in the spinal nerves. These spinal nerves, which exit the spine on both sides, from above the first cervical vertebral body to the sacral spine, consist of sensory axons carrying impulses to the spinal cord as well as the motor axons— both somatic and autonomic—transmitting the directions for action from higher up.

Note that I said that sensory axons run mostly in the spinal nerves; to be precise, I need to point out that some sensory axons from the viscera, the internal organs such as heart, the lungs, and the organs of the gastrointestinal tract, do travel to the spine in the two paired vagus nerves. These two nerves consist of parasympathetic motor fibers, which carry impulses away from the CNS, but also visceral sensory axons from certain internal organs. We will talk more about the vagus later.

If we continue to focus on the body below the head, sensory neurons—wherever they may innervate—the skin, the muscles, the internal organs—have their cell bodies, the central machinery of each cell, in the dorsal root ganglia, those nubbins of cell bodies that lie adjacent to the spinal cord on each side. The axons of these neurons extend to the end organ; there, the very tip of the axon forms what we call a sensory receptor, the microscopic place where the action begins. When stimulated, the axon tip sets off an action potential, the electrical current of a nerve cell, that moves quickly to the cell body in the dorsal root ganglion and then continues into the spinal cord itself, always toward the spine and central nervous system.

Now, if we start geographically on the outside, we need of course first to consider the sensory neurons whose axons reach into the skin. The receptors of the sensory cells of the skin tell the brain about three things: pain, temperature, and touch. It's important to keep in mind that each individual sensory nerve cell can respond to a single type of sensation; there are, consequently, sensory receptors that respond only to painful stimuli, neurons that relay information about temperature, and a third group that reacts only to touch and pressure on the skin. A pain receptor never sends back information about touch, for example.

The receptors of these various sensory nerve cells come in a great variety of shapes and sizes, specific to their function. The axon tips of pain neurons are quite simple, essentially free nerve endings, without any complicated microstructure. These receptors respond to either physical pressure or deformation that causes tissue damage, chemical toxins, or even electrical currents that can disrupt the cells of the skin. All these stimuli set off action potentials in the affected axon endings of the pain sensory neurons, potentials that travel to the dorsal roots and then up the spine again to the sensory cortex. Pain receptors let us know that something harmful is happening to us that needs to be acted on.

Receptors for touch and pressure are far more complex than the axon tips that transmit pain information. These nerve endings form complicated microscopic organelles, which I alluded to in a previous chapter, such as the intricate Meissner's and Pacinian corpuscles, which respond to events such as tissue stretching or pressure. Such activity sets off an action potential in these neurons, which travels back, as always, to the spine and ultimately to the sensory cortex of the brain. Pressure sensors alert the CNS that we're touching something, whatever that something might be—the hand of our lover, or the door of a crowded rush-hour subway car against which we are unceremoniously pushed.

There are specific sensory neurons in the skin that tell us about the ambient temperature of the world around us. Their receptors, like those of the pain nerves, are essentially the axon tips, which branch repeatedly but without forming a complicated organelle. Heat or cold sets off an action potential in the respective temperature-sensitive axons, which again ends up in the sensory cortex. It's amazing to me just how sophisticated these temperature sensors, like all sensory receptors, really are; they can distinguish instantly between the hot pot I like to talk about and a snowball, and all gradations in between. In a less dramatic way, our temperature nerves tell us about the temperature in the world around us, whether it is cold, hot, or just perfectly comfortable, and can monitor changes from millisecond to millisecond.

There is of course crossover, and sometimes sensory neurons, and their axons, of all three types will be needed to tell the brain about the subtleties of a single event. To return to the vision of your hand touching a hot pot, in such a circumstance pain receptors turn on, but so do those transmitting impulses about temperature and touch.

Remember, each single sensory nerve cell can transmit an impulse in response to only one type of sensation.

The sensory nerves of the muscle spindles send back information about the state of contraction, or relaxation, of every single muscle in the body, from the temporalis muscle of the forehead to the tiniest, most delicate muscles of the smallest toe of our feet. Though the intricate details are not relevant to our discussion, these spindles are really quite complicated little organelles spread throughout every striated "voluntary" muscle in our bodies, and they tell the brain what is going on with each of these muscles in each second of our lives. That's a lot of information, from several places. In addition, muscles also have abundant pain receptors that can tell the brain something isn't right, as any athlete who has ruptured a muscle, or who has just worked out too much, will know.

The sensory axons of the skin and muscles, whatever type of data they might be relaying, travel to the spine in the spinal nerves. As I have mentioned, things get somewhat more complicated when we start looking at our internal organs. Our viscera, as the scientists like to call the organs below the brain, are of course a heterogeneous group. There are the two lungs; the heart and the entire cardiovascular system with its network of arteries, veins, and capillaries; the gastrointestinal tract, with the esophagus, stomach, and small and large intestines; and the liver, gallbladder, and pancreas. Then there are of course the organs of the immune system, including the thymus and the spleen, plus bone, which scientists recognize as a complex and critically important organ system.

A great variety of sensory nerves connects to every one of these organs and organ systems, providing receptors for a variety of different types of information. Anatomists like to call sensory nerves that connect to different organs the visceral afferents, *afferents* meaning a nerve that carries impulses back to the CNS.

These neurons, and their axons, like those of the skin and muscles, come in a variety of different sizes and shapes and do a variety of tasks. Some are similar to those we have just discussed; others are completely unique, designed to tell the brain about the particular activities of a specific organ. All our internal organs have pain receptors, though some have far more than others, and like the pain receptors of the skin, these are simple arborizing, branching-free nerve endings of the axons. Like all other receptors, they respond to damaging (see Guyton 1956, 952) mechanical pressures and chemical toxins, and if somehow a plugged-in electrical cord ended up in your abdomen, they could respond to dangerous electrical currents, though this isn't something we generally would expect.

The gastrointestinal tract has a particularly rich supply of such sensory axons, as anyone who has had appendicitis or a gallbladder attack, or even a bad case of gas after eating too many beans, knows. Appendicitis, with its purulent excess of bacterial toxins, sets off a chemical warning; gas may also result from bacterial infection with its associated irritating chemical toxins, but gas itself, if it accumulates enough, also sets off the pain receptors responsive to excessive mechanical stretch. The heart too, like the gut, is rich in pain receptors: the pain of a heart attack can be excruciating. Medical students are taught that patients will describe the sensation that their chest is being crushed, as if an elephant were sitting right there; as ludicrous an analogy as this might initially seem, it is indeed the type of pain often described by heart patients.

Much of the pain of a heart attack is chemical in origin; with any myocardial infarction, to use the technical term, blood supply to the heart muscle itself gets blocked. The plentiful pain receptors in the cardiac muscle are deprived of oxygen while finding themselves overloaded with metabolic toxins that aren't being carried away from the heart muscle effectively. This is very irritating to these neurons and a sign of great danger to the brain; this is a pain that needs to be taken very seriously.

Our internal organs, particularly the abdominal viscera and the great veins such as the vena cava, do have receptors that can relay data on temperature back to the central nervous system. However, unlike the temperature nerves of the skin, which are sensitive to the ambient environment, the internal temperature sensors tell the brain about the body's core, or basic internal body temperature, and not the environment outside. This is an important point; though humans survive nicely in environments that range from the extreme cold of the Arctic to the heat of the tropics, our internal temperatures should, under normal circumstances, vary only slightly around 37 degrees Celsius (the classic 98.6 degrees Fahrenheit). Though ostensibly humans can do quite well running routine temperatures from about 95°F up to 99°F degrees, changes above the 106°F range or below the 95°F range for any length of time are not compatible with life. It is imperative, therefore, for survival, that the core temperature be maintained within a fairly narrow range, whatever the outside temperature may be. These internal sensors are therefore a very critical group of afferent nerves.

Many axons from these internal temperature sensors travel back to the spine, via spinal nerves, through the dorsal roots, to the dorsal spinal cord, and up the spine to end in the hypothalamus. Others travel with the vagus, the big nerve cable that wanders through the chest and abdomen, carrying both parasympathetic motor and visceral afferent axons. These vagus afferents also connect to the hypothalamus, which ultimately monitors and regulates internal temperature.

Mechanoreceptors, similar to the touch and pressure receptors of the skin, are found in most viscera, though they are particularly abundant in the lining of the gastrointestinal tract organs. This system is essentially a convoluted tube, beginning at the mouth and esophagus, continuing through the stomach and small and large intestines, and ending at the rectum. Here, of course, food enters, digestion occurs, nutrients and water are absorbed, wastes pass—all along a very active twenty-five-foot-long tunnel. Though the different parts of the digestive tract have different functions—the stomach starts the breakdown of food, which continues in the small intestine, where the absorptive process begins—in the colon, there is additional absorption of primarily water and electrolytes and the concentration of indigestible wastes.

Though the different regions of the digestive tube do different things, in structure the wall of this tube from start to finish has a very similar construction. On the inside of the tube, facing the oncoming rush of food and, depending on what region we're looking at, food in various states of digestion, lies a single cell lining of epithelial cells, called the mucosa. These are the basic lining cells of internal organs that I discussed rather at length in my book on the trophoblast and cancer. In the stomach, these cells secrete mucus to protect the lining, as well as acid and pepsin to begin digestion, and in the small intestine, they provide a whole range of enzymes necessary for digestion to occur. The lining cells of the small and large intestines do also secrete mucus, to lubricate the food bolus so it more easily moves along, but here, the epithelial cells also absorb water, electrolytes, and the range of nutrients—vitamins, minerals, trace metals, proteins, fats, and carbohydrates—that we need to stay alive.

This epithelial level, whether we're looking at the esophagus, stomach, small intestine, or colon, sits on, as all epithelial cells do, a basement membrane. Beneath this is the submucosa, a connective tissue layer through which run lymphatic and small blood vessels, into which move the microscopic nutrients. Beneath this lies an inner layer of what scientists call longitudinal muscle, which runs the length of the digestive tract, and outside this muscle layer is a second, circular layer, which circumscribes the digestive tube. These two muscle layers allow for the complicated muscular movements of peristalsis, which mixes food with the digestive juices and at the same time propels the food mass along. On the outside of the muscle is the serosa, a thin layer of connective tissue.

In my writings on the pancreas, I talked at some length about digestion from a more enzymatic, physiological perspective. But because now I'm talking about the nervous system, I'd like to consider the gut from a more neurological perspective. I think it's worth the discussion, because we are talking about the nervous system here, and because the gut is unique in terms of nerves and nervous activity.

When I was in medical school, though I wrongly and proudly tried deliberately not to pay too much attention to neuroanatomy during my first year, we were taught there is the central nervous system, of course, with its brain and spinal cord, and the peripheral nervous system, those nerves of the sensory and motor system (including the somatic and autonomic effectors) that reach out to all organs, tissues, and glands, from the skull to the toes. No one told us too much about the gut. In fact, I don't remember any of my first-year professors, in anatomy, histology, or neuroanatomy, paying much attention to the gut in terms of nerves. This was a mistake, though had these dedicated professors done otherwise, I probably would only have resented the extra load of information I would have been required to learn.

It was Langley, the great student of the autonomic nervous system, working at Cambridge while our friend Dr. Beard toiled north in Edinburgh, who first pointed out that in addition to the central nervous system and all its complex attachment, there really is a second nervous system, within the wall of the gastrointestinal tract itself, almost as complex as the brain. This system consists, Langley claimed, of neurons with their cell bodies not in the spine, or autonomic centers, or the dorsal roots, but in the lining of the gut itself, and their axons do not extend outside of the gut wall. It appeared to him to be a self-contained, complete-unto-itself nervous system, able to run itself, thank you very much, without help from the brain. This second system really controlled, Langley claimed, much of what goes on in the gut, from beginning to end, from movement of food in the esophagus, to digestion, absorption, and defecation.

We now know just how right Langley was. There is indeed a very rich collection of nerves within the gut itself that live entirely within the gut, just as he said. Oddly and interestingly enough, these nerves seem able to function independently of any input from the nerves of the brain, spinal cord, or autonomic system. The gut is influenced by these nerves, of course, and I have in several places alluded to the fact that the sympathetic and parasympathetic nerves control to some extent GI functioning, from chewing to digestion to defecation. This is true, and we will discuss this, but this very complex system can quite nicely operate on its own and tell the digestive tract to do the things it needs to do to keep us alive, such as secrete mucus, acid, enzymes, and other digestive aids and absorb nutrients. Autonomic input, as we shall see, helps, but the gut brain frankly can do it without any help.

We now know that there are more than 100 billion neurons in the nervous system of the gut that live entirely within the gut wall and, interestingly, use serotonin as their primary neurotransmitter. Neuroscientists have studied serotonin for years and appreciated its critical role in brain chemistry. It is, as simple a molecule as it may seem, the basis of an entire industry and the focus of the selective serotonin reuptake inhibitor (SSRI) class of antidepressants that are used by millions, that generate billions in profits, and that continue, for better or worse, to make front-page headline news. But what we don't generally realize is that 95 percent of all serotonin in our bodies is found not in the brain but in the gut nervous system! That, to me, is impressive and a sign that something important is going on there.

The cell bodies of these gut nerves congregate in two major regions along the length of the GI tract: between the inner longitudinal and outer circular muscles, and in the submucosa, right beneath the epithelial layer lining the inside of the GI tube. The plexus of nerves, as scientists like to call such things, in the muscle layers we call the myenteric plexus, and it controls the contraction of these muscles. The submucosa plexus, also known as Meissner's plexus (no relation to the skin corpuscles mentioned earlier by the same name) regulates the secretion of mucus and other digestive aids, as well as absorption.

These nerve collections, or plexuses, are a hot area of research in some circles. One of the great experts in gut neurology, Dr. Michael Gershon, wrote a wonderful, if under-appreciated, book called *The Second Brain*, an apt title for this very subject. I recommend it to anyone interested in the story of this nervous system.

I couldn't really talk about this class of gut receptors without letting you in on the secret of Dr. Gershon's second brain. These mechanoreceptors lie in the epithelial and submucosal layers and monitor distention and stretching of the gut, in response to the presence of food. Their axons do connect directly with neurons of both the myenteric and the submucosal plexuses, to let these nerves know whether there is anything moving down the tube and whether anything needs to be done—such as secreting mucus or enzymes, or absorbing nutrients. Yes, the myenteric and submucosal plexuses can take care of these things on their own, but the mechanoreceptors also send branches back to the spinal cord, as well as through the vagus nerve, to the brainstem and hypothalamus, so there can be additional input from higher up. Here, the autonomic nerves, as we shall see, do come into play and do what they are designed to do. We will discuss more about autonomic input to the second brain later.

There is another group of mechanoreceptors, or more specifically stretch receptors, that I believe warrants our close attention. These are the baroreceptors located in the walls of the large arteries of the chest and neck. Yes, some new terms: baroreceptors, where "baro" means pressure, are the sensory receptors of the circulatory system that relay information back to the brain about the second-to-second, moment-to-moment status of the blood pressure. This isn't a trivial job; earlier, when I opened my journey through the nervous system by following my rather mundane walk from my office to my workroom, I mentioned that the simple act of standing up can put the brain in jeopardy, unless the heart and the blood vessels of the body adjust accordingly to keep the blood flowing against gravity, to the brain, as I or anyone stands up. This response, really a reflex, which we don't need to think about but which keeps us on our feet instead of passing out on the floor, depends on the baroreceptors.

Baroreceptors are particularly abundant in two regions: the aortic arch of the chest and the carotid sinus of the neck. We hopefully remember the aorta from high school biology as the main artery that carries oxygenated blood from the left ventricle of the heart; just after this large vessel comes off the heart, it moves upward and then makes a gradual arching U-turn before traveling downward to bring blood to the chest, abdomen, and eventually, through its branches, to all the limbs and fingers and toes of the body. This U-turn area is the aortic arch, where we find a rich concentration of baroreceptors.

The carotids, one on each side of the neck, come off the aorta in the arch and then move upward, before dividing into the internal carotid, which feeds the brain, and the external carotid, which sends oxygenated blood to the muscles and skin of the skull. Just above the point where the common carotid, on each side, divides into the internal and external carotids is the carotid sinus, a small, dilated area with a large concentration of baroreceptors right in the arterial wall.

Baroreceptors, for all their importance, as we shall see, are quite simple in structure, basically like pain receptors, branching-free endings of axons. They are what neurophysiologists like to call stretch receptors, which respond to pressure, in this case, blood pressure. Their concentration in the aortic arch and the internal carotid is particularly appropriate, because from these specific positions, they can warn the brain of dangerous fluctuations in the blood flow of the systemic circulation as well as that to the brain itself. The carotid sinus baroreceptors are really the guardians of the blood supply to the brain, so essential for normal life.

The physiology of baroreceptors I always find particularly intriguing. They seem to be set, like a thermostat, to maintain a particular level of blood pressure that they read as "normal" for the body. Should pressure go above this level, even slightly, this increased force will stretch the arterial walls of the aortic arch and carotid sinus, and this stretching, however microscopic it may be, sets off an action potential in the baroreceptor and its axon. The axons from the aortic arch travel directly back to the medulla in the brainstem in the vagus nerve, which I have mentioned a number of times previously; this, remember, carries the main parasympathetic supply to the chest and abdomen, but also is the conduit for some sensory axons of the heart, blood vessels, and certain other organs. The carotid sinus baroreceptor axons travel back to the medulla as well, but as part of the glossopharyngeal nerve, the number IX cranial nerve mentioned in an earlier chapter.

Though the glossopharyngeal nerve is well known for its parasympathetic motor supply to the tongue and pharynx, it also carries back to the brainstem, as does the vagus, certain sensory neurons, such as those of the carotid sinus. Keep in mind the point, important as our discussion develops, that baroreceptors become active, that is, an action potential gets set off in them, when the blood pressure goes above the normal set point. This tells the brain that the blood pressure is too high. Should the blood pressure drop, the force against the aortic arch and carotid sinus wall drops, the stretch is less, and there is no action potential in these sensory neurons. No impulse goes back to the medulla, and there is no signal. The absence of an action potential from the baroreceptors warns the brain, specifically in the medulla, that the blood pressure is too low. A signal means too high; no signal means too low.

The baroreceptors connect, via their axons, directly to what we call the vasomotor center of the medulla. That's a fancy word for the two areas, one on each side of the medulla, that specifically monitor blood pressure. I always like visual images, and to visualize what the medulla actually looks like in cross section, I think of the way a moth would look if it were sitting on your wall with its head pointed upward and its wings spread: symmetric, but with an irregular outline, like the moth-like patterns I've seen in the Rorschach test psychologists have used in the past. Though I've never been much for moths, this is a good way to think about the medulla. In the upper section, say toward the head, of this moth-like image, toward the center, again, on each side, lie the mirror-image vasomotor centers.

I won't talk more about the baroreceptors at this point, but as you will see, they are of fundamental importance to the way the autonomic nervous system works. Before I move on to my discussion of autonomic anatomy, there is one more group of sensory nerves I would like to discuss, the chemoreceptors, which, like the baroreceptors, so greatly influence all autonomic function.

Chemoreceptors are free nerve endings of sensory axons found in the same places, in the walls of the aortic arch and the carotid sinus. They monitor and respond not to pressure, but to levels of oxygen, carbon dioxide, and hydrogen ions in the blood—the latter being the main acid ion in the body. When blood supply to these receptors falls, again from a set normal point, oxygen supply also drops, while carbon dioxide, the main gaseous product of respiration, along with acid wastes, accumulates. In this scenario, an action potential is set off in the chemoreceptor axon, which winds back to the medulla and ends, as do the axons of the baroreceptors, in the vasomotor centers of the medulla.

Like the baroreceptors, axons of the chemoreceptors originating in the aortic arch travel with the vagus nerve, while those of the carotid sinus make their way back to the medulla with the glossopharyngeal nerve. There, the incoming signal alerts the medulla that the blood pressure is too low. However, should the blood pressure be on the rise, the chemoreceptors sense an abundance of oxygen, and carbon dioxide and acid wastes are very quickly, in fact, too quickly removed from the blood. In this case, the chemoreceptors do not fire; there is no action potential and no impulse, no signal back to the medulla. The vasomotor centers read the lack of a signal; in this case, the information received is that pressure, and blood supply, is too high and too much.

We've been following the course of sensory receptors from the skin inward to the visceral organs, below the head. To sum up, wherever they originate, the sensory axons journey back to the central nervous system, mostly in the spinal nerves but also in the cranial nerves, particularly the vagus and the glossopharyngeal.

Let's think about the head for a moment. It is true that some of the sensory innervation of the skin and muscles of the head do originate from the first several spinal nerves exiting the cervical cord. In this respect, the region is no different from that below the head, with sensory receptors ending in the skin or muscles, the axons moving back to the cord in the cervical spinal nerves, with the cell bodies in dorsal root ganglia lying adjacent to the spine. In addition, a number of cranial nerves mentioned earlier carry sensory axons from both the head and below; I have alluded to this in my discussion of the glossopharyngeal and vagus sensory supply to the medulla.

I don't want to belabor the discussion of the cranial nerves, but some points are worth noting. As I have mentioned, these twelve nerves are quite a mixed group, with various and somewhat unique functions. Some are sensory only; some are somatic (or voluntary) motor only; some contain both somatic sensory and motor axons; others, in addition to whatever other axons run through them, house parasympathetic fibers. Several of the cranial nerves are highly specialized, carrying the impulses for the unique special senses (see Guyton 1956, 540) of smell, vision, hearing, equilibrium, and taste.

The olfactory nerve, cranial nerve I, lets us distinguish a rose from an onion and sends its axons to a specific sensory region in the temporal lobe, at the sides of the brain. The optic nerve, number II on the list, lets us see and winds back to the vision center at the back of the brain in the occipital lobe. The vestibular-auditory nerve, nerve VIII, ends in the hearing centers of the temporal lobe, and the glossopharyngeal, nerve IX, carries specific sensory axons from the posterior part of the tongue for taste. Remember also that the afferent axons from the carotid sinus also journey through this nerve to the medulla.

The trochlear and abducens, nerves IV and VI, provide the somatic motor supply to the small muscles around the eye, which allow for eyeball and eyelid movement and focusing. The muscle spindle sensory axons of these voluntary muscles journey back to the spine in these nerves as well, so these nerves are mixed somatic sensory and somatic motor. The trigeminal, nerve V, carries somatic sensory axons from the skin of the face and the teeth, as well as motor nerves to the voluntary muscles of the jaw. If you have a toothache, give credit to the trigeminal, the favorite nerve of the dental profession.

The facial nerve, nerve VII, is a complicated and busy nerve, consisting of somatic sensory, somatic motor, and parasympathetic motor axons. It seems to carry the afferent axons for deep pain from the face, as well as providing the motor input to most of the voluntary facial muscles, which allow you to frown if you feel pain or laugh if the pain has gone away. Axons from taste receptors serving the front part of the tongue also move in the facial nerve, as do parasympathetic motor fibers to a number of salivary glands in the mouth.

I have talked about the vagus nerve, nerve number X, many times: this provides the main parasympathetic supply to the organs of the chest and abdomen, but it also carries those important afferent axons of the aortic arch baroreceptors, as well as other sensory nerves from the viscera in those regions. It is indeed, like the facial, a very busy nerve.

The last two, the spinal accessory, number XI, and the hypoglossus, number XII, aren't quite as complicated. The accessory nerve supplies the somatic motor fibers to two muscles of the neck: the trapezius in the back and the sternocleidomastoid, the matched pair of neck muscles that let you bob your head up and down (should you choose to do so). Its sensory supply is also pretty simple, limited to the axons from the muscle spindles of these two nerves. Finally, the hypoglossus is purely motor, though I don't mean to diminish its importance; it serves the voluntary muscles of the tongue, which help you chew, move food down to the esophagus, and, importantly, help you talk. If this muscle becomes paralyzed, talk is no longer an option.

I don't intend to shower you with details, and my explanations have been, in the greater scheme of neuroscience, very cursory. I do hope that you at least have an understanding that the afferent nerve supplies to the central nervous system are extraordinarily varied and exquisitely specialized, allowing us to feel the gentlest of touches—a lover's hand, or a feather—to the worst dental pain. These sensory nerves let the brain know about temperature both outside in the world and inside our bodies; they let us smell, see, hear, and taste; they help us (through the muscle spindles) move; they let the brain know about blood pressure and the state of the gut . . . I could go on, but you get the point.

All this sensory information continually flows into the central nervous system, the spinal cord, and the brain. I'd like to review for a moment just where it all ends up. That will help us better understand how the autonomic system, when we get to it, works. It would be helpful, to keep things organized, to consider the body below the head first and begin, as I have before, with the sensory axons and sensory signals that originate in the skin, before working our way inward.

If we start with the skin, the afferent impulses, that is, the action potentials for both pain and temperature sensations, tend to follow the same pathway. They move in the respective axons traveling in spinal nerves, back to the posterior (back) half of the spinal cord itself. Pain can cause an instant reflex response, which involves interneurons and motor nerves only at the spinal level, without the need for instructions from higher up. In addition to whatever reflexes might be generated, the pain impulse is also relayed to a second set of neurons, which in turn transmit the impulse up the cord, to another set of neurons in the brainstem. From there, the impulse goes to the hypothalamus, then the thalamus, and ultimately to the sensory cortex areas responsive to pain, in the sensory strip of the parietal lobe.

Pain is a complicated sensation neurologically. Even if the cerebral cortex is removed, or nonfunctional, we can still feel pain. Special centers in the brainstem, particularly in the medulla and in the thalamus, will let us feel pain even without higher input from the cortex. The sensory area for pain in the cortex seems to let us know about the quality of pain—sharp like a knife, dull like a lead weight; aching, like a toothache, or excruci-ating, like a broken radial bone in the right arm (it happened to me three years ago). The brainstem and thalamus let us know there is pain and how much, but not the subtleties of what kind.

Interestingly, pain, even at the level of the brainstem and thalamus, tends to cause what physiologists such as Dr. Guyton call an arousal reaction, which keeps us alert, awake at night, and very much aware that we are in pain. This arousal does involve stimulation specifically of the posterior hypothalamus, through connections from the brainstem below and the thalamus above, and in turn arousal of the sympathetic nervous system. With the sympathetic nerves in high alert, no one is going to sleep.

Temperature impulses, like those of pain, can result in simple spinal reflexes, but they can also move up the posterior part of the spinal cord and then, like pain impulses, onward to the brainstem, hypothalamus, thalamus, and eventually to the sensory cortex. As with pain, we can sense heat and cold in centers in the brainstem and thalamus, without the need for cortical input, but the cortex adds infinite layers of subtlety. The brainstem and thalamus let us know it's hot or cold outside, but not much more; the cortex lets us know how hot, how cold, and how serious a problem the heat or cold really is, out in the world around us (remember, we're still talking about the skin, not the internal temperature).

The hypothalamus is very much involved in how we respond to temperature, both outside and in. Connections from lower down in the brainstem and from higher up, in the thalamus, travel to both the anterior and the posterior hypothalamus. As we shall see in some more detail later, the anterior hypothalamus, through its connections with the parasympathetic nervous system, is in charge ultimately of helping us adapt to higher external or internal temperatures, while the posterior hypothalamus—the center of sympathetic regulation—allows us to respond appropriately when the temperature, either outside or in, is too low.

Touch I always find a particularly interesting sensation, because it has so many varied shadings and we can distinguish them all so well. We have, as I have discussed, a host of different mechanoreceptors in the skin, each responsive to a specific type of touch or pressure. These afferent impulses move in the sensory nerves as do those for pain and temperature, traveling in the sensory axons of the spinal nerves to the posterior cord, up the spine, etc., ending in the sensory cortex. The lower centers of the brain—the brainstem, hypothalamus, and thalamus—do respond to touch to some extent: a dangerously heavy object on the toe sets off reflexes that don't need the higher brain, but again, the subtlety of sensation happens in the sensory strip of the cortex.

Only here can we tell where the touch, the pressure, is happening. If the sensory cortex is knocked out by a tumor, or a stroke, or surgery, we may know something is on our body, but we're not going to know where it is! The cortex lets us do this. It also tells us (see Guyton 1956, 546) about the amount of pressure an object is exerting: a gentle touch versus an oncoming bicycle, the weight of an object we've come across (think of a feather or a boulder dropped on your toe). The sensory cortex, and only the sensory cortex, allows us to determine the shape of an object we're touching—round, square, pointed, to name a few choices—and its texture—soft velvet, sandpaper, a rough sandpapery beard, newly washed hair. These distinctions happen only in the cortex.

We've already traced the pathway for a sensory axon traveling from the spindles of the voluntary muscles, and it differs only in quality from the journey of pain, temperature, and touch impulses from the skin. When we get to the internal organs, the viscera of the chest and abdomen, pain follows initially a somewhat different path. In the chest and in the gut, sensory neurons move back to the spine with the sympathetic motor axons, before reaching the spinal nerves and the posterior cord.

Entire textbooks have been written on visceral pain, that is, pain emanating from an internal organ, and much of Pottenger's text on the autonomic nervous system deals with visceral pain. For our purposes, it's important to know that pain from an internal organ can elicit reflexes at the spinal level, although the motor response travels back to the organ through the sympathetic motor nerves, because there is no somatic motor innervation to the gut (somatic nerves go only to voluntary muscle). These pain impulses also travel up the spinal cord, ending up first in the pain centers of the brainstem and thalamus, and then in the sensory cortex, where the quality and subtle degree of pain becomes evident. Visceral pain signals from the brainstem travel upward, and others move downward from the thalamus, to keep the hypothalamus informed.

The mechanoreceptors of the gastrointestinal tract, as we have discussed, respond to changes in volume of the GI lumen from the esophagus to the colon, and their responses are absolutely essential for normal digestion to occur. Digestion, however, is pretty much an unconscious process that really doesn't require much influence or input from above. It is true that higher sensory input from the smell, sight, or taste of food can start everything moving, triggering the secretion of hydrochloric acid, enzymes, mucus, etc., but most digestion, absorption, and elimination occurs as a set of reflexes that don't involve the cortex at all. A person in a coma, with no evidence of cortical activity, won't be able to swallow but beyond that can still digest food perfectly fine, if it is passed into the stomach through a tube.

With food present in the gut, at whatever level, the mechanoreceptors fire, and the reflexes begin. One set of reflexes occurs only within the nervous system of the gut itself, involving just the neurons of the myenteric and submucosal plexuses, and no other neurons at all. In this reflex, the impulses tend to travel only locally to both plexuses, through branches of the mechanoreceptor axon. When activated, cell bodies in the myenteric plexus then send motor neurons to the two muscle layers of the gut, which start contracting. Impulses to the submucosal or Meissner's plexus tell the epithelial cells to go into action; these cells release mucus to lubricate the food bolus and enzymes to aid in digestion.

In addition, the submucosal input tells the cells to start absorption, and quickly. The larger the food bolus, the larger the area of the intestinal tube involved, the more mechanoreceptors will be involved, and the stronger the reflex at this level. Peristalsis will be stronger and the secretion of enzymes and mucus more pronounced.

However, if the gut lumen is empty, with no food, no liquid, no waste, the mechanoreceptors are quiet, no action potential fires, and there is no signal. In turn, both the myenteric and the submucosal plexuses themselves remain quiet, the muscles relax, and the epithelial cells turn off. Digestion, appropriately, comes to a halt. All this can happen just at the level of the enteric nervous system.

Remember that in addition to this second GI brain, autonomic nerves, both sympathetic coming off the spinal cord and parasympathetic axons traveling through the vagus nerve, connect to the entire length of the GI tract, from mouth to anus. These nerves synapse on both internal plexuses of the gut, the myenteric and submucosal, as well as directly to the smooth muscle and epithelial cells of the mucosa. As I have already mentioned, the sympathetic and parasympathetic systems have completely opposite effects on digestion, the sympathetic nerves essentially turning it off and the parasympathetic system turning it on.

Importantly, mechanoreceptors not only send impulses to both internal plexuses of the gut but also, through branches of their axons, travel with the sympathetic nerves to the spinal cord and with the vagus axons to the medulla. These connections allow for another set of reflexes, at a higher level than the gut itself. If there is food in the gut, the mechanoreceptors fire, the myenteric and submucosal plexuses begin their work, and digestion proceeds. But in addition, impulses travel with the vagus nerve back to the medulla; there, signals that food is present turn on the parasympathetic centers, and a return signal through the vagus travels back to the gut and its two plexuses.

Parasympathetic action potentials make the myenteric and submucosal plexuses more active. Muscular contraction and epithelial secretion become stronger. But parasympathetic axons also end directly on the smooth muscle and epithelial cells of the gut, and these connections enhance still further the whole process of muscular contraction and epithelial secretion. And parasympathetic innervation allows the small arterioles that carry blood to the GI tract to dilate; this enhances both digestion and absorption of nutrients. Though digestion can occur without any parasympathetic input, it occurs much more efficiently with it.

If the gut is empty, devoid of food, water, and waste, the mechanoreceptors, the two enteric plexuses, and the muscles and epithelial cells are all relaxed. The absence of a signal from the mechanoreceptors also shuts off impulses from the parasympathetic medullary centers. The lack of a signal tells the sympathetic nerves that exit the spinal cord destined for the gut to turn on. In this scenario, the sympathetic signals inhibit both plexuses and, through direct connections to the muscle and epithelium, block still further both systems. Muscular contraction and epithelial secretion are blocked above and beyond what the enteric nerves have already started. Sympathetic impulses also cause constriction of all the arterioles feeding the gut, reducing blood supply, an effect that slows the metabolism of all organs of the GI system. Essentially, digestion comes to a complete and total halt.

Now, I would like to return to that other group of mechano-stretch receptors so crucial to understanding autonomic function, the baroreceptors of the aortic arch and carotid sinuses—and along with these, their first cousins, the chemoreceptors in the same location. Earlier I mentioned that when the blood pressure is high, the baroreceptors fire: their impulses from the aortic arch area travel back to the vasomotor center of the medulla via the vagus nerve, while action potentials from the carotid sinus journey with the glossopharyngeal. All this sensory input tells the medulla the pressure is high. If the blood pressure is low, the opposite happens: the baroreceptors are quiet, there is no action potential, and the lack of a signal lets the vasomotor centers know that the blood pressure is too low. With high blood pressure, the chemoreceptors turn off, and in this scenario the lack of an impulse tells the medulla that blood pressure is elevated. With low pressure, the receptors fire, and this impulse informs the medulla that pressure is too low.

Earlier, I referred to our friend Claude Bernard, the great French scientist, and his concepts about the internal and external milieu. In fact, as should be obvious by now, an enormous amount of information about the world outside and the world inside is making its way back to the central nervous system, in every millisecond of our lives. It is indeed a lot of information coming in, from all regions of the body and all manner of sensory receptors: somatic (from the skin and muscles), visceral (from the organs), and those of the special senses.

And all the information originating from below the skull makes its way to the brainstem, the medulla, pons, and midbrain, in essence, the first stopping point for impulses from lower down. Here in the medulla, we find specific regions that regulate many of the visceral organs of the body. Here are discrete centers for the cardiovascular system, for the lungs, for the bladder, and, to some degree, for the digestive organs. Incoming sensory information from a particular organ, say the heart or the gut, tends to be directed to the appropriate region—impulses from the baro- and chemoreceptors, for example, travel to the vasomotor centers, action potentials from the bladder to the region that controls the bladder.

It is true, as I remarked, that the hypothalamus exerts considerable control over the ANS, but it does so through connections that come down to the brainstem, to influence the autonomic nuclei. Anatomically, the autonomic system, both the sympathetic and parasympathetic branches, begins in the brainstem. It receives information from lower down and higher up, but it starts here.

I like visual images. If you were to slice a brain from front to back, so you're looking at one half opened up in front of you, the brainstem, hypothalamus, and thalamus together look like a parrot roosting, with its beak pointing toward the left, the tail curving out on the lower right. The hypothalamus would be the area around the beak, the thalamus the top part of the head. The brainstem would be the body below the head, including the tail. If you were to then take the brainstem and do a cross section, it would resemble the previously mentioned moth on your wall, with its head pointed to the ceiling: symmetric, irregular, like the Rorschach images of psychology.

In cross section, the brainstem, at each level, is symmetric, each side a mirror image of the other. So when I mention the vasomotor center of the medulla, for example, there is one on the right side and one in the same mirror image place on the left. This particular region is toward the central axis, and toward the head.

This area is of particular importance because it seems to determine, perhaps more than any other area in the brainstem, how the autonomic system behaves. It is part of an elaborate sensory receiving area, oval in shape, called the nucleus tractus solitarius, again with one on each side. Always keep in mind that the brain at all levels has two halves, one the mirror image of the other.

The nucleus tractus solitarius is a collection of neuron cell bodies extending through the entire brainstem, from the medulla, through the pons, to the midbrain. This is truly an extraordinary region, measured in millimeters in cross-section diameter, really quite small but able carefully and precisely and accurately to monitor incoming sensory information about blood pressure. It is a microcomputer of enormous sophistication, with an enormous task. I can't overstate how important normal blood pressure is for a productive, happy life; chronic low blood pressure can lead to the misery of chronic fatigue syndrome, and high blood pressure can end in stroke, with its terrible toll, kidney failure, and death.

Axons that have traveled from the baroreceptors and chemoreceptors of the aortic arch and carotid sinuses terminate on neuron cell bodies of the nucleus tractus solitarius (NTS) in the medulla. These NTS cells in turn send branches of their axons in several directions. First, some travel upward, to both the anterior and the posterior hypothalamus, and to the posterior pituitary at the base of the hypothalamus. Others travel to the lowest part of the medulla, just before it merges into the spinal cord, in a region which in the cross section is located in the lower outer part of the medulla, the lower outer part of the moth's wings. Here, the axons from the NTS connect to two very important regions; the first, the nucleus ambiguus, contains most of the cell bodies that form the parasympathetic input of the vagus nerve.

Other axons from the NTS terminate on cells in what we call the caudal ventral lateral medulla. This is a complicated way of saying that "lower outer" cells based in the caudal ventral lateral medulla send out axons that travel forward in the medulla to a second region called the rostral ventral lateral medulla. Here are yet another group of neuron cell bodies that have a job very relevant to our current conversation; these cells in the rostral medulla in turn send their axons back down the medulla, to the spinal cord itself, to end in a region of the spinal cord in the mid-outer section called the intermediolateral cell column. Here, finally, are the first neuron cell bodies of the sympathetic system.

Anatomy of the Sympathetic Nervous System

The somatic motor system and the autonomic motor system differ quite profoundly in many ways. In terms of what they do, the somatic system controls ultimately only the striated skeletal muscles, which allow for voluntary movement. The autonomic nerves, remember, control physiological functions that do not require conscious or willed input; specifically, autonomic nerves regulate cardiac muscle, all the smooth muscle, and all the glands in the body, wherever they may be. Through such connections and control, the autonomic system controls muscle activity and secretion in the GI tract and ultimately digestion itself, heart rate and blood pressure, bladder emptying, sexual function, and body temperature (see Guyton 1956, 697).

The somatic and autonomic motor systems differ in terms of the jobs they ultimately do, but they are also different in a very profound way in terms of their microscopic structure. If we stick to the region of the body below the head to make things simple for a moment, motor neurons along the length of the spine have their cell bodies in the frontal part, technically, the ventral horn of the spinal cord. Their axons exit the spine in the spinal nerves that exit the spine in pairs, one on each side of the spine, along its length. The somatic motor axons make their way ultimately to the target striated muscle. Though an individual striated muscle might be targeted by thousands of individual axons, there are no intervening nerve cells involved, however far away from the spine a given target muscle might be. The motor neurons that regulate the small muscles of the toes, for example, send their axons winding two to three feet out the back, down the legs, to the toes.

When an action potential moves down a somatic motor neuron to the synapse with the muscle fiber, the terminal part of the axon releases the neurotransmitter acetylcholine.

This is the product of acetate, produced during glycolysis, and the B vitamin choline. When it crosses the synapse and links up to the appropriate receptor on the muscle fiber cell membrane, it causes the fiber to contract. It is a very simple molecule, with a very large job, to stimulate voluntary muscles to contract—a job it does very effectively.

So, in the somatic motor system, an action potential moves from the cord to the muscle in a rather straightforward way, along a single nerve with its cell body in the spinal cord, its axon connecting to a single microscopic nerve fiber wherever in the body it might be. When we start thinking about the autonomic system, in terms of both the sympathetic and the parasympathetic branches, the situation is somewhat more complicated. In all autonomic nerves, whether sympathetic or parasympathetic, action potential signals move from the spinal cord, or in the case of the cranial parasympathetic nerves like the vagus, from the brainstem, through two consecutive nerves arranged in sequence.

The first nerve always has its cell body within the spine—or again in the case of the cranial parasympathetic nerves, in the brainstem—and the second nerve has its cell body along the route to the target tissue. It is the axon from the second nerve that tells the target tissue, either cardiac muscle, smooth muscle, or some gland, what to do. It's like a relay race, with the action potential signal being handed from the first to the second nerve. This is an important fact to keep in mind, as we begin our travels through the autonomic system: the somatic motor system is a single neuron system, whereas the autonomic system uses two neurons, in sequence.

Now, let's look in some detail at the sympathetic system. Anatomically, neuroscientists refer to it as the thoracolumbar system because the cell bodies of the first neuron of the two-neuron sequence live in the spinal cord only at the levels of the thoracic spine along its entire length, from the T1 vertebral body to T12, as well as at the level of the first three lumbar bodies. There are no sympathetic cell bodies higher up, in the cervical spine or in the brainstem, and none in the lower lumbar or sacral cord areas, just T1–L3. Of course, to perform its many complicated tasks, the sympathetic system receives action potential instructions from many levels higher up, including the brainstem, the hypothalamus, and even the cortex. I have made this point before. The sympathetic system begins with the cell bodies located only between T1 and L3.

In this length of the cord, the first sympathetic cell bodies are found specifically in the intermediolateral cell columns, one on each side of the cord. If you were to look at the cord in a cross-sectional view, these columns, each a mirror image of the other, are found in the mid-region of the cord, toward the outside. The axons of these neurons, like those of the somatic motor neurons, exit the spine with the spinal nerves—which, remember, also carry somatic sensory axons sending their signals back to the cord. Spinal nerves are, as you can see, a hodgepodge of activity.

The somatic motor axons keep on going in the spinal nerve, which eventually branches as it nears its target muscle. After leaving the spine, the sympathetic axons take a somewhat different route. Shortly after exiting the cord in the spinal nerves, the sympathetic axons then branch off to connect to the sympathetic chain of ganglia, which lie along each side of the spinal column. These are called paravertebral ganglia, because they are found alongside the vertebral bodies of the spine. Like so much of the nervous system, the ganglia really come in matched pairs, one on each side of the spine.

Ganglia, as I have mentioned before, are little round nubbins with the appearance of large beads that contain cell bodies of neurons. Though the cell bodies of sympathetic nerves are found in the cord from T1 to L3 only, there are sympathetic ganglia from the level of the cervical spine, down to the lower levels of the lumbar cord. In the region of the thoracic and upper lumbar spine, there are essentially paired sympathetic ganglia at each level of the cord. I say "essentially" because there really isn't always exactly a sympathetic ganglion at each level of the twelve thoracic vertebral bodies. There might be only eleven, or even ten.

Overall, there are generally three cervical sympathetic ganglia, eleven to twelve thoracic, and three to five formed from the lumbar nerves. These sympathetic ganglia do not live free but are linked to one another by connective tissue, to form the equivalent of a neurological string of pearls or, to be more mundane, a string of beads. The two sympathetic chains are quite visible during surgery or dissection and are often described just this way, as looking like a string of beads, again on either side of the spine.

The first set of sympathetic nerves is referred to as the preganglionic nerve because it originates in the intermediolateral cell column of the cord and sends its axons to the ganglia. Here, in the ganglia, a lot is going on. Axons from the preganglionic sympathetics arrive and branch, and then travel in several directions. Some axon branches move up and some move down the chain, within the connective tissue strings along the chain. Some of the higher thoracic sympathetic axons, for example, travel up to form the three cervical ganglia. There, these axons synapse with a second group of sympathetic cell bodies, called the postganglionic sympathetic nerves because their axons leave the ganglia.

These particular cells of the three cervical ganglia send axons up to the head and neck, where they end in a number of tissues. Some of these postganglionic fibers end in the ciliary muscle of the eye, which helps regulate the size of the pupil and, in turn, the amount of light that can enter the eyes. Other axons innervate the salivary glands in the mouth, as well as the various blood vessels in the head and neck. In addition, postganglionic sympathetic axons originating in the cervical ganglion travel into the chest, where they provide the sympathetic input to the lungs and to the heart.

But the preganglionic axons don't just branch up and down. In the ganglia in the thoracic and upper lumbar area, some of the branches stay at the level where they originate and synapse, right in the ganglia, with a group of postganglionic sympathetic neurons. These cells send out axons that course back to the spinal nerves and travel with the spinal nerves until they ultimately end in the blood vessels of the body wall and of all the four limbs. However, some of these preganglionic axon branches don't stop in the paravertebral ganglia, but move right through and move forward and toward the center of the body, to a set of ganglia that lie anterior, in front of the aorta as it travels down the abdomen, lying as it does in front of the vertebral column. These cell collections are called prevertebral ganglia, because they lie in front of the spinal column.

To sum up, certain preganglionic axons, or axon branches to be more precise, exit the spine with the spinal nerves and exit the spinal nerves to travel to the sympathetic chain ganglia but then move out beyond the sympathetic chain to end in the ganglia in front of the spine.

There are three such prevertebral ganglia, the celiac, superior mesenteric, and inferior mesenteric, which lie along the aorta at points where major arterial vessels branch off. The celiac ganglia, for example, lies right in the area of the celiac trunk, the aortic branch that divides into the hepatic artery, which feeds the liver; the splenic artery, which as the name implies brings blood to the spleen; and the left gastric artery, providing the blood supply to the stomach. The superior mesenteric and inferior mesenteric arteries largely feed the small and large intestines and the accessory digestive organs such as the liver and pancreas, along with the kidneys. These nerves also innervate the bladder and the genitals.

The axons that make their way to these specific three abdominal ganglia have not, remember, yet synapsed with any postganglionic cells. Here, in the prevertebral ganglia, the preganglionic sympathetic axons finally connect with a group of postganglionic sympathetic cell bodies. These cells in turn send their axons specifically to all the smooth muscle and glands of the entire digestive canal from beginning to end—the esophagus, stomach, and small and large intestines—as well as the accessory digestive organs. Sympathetic postganglionic fibers also connect to the urinary bladder and sex organs.

The sympathetic nervous system uses two neurons to send a signal and relies on two synapses. The first is located in the sympathetic chain or in the prevertebral ganglia, the point of connection between the preganglionic and postganglionic nerves. The second synapse links the postganglionic axon with the target muscle (cardiac or smooth) or gland. This is how, wherever it is working, the sympathetic system does its job. There is an advantage to such an arrangement. A single preganglionic nerve can synapse with multiple postsynaptic neurons, allowing for rapid spread of information from the central nervous system to the target tissues.

In the superior cervical ganglion, for example, it is estimated that each preganglionic nerve with signals meant for the smooth muscle of the iris synapses with approximately four postganglionic cells. The iris is a relatively small target area, and there is no need for a large input of impulses to achieve the desired end, pupillary dilation. However, in the ganglia that service the GI tract, it has been estimated that each preganglionic nerve synapses with up to 150 postganglionic neurons, allowing for a rapid and extensive spread of impulses (Mathias and Bannister 2013, 9). In the gut, this is of benefit because digestion is such a complex process involving a number of organs.

Interestingly, the system uses a different neurotransmitter at each synapse. When an action potential from higher up, say from an area in the medulla such as the rostral ventrolateral medulla, reaches a preganglionic sympathetic nerve body in the intermediolateral cell column, the sympathetic nerve fires, sending an impulse along its own axon. When the action potential reaches the axon tip located in a ganglion, the preganglionic nerve releases acetylcholine, the same neurotransmitter used by somatic motor nerves at the muscle synapse.

In the sympathetic ganglia, acetylcholine attaches to appropriate receptors on the postganglionic nerve and in turn sets off an action potential, in a relay, down its own axon to the synapse at the target muscle or gland. This is called the neuroeffector junction, because it is where the nerve causes its desired effect. There, the postganglionic axon tip releases the transmitter norepinephrine, also known as noradrenaline, which I mentioned in my earliest overview of the sympathetic system. Norepinephrine is made in nerve cells from the amino acids phenylalanine and tyrosine, commonly found in meat.

For the sympathetic nerves to do their work, the target cardiac and smooth muscle, or glandular tissue, must have specific receptors for norepinephrine, otherwise the neurotransmitter will just lie around doing nothing. It is its linking to a receptor that causes the end effect. There are two main subclasses of norepinephrine receptors on target tissues, called alpha and beta adrenoreceptors or adrenergic receptors, as a take-off on the word *adrenaline*. There are also a variety of subclasses of alpha and beta adrenoreceptors, but the details aren't essential for our current discussion. I just want to make the point that neurotransmitter receptor chemistry is quite elegant and sophisticated, with specific types of subclasses of receptors allowing for specific types of effects.

What we do need to consider, if only in a cursory way, is what norepinephrine does on target tissues. This will help us understand what the sympathetic system does in the human body. A good starting place would be the heart and the circulatory system, because the sympathetic nerves control so much of cardiovascular activity.

The heart itself is an interesting organ, because if you take out the heart from a living animal, as scientists did a hundred years ago, and place it in a nutrient liquid broth, it will continue to beat at least for a time even in the absence of any nervous system input. This happens because there are, in certain areas of the heart, collections of what we call pacemaker cells, a type of cardiac nerve cell that, without any input from anywhere else, can spontaneously and rhythmically send impulses through the heart muscles to cause muscle contraction. They are called pacemaker cells because they set the pace for heart contraction, the pulse we all know so well. In this regard, these cells are similar to the neurons of the enteric nervous system of the gut, which can keep the digestive system up and running with no outside nerve input.

Postganglionic sympathetic nerves from the three cervical ganglia directly synapse on these pacemaker cells, and when they release norepinephrine, the heart rate, the rate of cardiac contraction, goes up. Pulse, to use the common parlance, increases. Norepinephrine not only speeds up heart rate but also increases the strength of each contraction, so more blood is pumped out of the heart chambers with each beat. Think of the difference between gently squeezing a wet sponge in your hand and squeezing very hard. In the heart, this combined enhancement of rate and strength of contraction is how the sympathetic nerves increase cardiac output, the amount of blood the heart pumps per minute. This is important when blood flow must be increased.

In addition to this effect on the heart, sympathetic nerves reach the smooth muscles of all the small arterioles and small veins in every corner of the body, from the head to the toe. Postganglionic nerves from the three cervical ganglia supply the vasculature of the head and neck, as well as the lungs. Sympathetic neurons leaving the paravertebral ganglia of the thoracic and upper lumbar area connect to the arterioles and venules of the muscles and skin of the trunk, arms, and legs. The prevertebral ganglia—the celiac, superior mesenteric, and inferior mesenteric ganglia that lie in front of the aorta—supply the sympathetic input to the vessels of the internal viscera of the abdomen, including the entire digestive tract, with the liver, kidneys, and spleen. Sympathetic nerves, one way or another, reach everywhere.

Norepinephrine will have different effects on the vessels, depending on what area of the body we're looking at. In the skin, and all through the digestive system, the accessory digestive organs, and the kidneys, norepinephrine released from postganglionic sympathetic nerves causes contraction of the smooth muscles of the small arteries and veins. These smooth muscle cells surround the vessel lumen, much as a belt, so that their contraction essentially collapses the vessel, restricting the flow of blood to the organ. Veins, remember, carry blood back to the heart, after it has given off its oxygen and nutrients in the small capillaries of the tissues. Contraction of the smooth muscle in veins helps pump this blood back to the heart faster, much like squeezing a tube of toothpaste.

This combined effect of arteriole and venous constrictions tends to increase overall systemic blood pressure; when the arterioles contract, blood flows against increased resistance, which in and of itself will increase pressure. The added squeezing effect of the veins increases the blood volume returning to the heart. At the same time, sympathetic firing is also increasing the strength and rate of heart contraction itself, so you have increased blood volume flowing through smaller vessels. This means increased flow forces, the definition of high blood pressure. In a time of crisis, such as during physical stress or blood loss, such responses can be lifesaving.

In the skeletal or voluntary muscles, however, norepinephrine causes dilation of the arterioles and small veins, the exact opposite of what is going on in the gut. When the sympathetic system fires, blood tends to shunt away from the abdominal viscera and into the muscles. If we keep in mind that the sympathetic system tends to fire when we are under stress, this makes sense, because increased blood flow to skeletal muscles would bring in an enhanced supply of nutrients and oxygen, which in turn allow for increased motor activity—such as running, jumping, or defending oneself—something useful in a stressful circumstance. It would also make sense that blood flow would be diverted away from the GI tract, because in an emergency of whatever nature, digestion becomes a secondary concern.

And, though norepinephrine has opposite effects on the vessels of skeletal muscles as opposed to those of the gut, the overall effect of sympathetic nerve firing is to increase the blood pressure. The volume of blood vessels into the muscles is actually much less than that of the gut, so when, under the influence of norepinephrine, blood diverts from the GI tract to the skeletal muscles, the transfer isn't exactly equal. A greater amount of blood flows into a smaller volume of vessels, at a faster and stronger rate. Blood pressure will go up.

The increased blood supply isn't just a help for muscle activity; it is absolutely essential. During any type of physical activity, from twirling your thumbs to running up a mountainside, muscles contract. That's how we move, lift, walk, twirl, dance, jump, and fall. Obviously, some activities clearly involve more muscle contraction than others, but muscle contraction is always involved. When muscle contracts, the arteries, arterioles, and veins that lie in the muscle get squeezed, sometimes very strongly. That means that the arterioles bringing in oxygen and nutrients are facing a significant obstacle to delivering their goods, right where it is needed most, in the active muscle. It's like water moving through a garden hose lying on the ground with an elephant standing on the hose. The increased systemic blood pressure helps keep the arterioles and venules open, so blood can keep coming in and wastes can be efficiently carried away.

Earlier, I mentioned that even the thought of moving, before any movement has occurred, starts a cascade of events that dilates the arteries and veins in the specific muscles needed for the movement, and nowhere else. That's a very remarkable achievement, that blood supply could be so precisely and specifically directed, with just a thought. When the idea of a movement begins in the higher intellectual centers of the cerebral cortex—say, my idea to get up from my desk to start working on my book—the impulse that is the thought travels from the front lobe to the motor cortex, down to the posterior hypothalamus, to the nucleus tractus solitarius of the medullary vasomotor center, etc., eventually to the very preganglionic cell bodies of the intermediolateral cell column that control the blood supply to those specific muscles.

There is indeed that kind of precision in the brain's control of sympathetic activity. If more muscles are involved in the movement, more sympathetic nerves will fire. If you are running from a fire and virtually your entire somatic voluntary system is working very hard to save your life—even the muscles of your face that draw tight in a stressed frown—the sympathetic discharge will be total, not limited.

Muscle contraction itself, through the sensory nerves in the muscle fibers, feeds back to the nervous system and further stimulates the sympathetics. Any activity of the somatic voluntary muscle system activates the sympathetics, always, sometimes more, sometimes less, depending again on the extent of the movement and the number of muscle fibers and muscles involved. Even the slightest motion, such as scratching your face, stimulates sympathetic action at least to some extent. That's the only way muscles can work efficiently. There's no other way.

One more point about muscles. Norepinephrine, in addition to its effect on the blood supply to muscles, also has a direct effect on skeletal muscle fibers. Just as it does in the heart, norepinephrine causes these fibers to contract more strongly, leading to increased strength. Under stress, this too is a benefit, and it helps explain the stories of heroic strength of ordinary mortals in times of acute physical stress. I remember reading a newspaper account years ago, before I knew anything about autonomic physiology, about a man who was able to lift up the end of a truck to allow a child trapped underneath after an accident to escape. These things do indeed happen.

However, the sympathetic nervous system does not distinguish between a difficult physical challenge, such as the problem of a child trapped beneath a truck, and an emotionally stressful event, such as an impending final exam or a hearing before the medical board. In all stress, whether physical, emotional, psychological, or spiritual, the sympathetic system fires, and blood supply to muscles increases, as does muscle strength, tone, and tension. This can be a problem if, before a final exam, for example, you are trying to relax but the thought of what is to come keeps the norepinephrine flowing and the muscles tense and tight.

In a time of stress, it's obviously essential to increase the blood flow to the muscles. It's also absolutely critical to ensure a steady blood supply to the brain. Under any type of stress, whether physical or emotional or mental, we need to think fast, evaluate situations quickly, and make decisions forcefully. All this thinking requires, just as muscular activity requires, a rich supply of oxygen and nutrients. When the sympathetic system fires in response to whatever stress is looming, blood pressure goes up, and this translates into increased blood flow everywhere, including into the arteries that feed the brain.

Fortunately, the brain has a very extensive blood supply, and once the systemic blood pressure is on the rise, the sympathetic nerves don't really need to do very much to the brain arteries and veins themselves, just let the blood flow. This is exactly what happens. In the gut, the sympathetics cause vasoconstriction, and in the muscles vasodilation, but in vasculature of the brain, norepinephrine doesn't do much of anything. It leaves the circulation alone. The increased blood pressure into the extensive artery system of the brain does the job, without any additional tinkering by norepinephrine on the vessels needed.

In the muscles, norepinephrine, above and beyond what it does to the vessels, stimulates the fibers to contract. In the brain, above and beyond what it does to blood pressure, it stimulates the thinking areas of the cerebral cortex. It does so apparently both through a direct effect on the cortex, where it acts like an excitatory neurotransmitter, and indirectly, through ascending fibers in the brainstem that travel to the posterior hypothalamus. When the posterior hypothalamus turns on, it sends signals to the cortex that stimulate it into feverish activity. Our brain becomes awake, alert, and active, and thinking happens faster and faster—again useful in a time of stress. And yet this can be a problem, especially if you're trying to sleep before a final exam.

I would now like to leave the heart and its circulatory system and turn back to the gastrointestinal tract with its affiliated organs, to consider here the effect of sympathetic activity and its transmitter, norepinephrine. The digestive system is an interesting place for a number of reasons, but particularly because, as I have already shown, it has its very own complex enteric nervous system, its own second brain that controls much of what goes on within the digestive tube even without the need for consultation or input from higher up. I want to emphasize that the enteric nerves lie within the walls of the digestive canal from the esophagus to the anus, but not within the accessory organs, such as the salivary glands, liver, and pancreas. The traditional autonomic nerves of the sympathetic and parasympathetic system control these particular organs. The enteric system still regulates much of what goes on during digestion.

Langley, who named the autonomic nervous system and remains one of its great scholars, proposed that the enteric nervous system of the gut, which he identified, should be perceived as a third branch of the autonomic nervous system, along with the sympathetic and parasympathetic nerves. Although it can indeed function if all outside nerve connections to the sympathetic and parasympathetic nerves are cut, it is normally influenced significantly by these nerves and, of course, the brain above.

The digestive system is really remarkable when you think about it. Here you have this elongated tube, from the mouth to the anus, with several very extraordinary organs attached, whose job it is to take a variety of crude food stuffs ranging from tangelos to beef liver and turn it all into useful nutrients to support life—not a trivial directive. Though the digestive system, like any other area of human biology, can seem initially, even to a medical student, complicated and complex in its anatomy and physiology, it is helpful to think about what goes on there in its simplest terms, to get us started.

For all that goes in the gut, only three things happen in the tissues and organs themselves: secretion of a variety of digestive aids, smooth muscular contraction to mix and move digesting food along, and absorption of nutrients through the mucosal lining of the intestines once digestion has taken place. I deliberately don't include the actual digestion of food and its breakdown, because this happens in the lumen of the digestive tube, not in the tissues themselves. Here, I am thinking about what goes on in the tissues, not in the open space. Secretion in the digestive system is the job of the epithelial cells that line the GI tract, as well as the cells of the accessory organs, such as the salivary glands, the liver, and the pancreas. In the mouth, salivary glands release saliva, loaded with enzymes that begin the digestive process. In the stomach, mucosal cells secrete hydrochloric acid and pepsin, as well as mucus to protect the stomach lining.

The lining cells of the small intestine release a host of enzymes to continue digestion as well as hormones such as secretin and cholecystokinin that provoke the pancreas to start secreting bicarbonate and its enzymes. In response to cholecystokinin, the gall bladder releases bile to assist in fat digestion. All along the small and large intestines, the epithelial cells produce mucus to aid in the mixing of food and its movement along the length of the digestive canal.

Along the GI tube, or canal, from the esophagus to the anus—but again, not in the liver or pancreas—the enteric system can control, to a point, secretion, muscular contraction, and absorption. Its myenteric plexus specifically regulates muscular contraction, and the submucosal (or Meissner's plexus), as the name implies, lies right beneath the epithelial lining of the gut where so much secretion and absorption take place. These nerves regulate both these processes, but again only to a point. For the system to work really efficiently, and to perform with all the nuances that humans experience around eating, autonomic input is essential.

The sympathetic inflow to the digestive system begins with the axons leaving the superior cervical ganglia for the salivary glands. These particular nerves strongly inhibit the release of saliva and interfere with the initial processes of digestion in the mouth. When you feel a dry mouth under stress, you are experiencing the work of postganglionic sympathetic nerves.

When we arrive at the digestive canal itself, beginning with the esophagus and ending in the rectum, we find the preganglionic sympathetic cell bodies in the cord from the level of about T6 down to L3. Axons from these nerves pass through the sympathetic chain ganglion, to connect with the postganglionic cell bodies in the celiac, superior, and inferior mesenteric ganglia. Axons from these neurons in turn connect to the cells of the myenteric and submucosal plexuses, all along the length of the digestive tube, as well as directly to smooth muscle and epithelial cells, and to the arterioles that supply the entire length of the gut.

When the sympathetic system fires, and norepinephrine is released, the result is a generalized inhibition of GI function, from top to bottom. Salivation reduces, and the production of acid, mucosal enzymes, and hormones shuts down. The epithelial production of mucus also lessens. In the gut, norepinephrine relaxes smooth muscle. Muscular contraction—so essential for normal digestion—turns off, and interestingly, the epithelial cells are less able to absorb nutrients from the lumen.

The sympathetic nerves also reach directly to the acinar cells of the pancreas and the cells of the liver. In the pancreas, norepinephrine reduces both enzyme production and release, and in the liver, bile production shuts down. Importantly, blood supply into the GI tract, including the liver and pancreas, diminishes tremendously, affecting everything the cells do, from the manufacturing of enzymes to absorption. When the sympathetic system fires full blast, the gut, with its stomach and intestines and liver and pancreas, indeed shuts down.

Why would this be of benefit? If you're facing some type of physical or emotional stress that requires prompt attention, you want your blood pumping into the muscles, to provide for physical strength, and to the brain, for mental alacrity. Digestion just isn't that important. This also explains why, under stress, any type of stress—say cramming for a final exam in medical school—food, even the lightest of meals, feels heavy in the gut, like a brick. We'll often, in such a circumstance, experience indigestion, heartburn, bloating, and discomfort. Food, under stress, is not a pleasure.

The enteric system, as remarkable as it is, is really quite limited. It can respond to food in the gut, if it's there, but it really doesn't respond to much else. It lives in a very small universe, the world limited by the boundaries of the digestive tube. It can't for example respond to stress; it couldn't possibly be aware of stress without higher input. For it to respond to anything outside the gut, such as stress in the world, be it a child caught beneath a truck or a final exam, the enteric system requires autonomic input. Otherwise, it is like an autopilot—capable in some ways, but very limited in what it can do or respond to. The autonomic system gives the gut, so to speak, a higher purpose.

I have now described in some detail the actions of the sympathetic nerves on the heart, with its circulatory system, and on the GI system. These examples give us some idea of how the system operates. It is important to keep in mind always that sympathetic nerves one way or another go to every gland and every smooth muscle cell in the body, with enormous effects on all aspects of metabolism.

Though at this point I don't want to go into detail about the other activities of the sympathetic nerves, I thought several points warrant mentioning. In the eye, sympathetic firing leads to relaxation of the muscles and dilation of the pupil. This allows for a wider field of vision and for more light to enter the eye—both useful if you're in a stressful environment. Besides this, norepinephrine will inhibit the salivary glands, reducing the amount of saliva produced and released. With the general vasoconstriction norepinephrine produces in the vessels of the face, when the sympathetic system fires, we look pale.

In the lungs, norepinephrine causes relaxation of the smooth muscle that lines all the bronchi and bronchioles, the branching system of tubes that bring oxygenated air into the lungs and allow for exhalation of carbon dioxide. When the sympathetic nerves fire, the bronchi and bronchioles dilate, allowing more air to come in. This is important during stress, when increased physical activity will require an increase in oxygen intake.

In the liver, sympathetic nerves, and their transmitter norepinephrine, inhibit the release of bile and digestive juices into the small intestine. The liver is a great metabolic powerhouse, with many diverse and essential functions, all adeptly performed by its millions of hepatocytes. The liver is, for example, the body's main detoxification organ, where hepatocytes process, neutralize, and prepare for excretion all manner of metabolic wastes as well as environmental toxins and drugs. Liver cells can also store many B vitamins, including B12 and folate, as well as excess sugar as glycogen and extra fatty acids from digestion as triglycerides and cholesterol. In this way, the liver serves as a reserve supply for many critically essential nutrients that might be needed in a time of deprivation such as a famine or fast, or during a time of increased metabolism.

Branches of postganglionic sympathetic axons reach to every one of the liver's many cells. When the system fires, norepinephrine signals the hepatocytes to start breaking down the stored sugar and fats into glucose and free fatty acids, which they then release into the bloodstream. There, the glucose and fatty acids serve as a source of fuel for all the cells of the body, from the brain to the muscles of the toe—again, a benefit in a time of stress, because an increase in any type of activity, even thinking, requires increased fuel for the cells. Stress always involves heightened activity, either physical or mental or, commonly, both.

While this is going on, norepinephrine inhibits the detoxification activities of the liver cells. Under stress, we need energy fast, but detoxification can wait. At least keep in the corner of your mind that the sympathetic system tends to reduce kidney function and assist with sexual activity; I wouldn't want to leave that out.

Since the time of Langley, the sympathetic nervous system has been perceived as the fundamental "stress" nervous system, the system activated with any type of adversity, be it physical, emotional, psychological, or spiritual. It is the set of nerves that helps us deal effectively and efficiently with problems in our lives that must ideally be dealt with fast. It is, as we commonly hear of it, the "fight or flight" system, which in a primitive sense helps us protect ourselves or get away really quickly from impending disaster.

Stress comes at us of course from many directions and in many ways. Neurologically, the stress response can begin in the higher thinking centers. For example, a fire in our field of vision or a car out of control on Madison Avenue coming toward us begins with visual information translated into danger in the intellectual centers of the cerebral cortex. The sensory input can be limited initially only to what we see, even if we don't feel heat from the fire, and even if the car is a block away. This type of stress response begins in the brain.

Stress can begin as a signal from sensory receptors below the head without involving initial input from above. For example, if you feel pain, say if you step on a tack or touch a hot pan, the response begins with a reflex at the spinal cord and then works its way up to the autonomic centers in the brainstem and hypothalamus. Yes, with pain, we do become consciously aware in our intellectual cortex that something unpleasant is going on, but the response begins lower down. Regardless of where the danger is initially perceived, either high up in the cortex or lower down in the spinal cord, the result is the same: the sympathetic system fires. Sometimes it fires a little, sometimes a lot, depending on the extent of the danger or discomfort, but with any stress, it fires.

If you think about what the sympathetic system does, how it works, to me it isn't difficult to understand why it is so effectively suited to help us out of danger or unpleasantness. Guyton, the great physiologist, listed the series of events that occur whenever the sympathetic nerves fire in response to stress (Guyton 1956, 706), but you can figure out what happens and why it can be helpful from what we've already discussed. To summarize it all very quickly, when active, the sympathetic system causes increased heart rate and cardiac contraction, raising blood pressure. Blood vessels in the skin, in the entire digestive system and kidneys constrict, while those of the muscle dilate, allowing for shunting of blood to the muscles where it is needed for a potential physical response.

Norepinephrine directly, as we have seen, also increases skeletal muscle strength. In addition, with increased blood pressure, more blood goes to the brain, to allow for enhanced mental activity. Norepinephrine itself stimulates the brain at many levels into a greater state of alertness, for faster thinking and faster neurological response. Though digestion diminishes, liver cells begin releasing glucose and fatty acids into the blood, to provide an energy source for the increased brain and muscle needs. We can, overall, think faster, move faster, and move more strongly.

One final point I would like to make before we move on to the parasympathetic system: I have always found it interesting that the same sympathetic neurotransmitter, norepinephrine, can in one organ—say, the small intestine—cause the smooth muscle of the arterioles to constrict while at the same time and only microns away cause the smooth muscle lining the intestinal wall to relax.

It's an interesting concept, when you think about it, because smooth muscle, wherever you might find it, is very much the same in the way it looks and the way it works. Then, why should the same molecule, norepinephrine, have such a different effect in the same vicinity of the same organ?

The answer lies in receptor chemistry. Previously, I mentioned that for norepinephrine to have any effect, it must attach to a receptor on the target cell membrane. That's the only way any neurotransmitter does anything. These adrenergic receptors for norepinephrine, as they are called, are proteins in the cell membranes of cardiac, smooth muscle, or glandular cells, which extend from the membrane surface, where attachment of the neurotransmitter occurs, through the membrane, into the cytoplasm. Once norepinephrine connects to its receptor on the target cell membrane, the receptor protein changes its shape or, to be technical, undergoes a conformational change. This, in turn provokes a cascade of events in the cell cytoplasm that leads ultimately to the desired effect.

Earlier, I mentioned in passing that noradrenergic receptors are divided into alpha and beta groupings, which differ somewhat in their molecular structure. Though both alpha and beta receptors combine with the same transmitter, norepinephrine, they can at times evoke completely different responses within the cell.

Alpha receptors, for example, are found primarily in the blood vessels except for those that carry blood to the skeletal muscles, where instead beta receptors predominate. When activated by norepinephrine, alpha receptors cause smooth muscle contraction and, hence, blood vessel constriction. Beta receptors, in the vessels feeding the voluntary muscles, do just the opposite and cause the arterioles to dilate, allowing for increased blood flow at that site.

Beta receptors are the major receptor group in the lungs, in the heart muscle itself, in the smooth muscle that lines the digestive tract, and in the accessory digestive organs. Even beta receptors, which are subdivided into four different groups, can produce somewhat different effects in different organs. In the gut, along the intestinal canal, beta receptors, when activated by norepinephrine, cause the smooth muscle lining of the gut to relax. However, in the heart, beta receptors stimulate the heart muscle to contract with greater strength.

When norepinephrine combines with a receptor, the receptor will—depending on its type—stimulate one of two enzymes located on the inner cell membrane. The first of these, adenyl cyclase, catalyzes the production of cyclic AMP that most often leads to either contraction (in smooth muscle of the vessels for example) or secretion (in a gland). The second enzyme, guanosyl cyclase, if active, leads to the formation of cyclic GMP. Cyclic GMP generally has the opposite effect of cyclic AMP, causing relaxation of smooth muscle and decreased secretion of glandular cells. In this rather remarkable way, a single neurotransmitter, norepinephrine, can cause either excitation or inhibition, depending on how a particular cell reacts when it attaches to the surface receptor.

It's an amazing system, this sympathetic collection of nerves. Now, it's time to shift gears and move on to the parasympathetic system. Because we've already covered so much autonomic physiology, our foray into parasympathetic metabolism should not take all that long.

The Parasympathetic Nervous System

If we depend on the sympathetic nerves in times of stress and excitement, the parasympathetic system is more the workhorse of the body, responsible for such things as digestion, the absorption and assimilation of nutrients, and the processing and excretion of metabolic wastes—the more mundane, less dramatic aspects of metabolism. It is, as I like to think of it, the system of repair and rebuilding. Sympathetic nerves may help us survive in crisis, but the parasympathetic system reverses the damage.

And though, clearly, the two systems tend to provoke opposite effects in target tissues, in my earlier discourse, when I first introduced autonomic physiology, I made the point that the sympathetic and parasympathetic nerves work together, in every moment of our lives, to help adjust metabolism as need be for every challenge we face. Sometimes the sympathetic nerves will be more active, sometimes the parasympathetics, and sometimes both will be equally alert. It's a balancing act, with our benefit always the goal.

As is true for sympathetic nerves, impulses travel down the parasympathetic system along two neurons arranged in sequence: a preganglionic parasympathetic nerve, with its cell body in the central nervous system, connecting to a postganglionic nerve, which ends in the target cell or tissue and brings about the desired action. I want to emphasize that the parasympathetic and sympathetic nerves are quite distinct anatomically, originating in completely different locales and traveling down completely separate nerve routes to the end organs.

As we've discussed, preganglionic cell bodies of sympathetic nerves lie in the intermediolateral cell column of the spinal cord from the level of the first thoracic vertebra to the third lumbar. There are no preganglionic sympathetic cells anywhere else, hence its designation as the thoracolumbar branch of the autonomic nervous system.

The parasympathetic system is known as the cranial-sacral branch, in homage to the fact that its preganglionic cell bodies are housed in two very separate geographic areas: in the brainstem area, within the cranium, and in the sacral spine, the lowest part of the cord. There are no parasympathetic preganglionic cells whatsoever in the thoracic or lumbar spine.

Remember that preganglionic sympathetic axons originating in the spinal cord synapse onto the cell bodies of postganglionic sympathetic nerves located in the ganglia of the sympathetic chain, which are organized in a regular pattern on either side of the spine, or in the several prevertebral ganglia sitting in front of the aorta. In either case, the preganglionic sympathetic axons really don't travel very far from their point of origin in the spinal cord to their respective ganglia. Then, from these ganglia, postganglionic sympathetic axons travel, sometimes long distances, to the target tissue.

In the parasympathetic system, the situation is quite different. Parasympathetic ganglia, where the preganglionic parasympathetic nerve connects to the cell body of the postganglionic neurons, are located invariably either very near or in the end organ. In this case, it is the preganglionic axon that must travel a relatively long distance, at times several feet, before arriving at a ganglion, while the postganglionic route can at times be measured in microns or millimeters. Furthermore, sympathetic ganglia are quite big, the size of a pea perhaps, clearly visible with the unaided eye. Parasympathetic ganglia are quite variable in size, usually microscopic, hidden as they often are right in the organs themselves.

The cranial outflow of the parasympathetic system moves through four of the cranial nerves: the oculomotor (III), the facial (VII), the glossopharyngeal (IX), and the vagus (X). The preganglionic cell bodies for these nerves are located in very distinct areas of the brainstem, and each travels a very distinct route. The first three of these provide parasympathetic connections to limited areas in the head, and their overall contribution to parasympathetic physiology is minor. The preganglionic cell bodies for the oculomotor nerve begin in the midbrain, at the top of the brainstem, and then move through the skull toward the orbit of the eye.

There, just in back of the eyeball, the preganglionic axons synapse with the ciliary ganglion, which is by parasympathetic standards fairly large and visible to the eye. From there, postganglionic axons innervate the ciliary muscle of the eye; when the oculomotor nerve fires, this muscle contracts and the pupil constricts, reducing the amount of light that comes in to the retina. Other than this limited connection, the oculomotor nerve has no parasympathetic role.

The parasympathetic preganglionic component of the facial nerve originates in the pons of the brainstem, then travels a short distance in the head, and then branches and connects to several ganglia that provide postganglionic input to the tear glands of the eyes, the mucous glands of the nose, and most of the salivary glands. I use the phrase "parasympathetic component" when talking of the facial nerve because, as I have previously discussed, the facial nerve carries a variety of nerve fibers performing a variety of functions in addition to its parasympathetic axons. In this respect it resembles, somewhat, a spinal nerve.

The preganglionic glossopharyngeal nerves have their point of origin in the medulla. These parasympathetic axons then travel to the otic ganglion, which lies in the jaw near the ear openings, and which, like the ciliary ganglion, is fairly large. The postganglionic glossopharyngeal fibers innervate the parotid glands in the back part of the cheek, a pair of large glands that, in addition to producing saliva, seem to be involved in the immune defense of the mouth. Other than this connection, the glossopharyngeal has no parasympathetic role.

Though these three cranial nerves, the oculomotor, facial, and glossopharyngeal, are important in their restricted way, the vagus nerves are the real workhorse of the parasympathetic system, carrying as they do approximately 75 percent of all parasympathetic fibers in the body. Note that I use the plural, "vagus nerves," to remind us that the cranial nerves, like the sympathetic neurons, do come in matched pairs. Though I may speak of the vagus nerve, I am taking for granted that we understand there are really two of these.

Vagus preganglionic neurons arise in two separate nuclei in the medulla: the dorsal motor nucleus and the nucleus ambiguus, mentioned earlier. Not only are these two vagal nuclei separated geographically, but they are ultimately responsible for different tissues of the body. We find the dorsal motor nucleus at the top of the medulla, adjacent to, and more central than, the nucleus tractus solitarius, the center for much of the incoming sensory information that I discussed earlier. Here, in the dorsal nucleus, arise the preganglionic vagal neurons that eventually connect to postganglionic neurons with a very specific target: their axons synapse on all the various secretory cells of the chest and abdomen, a major undertaking to say the least. By secretory cell, I mean a cell that produces something important and essential for some metabolic process, be it mucus in the air passages of the lungs (that protects us against pollutants), hydrochloric acid in the stomach (for digestion), mucus along the lining of the digestive canal (for lubrication and protection), enzymes and insulin in the pancreas, bile salts in the liver—all those many and varied molecules we need to live.

I have earlier described the nucleus ambiguus as sitting toward the bottom of the medulla, on the outside, or to revert to my moth-on-the-wall analogy, at the back and toward the side of the wing. The preganglionic vagal outflow from this region specifically targets postganglionic parasympathetic neurons located in certain muscles in the throat, as well as, importantly, the heart. However, no vagal axons connect to any of the arteries, arterioles, venules, or veins in the body. This is in great contrast to the case of the sympathetic system, which reaches to the vessels in the chest and abdomen.

Of the twelve cranial nerves, only the vagus nerves leave the head region. After emerging from the medulla, they travel down the neck adjacent to the internal carotid arteries. They follow the course of these major blood vessels, literally clinging to them, right to the point of origin of the carotids at the arch of the aorta in the chest. From here, the vagi continue their journey along and down the aorta through the chest and diaphragm, one nerve trunk on either side of this great vessel, all the while sending off nerve branches destined for organs such as the lung and heart. The vagi pass through the diaphragm into the abdominal cavity, still following the course of the aorta. There, in the upper abdomen, much as the outermost rootlets of an old tree, the vagi divide and subdivide into a network of smaller nerves that continue on to the stomach, liver, pancreas, entire small intestine, first half of the large intestine, and kidneys.

I want to make a few points about the vagus nerves. In appearance, each vagus resembles a spinal nerve, clearly visible at surgery or during dissection, looking like a thick white-gray cord with a very tough connective tissue outer coating. Though it is correct to think of the vagus (or more correctly, vagi) as the main parasympathetic nerve of the body, it carries within it many axons that are not part of the parasympathetic system at all. It has been estimated that 85 percent of the axons of the vagus nerves are sensory in nature, carrying impulses back to the brainstem from the viscera. (Remember that the parasympathetic system, like the sympathetic, is a motor system, transmitting directions for action from the central nervous system.)

Baroreceptor and chemoreceptor afferent axons travel to the brainstem in the vagi and are examples of such a vagal sensory component. It's also important to keep in mind that though these sensory axons may physically course in the vagus nerve trunk, they are not part of the parasympathetic system. This is a motor system only.

Now, I want to consider only the parasympathetic axons in the vagal nerves. It's important to keep in mind that as the two vagus nerves take their wandering course through the neck, chest, and abdomen, a journey measured in many inches, the parasympathetic axons contained within are purely preganglionic in nature. There are no large cervical, thoracic, or abdominal ganglia where these axons end. Instead, these preganglionic fibers keep dividing and subdividing and subdividing again, until they ultimately reach the target organ itself, be it the lungs, heart, or viscera of the GI tract, and only there do these axons reach the end of the line. In the walls of these organs, each preganglionic axon synapses with a postganglionic cell, whose axon extends only briefly, usually at most several millimeters, before ending on the target cell. This is in sharp contrast to the preganglionic axons of the vagus, some of which are longer than twelve inches!

In the walls of the bronchi and smaller bronchioles, the air passages of the lungs, the postganglionic neurons terminate on the multitude of mucus-secreting and smooth muscle cells found there. Mucus is a critical component of our lungs, particularly today with pollution around us all, serving as it does as a trap for inhaled particulate matter and microorganisms, which can be expelled with coughing. Smooth muscle allows the air tubes to constrict or open wide, depending on the circumstances. We lose water vapor, for example, with each breath out. If we're dehydrated and the body needs to conserve water, constriction of the bronchi and bronchioles reduces the amount of air expelled with each breath, in turn conserving water.

In the heart, the postganglionic parasympathetic axons innervate the pacemaker cells primarily. Throughout the gastrointestinal canal—the esophagus, stomach, small intestine, and ascending and transverse colon—the postganglionic nerves originate in one of the two plexuses of the enteric nervous system. Those with cell bodies in the myenteric plexus send their axons to the two muscle layers of the digestive passageway, while those in the submucosal (Meissner's) plexus travel the short distance to the secretory epithelial cells, responsible for mucus, enzyme, and hormone production.

Above, I mentioned that the vagus nerves innervate the small intestine, as well as the first half or so of the large intestine. Here, where the vagus influence ends, the sacral component of the parasympathetic system picks up. (Remember, the parasympathetic system consists of nerves originating in both the cranium, like the vagus, and the sacrum—about as far apart in the central nervous system as you can get.)

The sacral preganglionic parasympathetic nerves, like those of the sympathetic system, have their cell bodies in the cord itself, in the first three sacral vertebral bones. Here, parasympathetic preganglionic neurons lie in the mid-outer and frontal part of the cord itself, an area somewhat analogous to the intermediolateral cell column of the thoracic and lumbar spine where the sympathetic preganglionic neurons begin. These cells, like those of the sympathetic system, do receive their instructions from higher up, particularly from the autonomic centers in the brainstem.

From the cord, the parasympathetic axons exit the spine in what are known as the pelvic spinal nerves, similar to the spinal nerves that carry sympathetic axons from the thoracolumbar area. In this regard, the sacral parasympathetic nerves follow a course more similar to that of their sympathetic cousins than to the cranial parasympathetic outflow.

The preganglionic parasympathetic axons travel in the pelvic nerves until approaching the target organ; at this point, the axons split off from the spinal nerves and journey until ending in the organs of the left abdomen and pelvis—the descending colon and rectum on the left, as well as the bladder and the sex organs (both male and female). In these tissues, these preganglionic axons—which have traveled a considerable distance—then synapse on the cell bodies of the postganglionic neurons. In the lower colon and rectum, these neurons, like those of the vagus, innervate the smooth muscle and epithelium. In the bladder and sex organs, the postganglionic axons connect to smooth muscle and, again, to secretory cells.

Earlier, I discussed the two different neurotransmitters released by sympathetic nerves. In the various ganglia, the preganglionic sympathetic neurons release acetylcholine, which sets off an action potential in the postganglionic nerve. This impulse causes the postganglionic axon to release a second transmitter, norepinephrine, at the synapse with the target muscle (cardiac or smooth) or secretory cell. Two different synapses, two different neurotransmitters.

In the parasympathetic system, things are a little simpler. All parasympathetic neurons, whether found in the oculomotor cranial nerve or in the sacral plexus, whether pre- or postganglionic, release only one neurotransmitter. In the synapses with postganglionic nerves, preganglionic axons, like preganglionic sympathetic neurons, secrete acetylcholine. In the connections to the end organ tissues, the postganglionic axons also release acetylcholine. Parasympathetic activity, whether in the ciliary muscle of the eye or in the rectum, depends on this rather small and in some respects simple molecule.

If we now look at the effects of acetylcholine on various cells and tissue, we will begin to understand just how the parasympathetic system works—and how it works together with the sympathetic nerves. In the heart, for example, acetylcholine released by postganglionic vagal neurons has a very straightforward action: it inhibits the pacemaker cells, slowing the pulse, and also reduces the strength of cardiac contraction. Parasympathetic firing, therefore, leads to a fall in cardiac output, meaning a fall in the amount of blood being pushed into the aorta and its offspring arteries. This effect helps reduce blood pressure.

Interestingly, parasympathetic nerves—unlike their sympathetic cousins—do not travel, except in a few select cases, to the blood vessels. One notable exception is the "blush area" of the face, where parasympathetic impulses, and acetylcholine release, cause vasodilation and in turn blushing. When the parasympathetic system is active, we often blush, even if we're not embarrassed. This is indeed a very limited effect; otherwise, parasympathetic axons do not connect to the various arteries, arterioles, venules, and veins. As a result, parasympathetic firing has little direct influence over systemic circulation.

Indirectly, it does indeed, however. Whenever the parasympathetic system becomes active, through the feedback connections in the hypothalamus, the sympathetic nerves invariably tend to be inhibited: with this reduced sympathetic tone, the smooth muscles in the various vessels relax, and the vessels will automatically dilate. With less norepinephrine circulating around, the skeletal muscles also relax. With the diminished cardiac output, overall we have less blood moving through wide-open vessels that are presenting less resistance. The result can be, if the vagal input to the heart is strong, a very rapid decrease in blood pressure.

As the pressure drops, blood flow to the brain will of course diminish. We become less alert, less mentally active, and tired. In addition to this, acetylcholine tends itself to have a sedating influence over much of the brain, adding to the effect of lowered blood pressure. All of this can be a good thing, a benefit when we are trying to rest or falling asleep, at times when a pounding heart, muscle tension, and an alert brain would be counterproductive.

As strongly as the parasympathetic system suppresses heart rate, cardiac contraction, cardiac output, and in turn blood pressure, it stimulates digestion, from beginning to end. In the gastrointestinal tract, when the parasympathetic nerves are firing, there is no relaxation, but much action. Here, in the gut, we have a living model of how a variety of signals, both from high up in the nervous system and within the gut itself, can influence autonomic activity.

First, I would like to think about what happens when we are hungry. Let's say it has been many hours since our last meal, breakfast. All the food from our morning meal has been effectively digested; the breakdown products, such as proteins, sugars, and carbohydrates, the vitamins, minerals, etc., have been absorbed into the bloodstream and either used in the metabolic processes of the body or stored away for use later. The body, with all its many complex activities, will use up glucose, the prime energy source for most cells, pretty quickly. Though glucose can be stored as glycogen in the liver and muscle, these reserves are fairly paltry, providing a supply that can be measured only in hours.

If time passes and we haven't eaten, glycogen will soon be gone. At this point, the adipose cells, the cells that store fat, start releasing free fatty acids, our main secondary source of energy. In addition, the body starts cannibalizing its protein stores in the muscles; certain component amino acids can be converted into glucose in the liver to provide an additional supply of blood sugar. We have all heard of people who have fasted for weeks, taking in only water; during such ordeals, our body is living off stored fat and protein.

Generally, after a few hours without food, the blood sugar starts dropping. In the posterior hypothalamus, a center for sympathetic control, certain sensory receptors, specifically designed to monitor blood sugar, sense the fall. These sensors turn on in a panic and send rapid-fire action potentials to the nearby sympathetic centers. Very quickly, the sympathetic system becomes active. At times, if we are very hungry, it becomes very active. We feel irritable, annoyed, and uncomfortable in our gut. Our pulse and blood pressure may go up, we become very alert, and we start looking for food.

We are in hunting mode, a purely sympathetic behavior. In our civilized lives, this may involve nothing more than opening the refrigerator, but we're in hunting aggressive mode nonetheless. While this is happening, reciprocally, signals from the posterior hypothalamus go cross-town and inhibit the parasympathetic nuclei in the anterior hypothalamus.

Once food comes within our reach, or even within the reach of our noses, the scenario changes dramatically. Remember, the smell and sight of food, before any food has reached our mouths, set off action potentials in the olfactory (I) and optic (II) cranial nerves, which send their messages to their specific sensory association areas in the temporal and occipital cortical lobes, respectively. In addition, the thought of food soon to be eaten, our vision of an expected meal, such as Thanksgiving dinner, sets up its own sensory responses within the frontal cortex.

All these different sensory impulses, from cranial nerves and from the highest intellectual centers (where thoughts of Thanksgiving dinner percolate), ultimately move downward, to the anterior hypothalamus. Now, the parasympathetic system has its revenge. Incoming signals about food turn on the parasympathetic centers, which in turn send signals down to the brainstem—and so on. The parasympathetic system now turns on, full bore—and the sympathetic nerves, having done their job and gotten us food, turn off. The search for food is indeed a sympathetic activity, but the digestion of food, and its enjoyment, is strictly parasympathetic.

When food enters the mouth, the taste receptors whose axons travel in the facial (VII) and glossopharyngeal (IX) cranial nerves now become active. Impulses travel quickly back to the respective facial and glossopharyngeal nuclei in the brainstem. The parasympathetic component of these two nerves becomes active, and as a reflex, signals fire back quickly to the salivary glands. Salivation commences, and copiously, if the food intake is grand. At the same time, signals from the sensory centers in the hypothalamus alert the dorsal motor nucleus of the vagus that something big is going on, that a meal is on its way. The vagal nerves turn on as well.

We have seen that vagal preganglionic fibers connect to postganglionic cell bodies located in the enteric plexus of the digestive canal, as well as those located in the pancreas and liver. The postganglionic fibers in turn reach all the smooth muscle cells that line the entire digestive canal, as well as the secretory cells of the stomach, intestines, first half of the colon, liver, and pancreas. Once the vagal nerves become active, the effect is enormous. Acetylcholine turns on the entire enteric system, and hydrochloric acid and pepsin start pouring out of the chief and oxyntic cells of the stomach, even before food has arrived. The epithelial cells of the duodenum, the first part of the small intestine, start releasing secretin and cholecystokinin into the blood; these two hormones, remember, stimulate the pancreatic production and release of both bicarbonate and the various pancreatic enzymes. Enterokinase from the duodenal mucosal cells will begin activating the pancreatic precursors when they hit the intestinal canal.

Acetylcholine stimulates all the smooth muscle in the gut to start contracting. The result is vigorous peristalsis, the rhythmic muscular movements of the gut. Much of this activity begins even before any food has made its way into the mouth. Up to that point, these responses in the gut occur only because of the sensory input about smell, and sight, and anticipation of food, that comes into the highest centers of the cerebral cortex. Once food actually arrives, first into the mouth, then downward and eventually into the small intestines, the effect becomes multiplied. Enteric reflexes become active, and this system moves into full gear. Though enteric nerves do respond to parasympathetic signals, food in the gut canal makes them react even more strongly. Secretion, smooth muscle contraction, and absorption at the epithelial layer become more efficient and more effective.

By the time the food bolus reaches the mid-part of the transverse colon—where vagal influence ends—most digestion is done. What are left at this point are mostly indigestible and unabsorbable waste, some water, and some electrolytes. Beyond this point, there is some uptake of water and certain nutrients, but the main job left is to move the waste material along the rest of the colon, and then out. Here, the sacral parasympathetic nerves take over this rather mundane and unattractive job. If these nerves don't respond appropriately—during stress, for example, when the sympathetic system is active and inhibiting parasympathetic firing—constipation results, sometimes terrible constipation. I remember a patient who came to me for treatment of constipation so bad that at times she would move her bowels once a month! Her sympathetic system was much too strong. Peristalsis, in her case, was virtually nonexistent.

After a big meal we, and other animals such as lions, often feel tired, though in a pleasant way. This is a classic sign of parasympathetic activity. With this system active, blood pressure drops, sympathetic activity diminishes, blood supply to the gastrointestinal tract increases, and blood diverts away from the muscle and the brain. Norepinephrine production is down; that of acetylcholine is up. The brain is less alert. We feel tired. Lions, classic parasympathetic-dominant, meat-eating animals, will rest for days after a big kill, rarely moving, their parasympathetic nerves on full time all the while.

Now that we've reviewed what parasympathetic nerves, and their transmitter, acetylcholine, do to the heart and the gut, a few more points need to be made about this system. In the eye, the oculomotor parasympathetic fibers, when active, cause the pupil to constrict, reducing the intake of light. This is beneficial when we're trying to rest and desirous of reducing the stimulating effect of light.

In the lungs, acetylcholine causes the smooth muscle to contract and the secretory cells to release mucus. As a result, the bronchi and small air passages constrict, reducing the flow of air in and out, while at the same time, mucus production increases. This can be a useful response if we're trying to reduce the intake of noxious pollutants, such as smoke during a fire, or seeking to prevent the loss of moisture. If the parasympathetic system reacts inappropriately strongly to small insults—such as harmless pollens in the spring—the result can be a serious case of asthma, complicated by excess mucus produced in a misguided attempt to rid the body of some perceived danger. Mucus plugs make asthma worse. In such a case, drugs that mimic sympathetic activity, such as adrenaline, can be lifesaving.

In response to norepinephrine, the sympathetic transmitter, liver cells release stored glucose and fatty acids into the bloodstream. When the parasympathetic system fires, its neurotransmitter acetylcholine signals the pancreas to release not only the important digestive enzymes, but also insulin from the beta cells. Insulin drives blood sugar and fatty acids into the cells, particularly at storage sites such as the liver and muscle. This is particularly important after a meal, when blood sugar levels tend to run fairly high and the excess sugar needs to be transported into the tissues. Insulin will do the job, generally nicely. If the parasympathetic system is too active, the pancreas will release too much insulin, and hypoglycemia results, with all its attendant discomfort. I find that my parasympathetic-dominant patients often are prone to hypoglycemia and the brain fog and fatigue that goes along with blood sugar drops.

In addition to this effect on stored liver sugars and fats, acetylcholine enhances hepatocyte detoxification processes. The liver acts as a large filter for all manner of metabolic wastes and toxins, which are processed, neutralized, and then prepared for release into the intestinal tract for ultimate excretion. Acetylcholine greatly enhances both the various liver detoxification pathways and the release of toxins from the liver into the intestines via the bile duct. When the parasympathetic nerves fire, the liver cleans out.

Parasympathetic nerves also enhance the work of the kidney, which we all know is another major detoxification/excretory organ. And the parasympathetic system, working jointly with sympathetic neurons, makes sex possible. Here, in this particular arena, both groups of nerves are equally important—a rare example in autonomic physiology when camaraderie takes precedence over reciprocal inhibition, and joint effort over one system dominating the other.

I hope you appreciate that, in so many ways, the parasympathetic system is the workhorse of the body, responsible for the digestion, the absorption, even the assimilation and utilization of nutrients. It helps keep toxins from coming into the lungs, and then helps the liver and kidneys effectively neutralize and excrete thousands of potentially dangerous metabolic wastes, environmental poisons, and drugs that can float through our bodies every day. It helps us rest at night, allowing rejuvenation from the day's stress and strain. If the sympathetic nerves and their transmitter norepinephrine help us survive in a crisis, the parasympathetic system and acetylcholine make it possible to repair the damage to our bodies such a crisis can bring. It's an extraordinary system, this autonomic collection of nerves, well planned, nicely organized, and very efficient in what it does.

The Sympathetic and Parasympathetic System: Two Examples to Make a Point

The Bible teaches us that blood is life. When Noah and his wife, and his three sons and their three wives exited the ark into a new and purified world, they were told by God that they now could eat "everything," meaning animal flesh as well as plant foods. Prior to the flood, humans were instructed to eat as vegetarians, touching no animal flesh ever. That restriction, at the dawn of a postflood world, had changed. Though he could now eat meat, Noah was specifically told he could not eat the blood, as Genesis 9 reported: "But flesh with the life thereof, which is the blood thereof, shall ye not eat" (Genesis 9:4, KJV). He could eat the muscles, the liver, the kidneys, even the brain—but no blood. Blood was so special that it could not be consumed.

A thousand years later, Moses described in Leviticus the dietary laws given him on Mt. Sinai for the edification of the wandering children of Abraham. He devoted a whole section, chapter 17, to the prohibition of blood eating. As Moses wrote of God's command, "And whatsoever man there be of the house of Israel, or of the strangers that sojourn among you, that eateth any manner of blood: I will even set my face against that soul that eateth blood, and will cut him off from among his people. For the life of a flesh is the blood" (Leviticus 17:10–11, KJV).

Blood is indeed life, and blood pressure keeps that life moving. So, it is easy to understand why our bodies have such a sophisticated set of mechanisms to keep blood pressure within a narrow range, to help ensure blood flows optimally. Though I have, in my discussions of the sympathetic and parasympathetic systems, outlined in some detail how these nerves help regulate blood pressure, I would like to spend a little more time on the subject. In this final review, I hope to be able to bring together previous lessons and show just how masterfully our autonomic, visceral efferent, unconscious nervous system works.

The autonomic system, which ultimately regulates blood pressure, is really quite remarkable. It can respond to changes in blood flow not only in a heartbeat, but literally between heartbeats, to keep blood pressure constant. The reactions of autonomic nerves can be very fast and, as Guyton (1956, 697) wrote, very intense. Sympathetic firing can double blood pressure when necessary within ten to fifteen seconds, and on the other hand, the vagus nerves when active can lower blood pressure so fast we can go from normal flow to one low enough to produce fainting within four to five seconds. That's a fast response, indeed.

I'd like to consider the case of high blood pressure first and then take a look at its counterpart, low blood pressure, and follow how both the sympathetic and parasympathetic nerves respond in each circumstance. First, I want to emphasize that I will be talking about a normal one of us, suddenly faced with a situation evoking hyper-, then hypotension. Later I will address the issues of pathological problems with blood pressure, that is, chronic hyper- and hypotension, either of which can lead to devastating consequences long term. For now, I am talking of normal variations of blood pressure, which provoke a normal and useful response.

There are a number of situations in which any of us normals can find ourselves dealing with a situation of elevated blood pressure. I myself, oddly enough for a physician, suffer from white-coat hypertension. Usually my pressure falls nicely within a very normal range, about 110 systolic, 70 diastolic (systolic is the pressure when the heart is contracting and squeezing out blood; diastolic is the resting pressure, the pressure when the contraction is done and the ventricles are filling with blood in preparation for the next contraction). However, if some other medical person comes at me with a blood pressure cuff, usually both pressures go up a good twenty points or more.

Doctors make me nervous, and what I am experiencing is my body's response to a perceived danger, threat, or stress. I want to be somewhere else, badly. My sympathetic nerves respond accordingly, firing freely. I've already outlined the drill: Norepinephrine, the sympathetic transmitter, increases heart rate, the strength of contraction, and cardiac output. The vessels in the gut and to the skin contract, reducing blood flow, while the vessels in the skeletal muscles dilate, and the arteries that feed the brain stay unchanged. The muscle contracts, tonically; digestion shuts off, my brain turns on, and my pressure goes up.

Any stress, real or imagined, frightening or laughable, does the same, again, of course, sometimes more strongly, sometimes less strongly. Any stress, through all the connections we have discussed before in detail, will push up the pressure. In addition to stress—physical, mental, or emotional—certain drugs, such as adrenaline and, yes, norepinephrine, will raise pressure. Physicians have available to them a host of medications that mimic norepinephrine and evoke a sympathetic effect. Such drugs are useful in acute life-threatening situations such as shock or heart failure, when the heart does not pump strongly enough and blood pressure can bottom out with very unpleasant consequences.

These sympathomimetics, as they are called, include such medications as dobutamine and isoproterenol, which have been used for years in most intensive care units around the world. Much of what we know about the body's autonomic response to high blood pressure dates from studies done in the 1950s and 1960s, when scientists would inject norepinephrine intravenously into "normal" volunteers and watch what happened.

In my particular embarrassing case of white-coat hypertension, the stress is imaginary: my own doctor is a wonderful and kindly man, whom fortunately I have needed to see only rarely over the years, for very minor issues. There is no real threat and no need to keep the pressure high for long. My mind knows this and responds accordingly, generally very quickly. If my doctor repeats the blood pressure testing within thirty seconds, usually the levels are down to my baseline normal. The response and regulation is in this case very fast. Of course, if the stress were real, and truly a danger, and truly frightening—say an oncoming forest fire, for example—the stress might be prolonged; the brain will know this and know it must keep the pressure high until we are out of danger and can relax.

Whether the stress is real or only perceived, physical or emotional, short term or long, the response works the same way. The response begins with the baroreceptors, those pressure receptors in the walls of the aortic arch and carotid sinus I discussed at some length earlier. Yes, the chemoreceptors are also involved, but for my personal example, I am going to restrict the discussion to the baroreceptors, because they are of more importance in the particular example mentioned above (my white-coat hypertension).

Baroreceptors are tonically active at a low level, their activity set to keep pressure at a precise normal number, say 120/80. They will respond to even slight changes either up or down, to bring the pressure back to the preset "normal." Overall, baroreceptor firing increases in response to high blood pressure, and their signals inhibit the sympathetic system, in effect lowering blood pressure. With low blood pressure, baroreceptor activity lessens, the inhibitory effect on sympathetic nerves is lifted, and blood pressure goes up.

In my case, with the nurse approaching with the cuff and my systolic and diastolic pressures going up twenty to thirty points, the increased force of blood flowing through the aortic and carotid arteries causes stretching in both the aortic and the carotid receptors. When they stretch, these sensory nerves become more active. Keep in mind that baroreceptor activity increases when the pressure goes up. Impulses travel in the vagal nerve, for the aortic receptors, and in the glossopharyngeal, for the carotid axons, back directly to the nucleus tractus solitarius (NTS).

This nucleus is the small area in the central upper part of the medulla that serves as a reception center for much incoming visceral sensory information. In the tractus solitarius, axons originating in the baroreceptors synapse on neuron cell bodies that specifically handle information related to blood pressure. Here, interestingly, the baroreceptor axons release the neurotransmitter glutamate, known as an excitatory transmitter because it stimulates activity; that is, it causes an action potential in the target cell.

These NTS neurons connect to two different areas in the outer lower medulla I have mentioned before: the caudal ventrolateral medulla and the nucleus ambiguus. The caudal ventrolateral medulla (CVLM) is an interesting place. It sends axons forward in the medulla to the rostral ventrolateral medulla (RVLM), which is really the center, in the medulla, for sympathetic control. The RVLM tends itself to be tonically active, and it really functions as a pacemaker for sympathetic activity. Its own axons move down the brainstem to the spinal cord, where they synapse directly on the sympathetic preganglionic cell bodies located in the intermediolateral cell column.

Under normal circumstances, without any presenting stress or stressor, the RVLM is continually active in a low-grade way, sending weak signals to the sympathetic nerves to keep the system active, though weakly. This effect prevents blood pressure from dropping to zero.

The nucleus ambiguus, on the other hand, contains the cell bodies for the vagal preganglionic parasympathetic nerves that go down the brainstem, eventually reaching to the heart. This nucleus is essentially the parasympathetic cardiac center.

When an excitatory glutamate signal hits the NTS, the target neurons themselves become active, meaning they start sending off action potential signals to both the caudal ventrolateral medulla and the nucleus ambiguus. At the CVLM, the NTS axons themselves release glutamate that excites the CVLM. When these nerves in the CVLM turn on, however, they release the inhibitory transmitter GABA, which essentially inhibits the rostral ventrolateral medulla nerve cells. When the CVLM is active, the RVLM is not. When the rostral ventrolateral medulla is quiet, the sympathetic nerves go still.

When the NTS is excited, the input to the nucleus ambiguus is also excitatory, meaning the NTS axons release glutamate there. When the vagal cell bodies in the nucleus ambiguus are hit with such a jolt of activating impulses, the vagal parasympathetic nerves to the heart turn on. The signal travels to the postganglionic vagal nerves in the cardiac wall, which then flood the heart muscle with acetylcholine.

We have diminished sympathetic activity and heightened vagal reactions. You know the rest. Heart rate slows, cardiac contraction and output lessen, vessels to the gut and skin dilate, the muscles relax, and we feel more relaxed. Importantly, blood pressure goes down toward normal, all happening at times within a millisecond. By the time my doctor has redone the pressure himself, in my case it is usually normal. It's a good system, usually, bringing down pressure appropriately to avoid the dangers and damages that high blood pressure can bring.

Fortunately or unfortunately, the baroreceptors work best for this type of millisecond-by-millisecond monitoring and adjusting of changes in blood pressure as we go through a typical day. However, if the day is not normal—perhaps we are subjected to bad stress that doesn't go away quickly—the brain perceives that it's a good thing to keep the pressure high, and keep it high it does. Excitatory signals travel from the cortex to the posterior hypothalamus to the RVLM, overriding the inhibition from the NTS. The sympathetic nerves stay on, norepinephrine floods the body, and the pressure stays high—for hours, days, even for weeks or years if the stress never relents.

When the stress continues without letting up and the pressure stays high, the baroreceptors accept that the elevated pressure is now the norm. After several days, they become less active, providing less inhibition to the sympathetic system, even though the pressure remains high. That is a problem, and chronic hypertension, "essential" as we doctors like to call it for some odd reason, as it isn't essential at all, has just reared its head.

Depending on the study, it has been estimated that anywhere from one-fifth to one-half of all adults in the United States suffer some level of elevated blood pressure. Yet, despite public education campaigns, aggressive screening, and improvement in treatment approaches, it remains a major killer here and a major factor in the epidemic of strokes, kidney failure, blindness, heart attacks, and heart failure that pervades our country. It is a problem to be taken very seriously, a potential problem for many of us. Yet despite the enormous research money invested, and the many bright minds who have spent their lives studying hypertension, in the great majority of cases, the "cause" is "not known."

Low blood pressure, or hypotension, can, like elevated pressure, occur for any number of reasons. Dehydration, mentioned in an earlier chapter, is one such circumstance and a very common one, particularly in dry, hot climates in summer. Simply put, if water loss is excessive and water intake inadequate, overall body water stores fall, and with them goes blood volume—because blood is mostly water—and down goes pressure.

Dehydration is a common cause of orthostatic hypotension, that is, the sudden onset of very low pressure that happens when we stand from a sitting or lying position; the dizziness, spaciness, even loss of balance in such a situation have happened to many of us. The symptoms happen because not enough blood is getting to the brain. I have a patient, a superb athlete, who competes routinely in various well-known marathons and triathlons. During one recent Boston Marathon, about two-thirds of the way through, he suddenly became dizzy, had to slow down, and fainted. He came to within seconds, but he was helped to the first aid tent, where the physician ordered intravenous fluids.

In hospital emergency rooms, blood loss is a potentially dangerous cause of low blood pressure. If there isn't enough blood volume, there isn't going to be adequate pressure, period. Drugs, too, can lower blood pressure, as all of us know. I don't know the exact number, but certainly tens of millions of Americans have been prescribed medications to lower blood pressure. These drugs can work, sometimes too well, and lead to low blood pressure with its attendant problems—dizziness, fatigue, depression, spaciness, etc.—that can make patients stop taking the drugs. It doesn't feel good when the brain becomes blood starved.

One winter, about five years ago, I was walking with a friend on Madison Avenue near my office and suddenly experienced dizziness and a slight loss of balance. I had to stop walking for a second, until I regained my composure. The symptoms passed but periodically recurred over the next several days. I realized that despite my warnings to patients about the need to drink large amounts of water each day to avoid dehydration, I was myself fluid depleted: I had been working very hard, long hours with very ill patients for months, and I had just gradually, without even thinking about it, cut back on my water intake. When I realized what the problem was, I began my usual seven to eight glasses of water daily, with quick resolution of the symptoms. Dehydration is certainly not pleasant, though the body works hard to minimize its effect.

In such a situation, though certainly not life threatening like acute blood loss after an accident, the body works hard to keep the pressure up. With hypotension, the flow forces in the aortic arch and carotid sinus are reduced, causing little or no stretch in the aortic and carotid baroreceptors. When there is reduced stretch, there is reduced baroreceptor firing, and fewer impulses go up to the tractus solitarius in the medulla. Baroreceptor axons release less glutamate in the synapse, so the vasomotor neurons in the tract remain themselves quiet. In turn, fewer signals, that is, fewer action potentials, flow to the caudal ventrolateral medulla. The nerve cells there also remain neurologically more silent.

Fewer inhibitory signals travel to the RVLM, and less GABA appears in the synapse of that nerve center. Without such inhibition, the RVLM neurons start firing more freely and more strongly, releasing copious amounts of glutamate down in the intermediolateral cell column. Sympathetic neurons, their inhibition lifted, become more active. Heart rate, cardiac contraction, and cardiac output increase; blood is shunted away from the gut and skin to the muscles and brain, etc. Blood pressure goes up, quickly.

In summary, when the pressure is high, the baroreceptors become more activated, and their firing has the overall effect of inhibiting the sympathetic system and turning on the parasympathetic nerves, to bring pressure back down toward normal. When pressure is low, the baroreceptors become less active; their inhibitory effect is gone. The sympathetic system turns on and the parasympathetic turns off, in an attempt to raise blood pressure.

As I've earlier remarked, the brain has a remarkable ability to control the intensity, the degree of firing in both sympathetic and parasympathetic nerves. If the dehydration is minimal, as it was in my case, and the blood pressure effect slight, the sympathetic system will be slightly activated. If the dehydration is severe and the pressure drop significant, then the sympathetic nerves will fire powerfully and repeatedly, trying to keep the pressure up. A strong sympathetic response can be lifesaving in a situation where there has been significant blood loss, for example.

In my illustration, I am talking about a normal physiological response to a common problem. Like high blood pressure, low pressure can also become chronic, debilitating, and life altering. Admittedly, we don't think about chronic low blood pressure as a serious medical problem. There are no public awareness or screening programs in place, no groups or organizations that I know of to champion its cause. As a public health issue, hypotension seems to be quite far down the list of problems we need to address, lagging far behind, for example, cancer, heart disease (including, of course, hypertension), stroke, and diabetes.

It's difficult to find accurate statistics on the prevalence of chronic hypotension. The latest version of *Harrison's Principles of Internal Medicine* (15th edition) has a long and comprehensive section on hypertension, but only scattered references to the opposite condition, low blood pressure. No one seems to know how common it is, or even to care very much about finding out. One would think, for all this indifference, that hypotension is hardly a serious medical problem at all.

I believe it occurs very commonly and is, despite its shunning by the medical world, a common source of disability. Furthermore, I believe that it is often the cause of chronic fatigue in general and the chronic fatigue syndrome (or more correctly, CFIDS, chronic fatigue with immune deficiency) specifically.

It is estimated, according to *Harrison's* (Braunwald et al. 2001), that fully 25 percent of all patients who seek a doctor's advice in a general medical office or clinic come because they are chronically tired. Though of course there are many reasons why someone may feel tired—poor sleep, low thyroid function, anemia, to name but a very few—most often no cause can be found, no source for the fatigue. Patients are told to get some rest, to avoid stress, and to sleep more, but often the advice doesn't work.

Many of these patients suffer from chronic fatigue, which can go on without a break for years and seems unrelated to the usual causes of fatigue such as anemia or hypothyroidism. Over the past fifteen or so years, so many patients, many of them young, educated, and previously vigorous, have started appearing in doctors' offices around the country complaining of fatigue so bad that many could not leave their houses for days. A small group of doctors began to believe they were witnessing a growing problem, which they labeled chronic fatigue syndrome.

For years, CFS, or CFIDS, was a disputed diagnosis in the medical world, considered by many to be a nondisease. Recently, the problem has received medical respectability and can now be officially diagnosed as a real illness based on a list of criteria published by the Centers for Disease Control (CDC) in Atlanta, Georgia. Primarily, to the CDC, chronic fatigue syndrome means unrelenting fatigue and exhaustion that is not the result of exertion and not relieved by rest. There are other requirements that must be met for the diagnosis to be established, but the fatigue and exhaustion are the major symptoms the patient must have. Currently, epidemiologists estimate that there are about one thousand to three thousand cases that satisfy the criteria per one million US citizens.

Chronic fatigue, whether formally diagnosed or not, is a pervasive, at times unrelenting, insidious, invidious problem that can wreck marriages, careers, and lives. I have one patient who had been to many doctors over a period of several decades looking for an answer to her chronic devastating illness, with no success. Several different internists had referred her to various psychologists and psychiatrists, again with no effect. She was labeled lazy, a malingerer, mentally ill, and as having a personality disorder. She had none of those things. She had chronic fatigue, fatigue so bad and so endless it had affected every aspect of her life. At one point, she said she envied my cancer patients, because their disease was easily identified, their struggle very basic: they either get well and get on with their lives, or "it's over." (She is now doing well, thankfully, and has, as she says, "The newest and best lease on life someone could have.")

Though our office is known primarily as a place to get cancer treatment, we routinely receive desperate calls, letters, and faxes from the victims of CFS, wondering whether we can help them. Usually, they've been to many doctors, who give a variety of diagnoses, and who don't do very much.

Recently, as the problem has achieved respectability, doctors have begun to address, in all seriousness, what can cause an otherwise healthy patient who had previously been living a normal, productive life to become so disabled with fatigue that leaving the house becomes at times impossible. A good percentage of chronic fatigue sufferers are now known to have chronic low blood pressure, and with such patients, blood pressure-elevating drugs have been very useful, at times turning patients back to good health.

Chronic low blood pressure isn't to be taken lightly. It means that not enough blood gets to the brain, chronically, particularly when you stand or are standing, and the vascular system must fight gravity to get adequate blood and, with it, oxygen and nutrients to the hungry brain. Chronic low pressure can mean chronic brain fog, fatigue, diminished concentration, decreased memory, dizziness, nausea, and balance and coordination problems—anything that can happen when the brain isn't getting what it needs to function optimally. Low blood pressure may not kill, the way high blood pressure does, but it can make life not worth living.

We find in many of our chronic fatigue patients weak sympathetic tone, and their symptoms seem to have begun after a period of prolonged stress. Though in a stressful situation, generally the sympathetic system fires and pressure should go up, in this group of patients, the sympathetic nerves seem inherently weak, and when pushed, they turn on but quickly burn out. The sympathetic system blows a fuse. In my discussion of high blood pressure, I pointed out that baroreceptors are superb short-term monitors of blood flow, but if the hypertension persists beyond a few days, they can begin to accept abnormally high pressures as normal. The same is true with low blood pressure that continues beyond a few days: the baroreceptors can start accepting an abnormally reduced pressure as acceptable.

I believe the usual scenario with such patients begins with an episode of stress that tires out their sympathetic system, leading to persistent low blood pressure. After a few days of this, the baroreceptors reset so that they interpret even significantly low pressure as perfectly fine, and should the pressure rise above this low level toward normal, the baroreceptors turn on strongly to reverse the increase. In a state of chronic hypotension, they do not turn off as they should, to release their inhibiting impulses to the sympathetic nerves. The sympathetic system stays quiet, even when it should be firing vigorously. Blood pressure stays low, and fatigue becomes predictably endless.

I would like to discuss briefly one final illustration of how the autonomic system works before we move on. I could choose from any number of interesting phenomena—consider low or high blood sugar, for example—but a very brief discussion of how the autonomic system regulates our body temperature might yield some useful insights into these nerves that I, at least, find so remarkable.

On first glance, our ability to respond effectively to great extremes in ambient temperature might seem a rather dull and perhaps esoteric footnote to neuroscience. But when we think about it more closely, very quickly we should realize how important this quality has been to our own history. Humans, more so than most if not all other animals, have a remarkable ability to adjust and survive and thrive in a variety of climes, from the extreme Arctic cold of the Eskimos, to the torrid heat of the African savannah or the tropical rain forests. If our bodies did not have the facility to adapt, and adapt very effectively to such variations and extremes in heat and cold, our expansion into the corners of the Earth would have met with disaster and defeat.

Our survival in difficult temperature extremes certainly makes for good television. Though admittedly I have little time for any activities other than dealing with life and death on a daily basis, in my previous life as a journalist I was always somewhat of a history buff. I have been particularly an amateur student of great adventurers in difficult places such as Stefansson, the meat eater from Harvard who lived with the Eskimos, and Shackleton, the great English explorer.

Shackleton's trip to the Antarctic in the early years of the last century ended up in near disaster, as many of you already know. He and his crew were forced to abandon their square-rigged ship after it got stuck in an ice floe in the middle of nowhere, hundreds of miles from the nearest settlement. In a desperate move, Shackleton successfully led a small group in a whaleboat across treacherous waters, through brutal cold, to safety and help. His crew was eventually saved, with minimal loss of life. It was indeed a great victory over the forces of nature, particularly the forces of cold winds, icy rains, and ice. Even I found the recent TV miniseries dramatizing this adventure riveting, perhaps because it was real, and a story far more extraordinary than any fiction.

There are, of course, equivalent stories of heroic treks across, and survival in, places of great heat, such as deserts and rain forests. My father, who served his country in Asia during WWII, reported to me that it was absolutely true that in the middle of a hot day in India, one could fry an egg on a stone just from the absorbed heat!

Without an extraordinary capacity to adjust to temperature, human history and certainly at least some TV would have been, I suspect, much duller. Of course, most of us never will experience the extremes of Antarctica or the tropics, but in any given day, we will generally be exposed to frequent temperature changes. Our comfort would be less if we were not able to adapt so quickly and so well. Think of summer in New York, moving from an air-conditioned office to the hot street in August, and back to an air-conditioned apartment. We may be a little uncomfortable walking up Madison Avenue when the temperature is 98°F, but most of the time, we feel fine and are able to go about our business without restraint.

It is the autonomic system that saved Shackleton and his crew, and it is the autonomic system that allows us to survive with a certain degree of comfort in most earthly temperatures. It is the autonomic system that allows the body to adjust as it does, to heat and cold, and it is our autonomic system that allowed us humans to journey far and wide to the four corners of the Earth.

This is all quite remarkable when we realize that we humans can survive only when our internal temperatures stay within a limited range. Though we can live for brief periods of time with body core temperatures around 90 degrees Fahrenheit on the low side and 107 or so on the high side, for normal healthy functioning, temperature needs to stay in the range of about 97 degrees up to 99.5, with most of us falling on a day-to-day basis between 98.0 and 98.6 degrees. This is a narrow range indeed. Fortunately, our temperature regulatory mechanisms are so efficient that we can be exposed to an extraordinary range of outside temperatures, with little internal variation. Guyton (1956, 822) reported that a nude human can withstand temperatures from 55 degrees up to 130 degrees with little change in the core temperature.

We generate heat, in every second of our lives, through the mundane processes of cellular metabolism. Most heat is generated in several organs: the brain, liver, heart, and, when contracting, muscles. We can lose some of the heat we generate through breathing, but by far the greatest losses occur through the skin, by direct transfer of heat into the environment, known as radiation, an apt description, or by the evaporation of sweat on the skin. Heat moves from the internal organs and muscles to the surface via the blood, which among its other talents is an excellent medium for carrying heat energy.

Our bodies have a number of ways of reading, so to speak, the ambient temperature. Remember, there are temperature receptors in the skin, one group responding to heat, another group to cold. Their function is, understandably, to respond specifically to environmental temperatures. In addition, both heat and cold sensors are found in certain internal organs, particularly the spinal cord and the abdominal organs. These report specifically on the core body temperature. Of course, our internal body temperature will ultimately reflect what's going on in the ambient environment, though less directly.

All of this sensory input, from both the skin and the internal viscera, travel back to the central nervous system, particularly to the hypothalamus, which has ultimate responsibility for maintaining a constant, steady, livable internal temperature. Here, information from the heat sensory neurons ends up in the anterior hypothalamus; signals from the cold sensors go to the posterior hypothalamus. In addition, the hypothalamus has its own set of heat and cold receptors, to complement the peripheral input.

Like the baroreceptors for blood pressure, the hypothalamic temperature centers tend to be set at an ideal normal. Any deviation, even a tenth of a degree, sets off a series of responses, to ensure that the internal temperature, whatever the environment around us may be doing, stays steady. If the ambient temperature changes even a few degrees, the response can be rapid, within seconds.

Cold, even a slight drop in temperature, activates the cold receptors in the skin; impulses travel back to the posterior hypothalamus, which, remember, is a center for sympathetic control. When the signals that the temperature is dropping arrive here, the sympathetic center turns on—and inhibitory signals are sent across to the parasympathetic nuclei in the anterior hypothalamus. You know the drill: yes, pulse and cardiac output increase, but, importantly, there is vasoconstriction in all the vessels of the skin. This means significantly less blood flow to the skin and, as a result, significantly reduced heat loss.

It has been estimated (Guyton 1956, 823) that, depending on the state of constriction or relaxation of the skin vessels, from near 0 percent to 30 percent of the total cardiac output can flow to the skin. That translates into quite a range of potential heat loss (or heat conservation) that scientists say can vary eightfold, from virtually minimal to very high levels. In extreme cold, the peripheral blood flow shuts down to almost nil, meaning very little heat transfer from the internal organs and minimal loss of internal heat.

That's a start. When the sympathetic system fires, in addition to peripheral vasoconstriction, its neurotransmitter norepinephrine causes an overall increase in the metabolic rate in most tissues and organs. From this effect, heat production can go up 10 to 15 percent. Furthermore, as you might remember from an earlier discussion, the anterior pituitary is directly connected to the posterior hypothalamus and comes under its direct control. When the cold sensors and centers in the posterior hypothalamus turn on, they also send signals to the anterior pituitary to release a hormone that in turn stimulates the thyroid gland to release its hormone, thyroxin.

Thyroid hormone, along with norepinephrine, is a key stimulant of overall cellular metabolism. With increased amounts of thyroxin circulating in the blood, the metabolic rate can go up considerably, and with it, heat production. It has been estimated that Eskimos secrete considerably more thyroxin, and in turn have a higher metabolic rate than those of us who live south of the Arctic Circle. This is one way they traditionally survived so well in their difficult and very cold land.

Finally, when we are cold, we shiver, and when we shiver, we generate heat. There is a shivering center in the posterior hypothalamus that turns on when the internal temperature falls below the set point for acceptability. When active, these shivering neurons send signals down the spine to the anterior horn, where we find the somatic motor neurons that go to all voluntary muscles. These nerves become active throughout the body, causing a continuous increase in the basal muscle tone and producing low-grade repetitive contractions. This motor activity produces heat.

If the temperature around us should go up, we are witness to the opposite chain of events. The heat sensors located primarily in the skin, but also to some extent those of the internal viscera, become active and send impulses back, this time to the anterior hypothalamus. Here, the elevated temperatures also stimulate the heat sensors located within the anterior hypothalamus. All this sensory information about heat turns on the parasympathetic system (with reciprocal inhibition of the posterior hypothalamic sympathetic centers). With the sympathetic nerves turning off, we have vasodilation, not constriction in the skin, with—if it is really hot—considerable diversion of the total cardiac output to the periphery.

Heat loss through the skin surface can increase substantially, up to eight times the amount lost when the vessels are completely constricted. In addition, the release of the parasympathetic transmitter acetylcholine stimulates sweating, and its evaporation can lead to a major loss of heat. Guyton reported that when the core body temperature goes up just a degree, sweating increases to the point that ten times the overall basal body heat production will be lost in evaporation. That's much heat, indeed.

With the sympathetic nerves inhibited and the parasympathetic system turned on, basal metabolism in all our cells slows down and, in turn, so does heat production. The anterior hypothalamus specifically inhibits the release of thyroid stimulating hormone from the anterior pituitary, so the thyroid secretes less thyroxin. This too, lowers the rate of cellular metabolism and cellular heat production. Interestingly, when the anterior hypothalamus is active, it specifically inhibits the shivering center in the posterior hypothalamus.

With the sympathetic tone and norepinephrine secretion already reduced, the muscles become very relaxed. If it is really hot, and the parasympathetic system is really turned on, we will become relaxed in every way. It is not strictly cultural that in the days before air conditioning, in Latin American countries such as Mexico, an afternoon nap traditionally was a normal part of the hot day. With the sympathetic system off and the parasympathetic nerves on, no one was going to feel like doing much of anything.

So, when we are cold, the sympathetic system turns on, and the parasympathetic nerves turn off. When we are hot, we have the opposite, high parasympathetic and low sympathetic tone. Of course, as always, the responses of each system can be very precisely graded, depending on how cold or how hot it is outside. Now you understand why, if it's cold, you shiver, and if it's hot, you need to take a nap.

Though all this autonomic physiology is interesting—or at least I hope you think so—we must now reconsider the point that in my work, in my approach to patients, I believe that certain people have an inherently strong sympathetic nervous system and a correspondingly weak parasympathetic, and others have a strong parasympathetic system and weak sympathetic collection of nerves. I believe much disease occurs as a result of such innate autonomic imbalance, and with my therapy, I am always trying to bring the two systems into balance. That's the core of what I do, the basis of my treatment.

Just how strong is the scientific justification for what I do in my office today? Kelley in his own thinking relied heavily on Pottenger and a few other alternative-type practitioners such as Royal Lee, who proposed various systems of autonomic dominance. Is there a more solid scientific foundation than this, than a few researchers on the fringes of acceptability? The answer is a definite yes. That answer requires that I take a step back in time, and look again—just as we did when I discussed our use of pancreatic enzymes in other books—at history, medical history. In there are answers even Dr. Kelley seemed not to know.

The Autonomic System in History, Pavlov's Dogs, and Dr. Funkenstein's Autonomic Types

For students wishing a more detailed introduction to the autonomic nervous system throughout history, see Dr. Tansey's excellent review in *Autonomic Failure* (1999), fourth edition, beginning on page 23.

Remember, although the term "autonomic nervous system" wasn't used until it was coined by Dr. Langley of Cambridge University in a paper he presented in 1898 in the *Journal of Physiology*, scientists had been aware of the autonomic nerves since the time of Greece and Rome. Galen, the great Roman physician and anatomist, first described what we would call the sympathetic chains and ganglia in the dissected bodies of animals such as pigs and apes. At that time, and well into the Renaissance, scientists such as Galen were strictly forbidden from dissecting human corpses, but he does seem to have observed, according to Dr. Tansey, the sympathetic system in the living bodies of wounded gladiators whom he served as physician. Galen correctly believed that the sympathetic nerves arose from the brain, though his knowledge of their physiology did not go much further than that.

Galen was, to medicine, a man who could do no wrong, and though he never dissected a human body, his concepts of human anatomy were held as literal law for a thousand years. It wasn't until the sixteenth century that the religious and secular prohibitions on human dissection were finally lifted, though, strangely, for some time Galen's thoughts still reigned supreme. I remember reading years ago that during anatomy classes in Italian medical schools even at the time when dissection was allowed, the professor—who would never touch the cadaver—would read Galen's "truths" to the students, even as they did the actual cutting. Galen's words were still thought of as supreme, even when the observations contradicted his propositions!

Many of Galen's ideas of human anatomy were derived from his dissections of apes, and he assumed that human anatomy was no different. It is. The ape liver, for example, has five lobes, the human four. No matter, the students were told. Galen was right, and the cadaver was wrong! So much for science and the acceptance of new ideas.

Things began to change during the seventeenth century, the age of scientific enlightenment. The great English anatomist Thomas Willis (1621–1675), able to study human specimens, first described and named the vagus "wandering" nerve. In experiments on living dogs, Willis noted that when the vagus branches to the heart were cut, the heart "fluttered." In addition, he performed detailed dissections of the sympathetic chain and proposed, rather correctly, that the various sympathetic ganglia were "small brains," a thought later supported by his intellectual successor, Jacobus Winslow (1669–1760).

To Winslow goes first credit for using the term "sympathetic" in his descriptions, so the term goes back well over two hundred years. Importantly, as Dr. Tansey reported, the French anatomist Francois Xavier Bichat (1771–1802) differentiated between the voluntary "somatic" nervous system and the "visceral," or what we would today call the autonomic nerves. That was a proposition of, at least in our story, monumental proportions.

Despite the work of such brilliant scholars, knowledge of the autonomic nervous system and how it worked was still very elementary until the nineteenth century, when the widespread use of microscopy enormously aided studies of nervous system anatomy. During that century, a large number of scientists devoted their lives to unraveling the mysteries of the nervous system and the autonomic system in particular. The English researcher Benedict Stilling (1810–1879) first suggested the term "vasomotor" to describe sympathetic fibers to the arterioles of voluntary muscle, and the great physiologist of the nineteenth century, Claude Bernard (1813–1879), first reported that when the sympathetic nerves were cut, the blood vessels dilated—an important observation. Dr. Edouard Brown-Sequard noted that when the cut ends of sympathetic nerves were stimulated with an electrical current, the vessels constricted. Dr. Charles Sherrington (1857–1952) did much to uncover the mysteries of reflex responses and first used the word "synapse" to describe the connection between a nerve and its target cell.

Throughout much of the nineteenth century, our knowledge of autonomic anatomy and physiology increased in small bits and pieces, rather than by leaps and bounds. At least that was true until the extraordinary Cambridge physiologists Walter Gaskell (1847–1914) and J. N. Langley (1852–1925) came onto the autonomic scene. These two men, working together at Cambridge, devoted their lives to untangling the complex mysteries of the autonomic nervous system.

Gaskell first emphasized the involuntary nature of "autonomic" function and was the first to clearly define the antagonist activities of the sympathetic and parasympathetic systems in the visceral organs they innervated. Langley was particularly devoted to studying the nature of the "chemical transmission," what we would call today neurotransmitter chemistry, at the synapse. Overall, these two unusual men took the pieces of information that had been accumulating for some two hundred years, went light years beyond, and put it all together into a comprehensive vision of autonomic action and the critical importance of the system to life as we know it.

In 1849—when Gaskell was two years old, and three years before Langley first saw the light of day—far removed from the intellectual centers of Paris and Cambridge, Ivan Petrovich Pavlov (1849–1936) was born in Ryazan, Russia. Of course, we all know the name Pavlov. Pavlov and at least the rudiments of his work have become such a part of our colloquial lexicon that I doubt few if any reading this have not at least heard of him.

Most of us know the basics, that Pavlov took dogs into his lab and put food in front of them, and they salivated. Then each time the animals were to be fed, before putting out the food, he would ring a bell. After a certain number of bell ringings, he would ring the bell but not provide the food. The dogs salivated nonetheless, their brains having been conditioned to understand that bell equals food, and food means saliva.

We've all heard the story, a provocative example of how the brain can be tricked. To most of us, the tale has a negative, even sinister connotation. For years, until I studied Pavlov's work, it did to me. We use the term *Pavlovian* often to imply deceit, manipulation, and mind control. Few of us truly appreciate just how important Pavlov's work really was, to psychology, to medicine, to psychiatry particularly, and to autonomic physiology.

Pavlov was a most interesting man, like so many of the great minds working at the end of the nineteenth and beginning of the twentieth centuries—at the same time Gaskell and Langley were in the middle of their own revolutionary careers. His life was hardly a straight line. The son of an Orthodox Russian priest, in his early student years Pavlov showed no interest in science, and in fact as a teenager began preparing for the priesthood himself. However, while pursuing his religious vocation, he became increasingly excited by the work being done in physiology and medicine both in Russia and abroad and, midstream, he decided to abandon his priestly studies and switched to natural science.

Through a circuitous route, he finally ended up in medical school, eventually receiving his medical degree at the ripe old age of thirty-four—old by standards then and now (I was thirty-five when I got mine). Though we think of him as a psychologist, his interests throughout his life focused on physiology, particularly digestive physiology—and, important for my story, the nervous system and the gut. His first published paper, which won him his first of many awards, dealt with the nerve input to the pancreas. His doctoral thesis presented in 1883 was entitled "The Centrifugal Nerves of the Heart," and it reported on his investigations of nervous system stimulation of the heart, that is, of course, the sympathetic nervous system influence. To his great credit, he was the first to codify the autonomic control of the heart and its circulatory system.

Pavlov's star rose quickly. In 1890, he was selected to head the department of physiology at the Institute of Experimental Medicine, which he continued to direct for the next forty-five years, until his death in 1936. There, he continued his studies of the digestive system and the nerves that control it. Though czars would come and go, though revolutions would traumatize his land and Leninism and Stalinism would seek to make science a slave of the state, Pavlov was so revered by all, and attained such international recognition, that he was generally left alone to do his work. Both czars and tyrants supported his work handsomely. He was a true Russian treasure, and everyone seemed to know it. The Communists hailed him and his work as being of enormous significance for the working class of the whole world.

With great, patient diligence, Pavlov and his group in Leningrad developed a number of research techniques that helped change the course of physiology. Anatomy is the science of where things are in the body, its geography; physiology is the science of how things work in us, the mechanics of life. Prior to Pavlov, physiologists could only deduce what was going on inside of us, say, inside the stomach, by dissecting and studying dead specimens—something not very physiologic, to say the least. No one before had quite figured out how to study the internal glands and organs in a living animal. Much imagination was involved, and what was imagined to be happening was wrong.

Pavlov, however, solved the problem, quite nicely. He was the first to show how useful fistulas could be for the study of GI function. These are simply surgically created channels that allow the observer to gain access in laboratory animals to the internal organs, such as the salivary glands, the stomach, and the intestines. Small tubes could be inserted into such channels, to retrieve secretory products, such as saliva from the salivary glands, or hydrochloric acid from the stomach. These fistulas, and the related "pouch" technique that Pavlov also invented, enabled scientists to witness what was going on during digestion, as well as retrieve an endless supply of digestive juices for analysis and study. Such techniques are still in use today.

During a ten-year period, from 1891 until 1900, Pavlov did much to uncover just how the nervous system, the sympathetic and parasympathetic nerves, controls digestion from beginning to end. For this work, he received the Nobel Prize in Medicine and Physiology in 1904, at the age of fifty-four, rather young for this ultimate honor. His investigations of digestive physiology led him in a new and challenging direction, into the realm for which he remains best known, that of the conditioned reflex.

Some terms need to be defined simply. An unconditioned reflex, whether one is thinking about dogs or people, is a normal, untrained reflex response that doesn't require conscious thought or decisions and that happens in a normal life setting. For example, if you hear a loud noise, you jump. A dog sees food, and saliva starts to flow. The noise or the food is an unconditioned stimulus; the jumping or the salivating is an unconditioned response. No training, no conditioning, is required.

These things happen automatically, normally, as reflexes, because our nervous systems, and those of dogs, are designed to make them happen these ways for our own safety or benefit. It's useful to jump at a loud noise, or salivate when food appears—particularly if you are hungry.

On the other hand, a conditioned reflex is a trained, or conditioned, response that isn't necessarily useful or to our benefit. Sometimes, they can be to our harm. The classic example, for which Pavlov seems forever to be remembered, is that mentioned earlier, the case of a dog trained, or conditioned, to salivate not at the sight or smell of food, but at the ringing of a bell, an occurrence that normally has nothing whatsoever to do with food.

Bell ringing, at least if not loud, is essentially a neutral stimulus. If unusually loud, of course, it might stimulate jumping, but the bell ringing that went on in Pavlov's lab was mild, nonthreatening, and nonirritating. It was just a mild bell that normally his laboratory dogs ignored. It evoked no reflex of any kind, hence the term *neutral stimulus.*

However, the dogs could be trained over time to respond to the bell as if it were food, even in the complete absence of food. This was a conditioned reflex, a trained response. The dogs were trained, or conditioned, to respond to the bell as if it were food. The bell ringing reaction isn't particularly detrimental to the animal, just a waste of saliva and, perhaps in the trained dogs, a cause for disappointment because they had been taught to expect food with the bell.

In his studies, Pavlov learned that he could design conditioned reflexes that could be less pleasant and have a detrimental effect on an animal. In one series of experiments with dogs, Pavlov first trained the animals to, in response to a bell, jump on a table where they would then be fed. That was simple enough: the bell would ring; the trained, or conditioned, dogs would automatically—without thinking—jump on the table.

Then he added another step. The bell would ring, the dogs would jump on the table and receive an unpleasant electrical shock, and then food would appear. After several shocks, the animals would not jump on the table, no matter how hungry they felt. Instead, now when the bell rang, some dogs would become restless and aggressive, and some would howl. Others would become very passive, appearing frightened and anxious. It got to the point that the animals would struggle when brought from their kennel to the room where the bell ringing experiments took place.

As time passed and the experiments continued, the animals, even in their kennels, away from the experimental room, would behave abnormally. Some appeared aggressive, to the point that they would attack the handlers sent to bring them to the experimental room. Others became unusually shy, less social, and more withdrawn. If placed in the same cage with a "normal" dog, they would refuse to eat. Though different dogs might exhibit a different set of behaviors—some becoming more aggressive and others more passive—the behavior was generally, Pavlov observed, neurotic. The confusion over what the stimulus—in this case, the bell—meant produced in the animals mental illness.

He designed a serious of similar experiments with dogs, cats, and even sheep. Pavlov learned that he didn't have to use a painful stimulus to evoke neurotic behavior. He found with dogs that he could establish a more complex feeding-conditioned reflex, in which the dogs were trained to understand that food appeared only when a ring sound occurred at a particular pitch, but not at other pitches. The animals learned to respond to only that particular pitch, which to them meant food, and would then ignore other notes.

If Pavlov presented a series of ringings that were so close together in pitch that the animals couldn't distinguish which one meant food and which didn't, neurosis would raise its head. The animals became restless and irritable and appeared confused. Some again became very aggressive, others very passive. They resisted leaving the kennels, just as they did in anticipation of the electric shock experiments. Some animals even began reacting just at the site of the handler who normally led them to the experiment.

The point of all this is that a really benign stimulus, a neutral stimulus to use the technical term, a series of musical notes, led to mental illness in these poor dogs! Pavlov assumed it was the conflict created by a stimulus such as a bell that had meant comfort but now was meaning pain.

Of course, I am summing up years of experimentation briefly, but all this meant much to Pavlov, about dogs' behavior and about human behavior. Pavlov came to believe that much of our behavior consists of little more than such conditioned reflexes complicating unconditioned responses—not, as Freud would say, complex meanderings and confusions based on subconscious trauma. It was all a trained reflex of one sort or another, either positive or negative.

For example, a parent—who should mean food and warmth and comfort—might become associated with pain if there has been abuse of one sort or another. Thus, in the Pavlovian world, where a conditioned response that should mean something pleasant such as food or comfort becomes complicated by a painful stimulus, mental illness is going to happen. He saw it in whatever species of animal he worked with. He assumed the same in us.

Of course, these reflexes he studied were, for better or worse, all basic autonomic reflexes that are meant for our well-being, such as our physiological response to food. In the case of neurosis, they were good reflexes, meant to serve a comfort or survival function, gone bad. The responses, even if neurotic, were still reflexes; the animals who were trained that a bell meant a shock as well as food didn't consciously think about what the bell meant; they responded automatically with fear and anxiety. What should be a pleasant experience, eating, had become for these animals a nightmare.

What intrigued Pavlov was that different dogs responded differently to the training procedures. Some, as I've mentioned, became very aggressive, hostile, and even violent to the handlers and other dogs. Others became very passive and withdrawn and would refuse to eat, sitting in their cages for long periods of time without moving. These dogs were almost unresponsive.

Interestingly, Pavlov found that not all dogs were susceptible to developing neurosis; in fact, no matter how extreme the negative stimulus, some dogs simply didn't demonstrate any long-term effects of the training. They certainly would react when being buzzed or confused, but the reactions were short lived. Once in the kennels, they seemed like perfectly normal and happy dogs.

Pavlov eventually divided his dog population into four groups, based on their underlying personality and capacity to form neurosis. Type I were very aggressive and difficult to restrain, easily excitable, even before the experiments began. When confronted with painful or confusing conditioned stimuli, they quickly developed experimental neurosis of the very aggressive, violent type. These were the dogs that, after a period of training, would attack their handlers, who were attempting to bring them to the experimental room.

Type IV, Pavlov reported, tended to be very frightened and nonaggressive, again even before the experiments began. These animals did not socialize well and were easily intimidated by other dogs in the kennel. These, like Type I, proved very susceptible to negative training and, when exposed to negative stimuli, became even more withdrawn, to the point at times of catatonia. They would refuse to eat or move, and at the sight of a handler, they would freeze in fear. They would never show any aggression.

Types II and III were happier dogs, appropriately tough and aggressive if attacked and showing very little fear and anxiety. They socialized well and were neither shy nor overly dominating to other dogs. Interestingly, these "well-balanced" dogs could not be trained to respond to a conditioned stimulus, either positive or negative. Psychologically sound dogs, to use that term, could not be induced to develop neurosis even under the most trying of circumstances; they might not be happy if shocked, but they didn't develop mental illness. They withstood the pressure, the stress, and the training well, and then went about their business as if nothing important had happened.

Pavlov wasn't sure why dogs had different personalities, or why the different types responded so uniquely to conditioning training. It was an important observation, as we shall see.

The next stop in our historical journey brings us to the late Dr. Daniel Funkenstein, a psychiatrist by training, who for years was a professor at Harvard Medical School until his death in 1994. Beginning in the late 1940s, Dr. Funkenstein began investigating the role of autonomic activity in mental illness—an effort that would occupy the better part of the next thirty years.

I had the opportunity to meet Dr. Funkenstein, under the most unusual of circumstances in the fall of 1969, when I was a senior at Brown. Though I was an English major, I had completed the usual premedical requirements and had applied to medical school. It was a very confusing time for me. I had started the previous summer of 1969 with great expectation. One of my professors at Brown had offered me a position for the summer as a research assistant in his laboratory at the great Marine Biology Research Center at Woods Hole, Cape Cod. Woods Hole was a common summer destination for biology professors, because it offered a place to do top-notch research in a rather serene vacation paradise.

It took only a week at Woods Hole to feel I had made a mistake. The work was dreary, dull, and boring. The professor was an invertebrate biologist by trade, and much of our work was very routine, analyzing the color patterns, evaluating—I don't even remember now, but it seemed we were trying to unravel the biochemistry of crab pigments. My professor, who seemed bored himself with his own work, spent much of the time at the beach or hosting barbecues, leaving his assistants to run his tedious experiments. My fellow lab workers, all premeds, seemed to be there only because they all knew it would look so good on their application to have spent a summer at Woods Hole.

Unfortunately, I never tended to think so practically, and after a week I began to feel restless. The great intellectual experience I had rather naïvely anticipated was not going to happen. As the days passed, I grew more restless, more bored, to the point that I dreaded going to the lab. I spent my off time reading not science, but Hemingway and Fitzgerald, and the "artistic" impulses that had periodically plagued me began to rise to the surface.

If this was science, I didn't want it, I remember thinking to myself. I began to question whether I really was by temperament suited for a research, or even a medical career. I remember reading in the lab Hemingway's *A Moveable Feast*, his stories of his youth in Paris, and Durrell's *Alexandria Quartet*, filled with its exotic locales and magic and mysticism. I remember my yearning to be anywhere else but Woods Hole, Massachusetts, studying fiddler crab pigments.

During my stay at the Cape, I shared a room in a boardinghouse in town with another research assistant, whom I hadn't previously known. The manager of the boardinghouse thought we would get along and threw us together. We did get along, quite well, though he seemed much more interested in his work than I was in mine. His father was a very famous novelist who, during the 1950s and early 1960s, had written a series of critically well-received and financially successful novels. One had been made into a highly regarded movie starring Gregory Peck.

I had read several of his books and seen two of the movies based on his novels. His more recent work was not thought to be as good, nor did it sell as well, but nonetheless, to me, the fact that, out of all the hundreds of people who made their way to Cape Cod, I would end up sharing a room with the one student whose father was a novelist seemed to me a sign from heaven.

After about six weeks, I walked into my professor's office and announced I was quitting. He look dumbfounded, even hurt. I think my decision took him completely by surprise. I know he wasn't happy, but in my defense he had done nothing to make the stay anything but drudgery for us, or at least for me.

My parents, in their usual patient way, were very understanding, though they suspected that my laudable goal of a medical career might be tumbling apart. With their support, I ended up spending the rest of my summer in Mexico with my father's family, most of whom lived at the time in Mexico City. In those days, Mexico City was a vibrant, safe, thriving city, filled with hope for the future, a city dominated by art and culture and music. Colorful murals were everywhere, most often depicting the democratic revolutions of the early twentieth century, when a series of military dictatorships were repeatedly fought and finally defeated.

I spent most of the time there with my cousin Juan José, considered a cultural icon in Mexico even then, the finest jazz pianist ever to come out of that country or even Latin America. He was a superb musician, a wonderful man, gentle, kind, shy, almost embarrassed by his fame. So often, we would be walking down the street in Mexico City, and he would be stopped by adoring fans. He would smile shyly, as if he didn't deserve the praise.

The climax of the summer came when Juan José was guest soloist with the National Symphony of Mexico, playing Gershwin's *Rhapsody in Blue* at the Palacio de Bellas Artes, the large concert hall in the center of the city. He played beautifully and flawlessly and received a standing ovation that would not stop. I was so proud of him. I use the past tense, because just as I have been writing this book, Juan José suddenly died of advanced cancer, two weeks after he was diagnosed. There had been no prior symptoms, no signs. One day he couldn't get out of bed, and two weeks later he was dead in a Mexico City hospital. There wasn't even time for proper good-byes.

In 1969, he was very much alive. He was a little older than I was, and a cousin, my blood, as well as a successful artist. He was all I needed to convince me when I returned to Brown in the fall that I needed to follow my heart and do what I had long wanted to do: go off and be a writer, live in wonderful exotic places, and write long and passionate novels. I still applied to medical school that fall, but it was a half-hearted attempt. My senior-year biology courses I found, after the summer with my cousin, intolerable. The literature courses I was taking—the modern novel, for one—I relished.

I met Dr. Funkenstein in November, I believe, of 1969, because he served on the admissions committee at Harvard Medical School and was assigned to interview me. When I learned I was going to be interviewed by a psychiatrist, my heart dropped. Dr. Funkenstein's reputation had long preceded him. Of course, all premeds at Ivy League schools dream about going to Harvard Medical School, for good reasons, because its reputation is of course stellar. Dr. Funkenstein was infamous as the most difficult interviewer at Harvard, or perhaps at any medical school in the country.

The stories were legendary: Dr. Funkenstein asking a student to open a window that had been locked shut, so he could observe how the applicant handled the difficult situation. Dr. Funkenstein arriving forty-five minutes late for an interview appointment, deliberately. Dr. Funkenstein sitting across the desk at an interview, saying nothing. I don't know how many of the many stories I heard were real or not, but he did have a terrifying reputation.

The Dr. Funkenstein I met was nothing like what I had heard. From my application essays, my English literature major, and my family background, he knew of my interests in the arts, and we started at once talking about art, literature, and music. He was obviously very smart, very quick, evidently knowledgeable in a variety of fields other than his own. He was animated and lively. I remember him so well, in his office at Harvard, about 5'10", balding, I estimated in his early sixties at the time.

He seemed to like me immediately. He wanted to know all about my summer in Mexico with my cousin and whether my cousin ever played classical music (he did). He wanted to know about my grandfather, the Mexican revolutionary and well-known cellist. He wanted to know about my interest in Hemingway and Durrell, as well as my own interest in writing. Of course, we also talked about medicine. I remember liking him so much, and trusting him at once, that I told him the truth: that I saw medicine as a wonderful thing, a noble profession, but the reality of science seemed so oppressive.

He agreed with me, that much of research and much of scientific study was ritual, routine, boring—but not all. We talked about some of the great American thinkers, such as William James, who had gone through and taught at Harvard, who themselves had found the actual process of studying medicine very difficult. We talked about doctors who had become writers, such as Keats, and Chekhov, and Celine, and William Carlos Williams.

He told me the admissions committee wanted me at Harvard, but they were concerned that I might just give up medicine to pursue writing. Michael Crichton, the extraordinarily successful writer, had, at the time, recently graduated from Harvard before deciding to give up science completely to move to Hollywood and write his popular novels and screenplays. The admissions committee felt it had been a waste of a Harvard Medical School education. They wanted to produce leaders in medicine and science, not leaders in the literary world.

Dr. Funkenstein, who knew Dr. Crichton well, said his colleagues felt "burnt" by what had happened. I could tell that Dr. Funkenstein did not necessarily agree that there was a problem if a Harvard Medical School graduate achieved fame in a field other than medicine. I think he was proud, by the way he spoke, of Dr. Crichton.

As it turned out, I decided not to go to medical school at that time. I wrote Dr. Funkenstein a note, telling him how much I had enjoyed meeting him, but that a medical career was not something I was going to pursue. I spent the remainder of my senior year studying literature and beginning my first attempt at fiction. I never forgot Dr. Funkenstein, but I also never expected that decades later his research—which we barely discussed at my interview—would prove so important to my work as a physician and scientist.

As I understand his life now, when I met Dr. Funkenstein in 1969 he had already published a series of pioneering and extraordinary papers detailing his work on autonomic physiology. He had already spent twenty years meticulously studying autonomic responses in both normal volunteers—usually Harvard University students looking to contribute to science or make some extra money as a research subject—and patients suffering from a variety of psychiatric disorders.

In his papers such as "Autonomic Nervous System Changes Following Electric Shock Treatment" (1948), "Autonomic Changes Paralleling Psychologic Changes in Mentally Ill Patients" (1951), and "Norepinephrine-Like and Epinephrine-Like

Substances in Psychotic and Psychoneurotic Patients" (1952), Dr. Funkenstein outlined a new model of mental disorders that was based on abnormalities in autonomic nervous system activity. It's interesting that early in his career, Dr. Funkenstein's interest would develop in this way, because most investigators in the mental health field seem proudly determined to ignore completely the autonomic system in their pronouncements and in their theories. Funkenstein suspected such disregard was a mistake.

His achievements, though apparently ignored or forgotten by most of his colleagues, were many. One of the most important was his design of a simple test during the 1940s to measure autonomic system function. This may seem like an unremarkable accomplishment, but prior to Funkenstein, there really weren't simple, accurate, reliable methods to test the responses of the sympathetic and parasympathetic systems in a controlled, scientific environment. Any good research effort requires that you be able to measure what you're testing, and for the autonomic nervous system, that had been a major obstacle.

Funkenstein's approach was simple but elegant. Scientists by the 1940s already knew that the sympathetic and parasympathetic nerves regulated blood pressure, sympathetic activity pushing it up and parasympathetic firing pushing it down. This was well documented. During the 1940s, hypertension was already being recognized as a common problem, and in fact President Franklin Roosevelt had died suddenly from a stroke brought on by persistent hypertension. Researchers had already developed a few drugs that seemed to lower high blood pressure, and Funkenstein focused his attention on these.

He eventually decided to study the effect of the medication mecholyl, an antihypertensive medication already in clinical use. The drug wasn't very convenient to use, because it had to be injected intramuscularly, but it was one of the first drugs that consistently could be used to reduce dangerously high pressure. It seemed to work not on the heart or brain, but on the peripheral arterioles, causing them to dilate. With this, the resistance of the small vessels to blood flow was reduced, and additionally, blood could more easily pool in the vasculature. The result was less blood returning to the heart, blood being pumped against lowered resistance, and lowered blood pressure.

No one before Funkenstein had tested the drug in populations with normal blood pressure, but Funkenstein suspected that if the drug were given to such individuals, the pressure would indeed drop, but then the baroreceptors would turn off, reducing their inhibitory action on sympathetic firing. The sympathetic system would kick in, in an attempt to override the drop in pressure, and bring the pressure back up to normal.

Funkenstein suspected that an individual's response to mecholyl—how quickly and how much the blood pressure dropped, and how quickly it returned to normal—might tell him something about the relative strength, or weakness, of the sympathetic and parasympathetic system. He was, as it turned out, prophetically right.

In a series of experiments beginning in the late 1940s, Dr. Funkenstein and his colleagues repeatedly gave a standard dose of mecholyl to hundreds of normal volunteer subjects, as well as patients with psychiatric disorders, and tracked carefully the effect of the drug on blood pressure. Invariably, Funkenstein observed that responses and responders in both the normals and patients tended to fall into three distinct groups, even though the dose of the drug was always the same. In Group I, as Funkenstein labeled the subjects, the blood pressure would drop slightly from the baseline reading, then quickly, within three to five minutes, come back to the original level and then shoot above the baseline.

In Group II, there was a greater drop in blood pressure, before the level would gradually, within about five to eight minutes, return to baseline. In these subjects, there was no overshooting; the pressure returned to the original level and stayed there. In Group III, the pressure dropped to very low levels, then stayed there, never, even after fifteen minutes, returning to the original baseline. In test after test, Funkenstein saw the same three groups of responders, each reacting to the same dose of the same drug very differently!

Funkenstein assumed, correctly, that subjects falling into Group I had a very strong sympathetic nervous system and a correspondingly weak parasympathetic. That would explain the minimal drop in pressure, the rapid return to normal, and the overshooting. He suspected the overshooting resulted because the inhibitory effect of the baroreceptors on the sympathetic system was very weak, so that when the pressure dropped and the baroreceptors turned off, there would be an excess of sympathetic firing.

Subjects in Group II, Funkenstein believed, had a more balanced autonomic system, with the sympathetic and parasympathetic systems equally as strong, equally as responsive. When the pressure dropped, the baroreceptors would tone down and sympathetic inhibition would be reduced, but not excessively so. The pressure would appropriately return to normal but not overshoot. In Group III, the sympathetic system was unusually weak, and the parasympathetic system strong, so when the drug pushed the pressure down, the sympathetic system would not kick in and there would be only a gradual and slight rise in pressure toward the baseline, though it never went back to the starting point.

Funkenstein labeled his Group I as sympathetic "hyper-responders" and his Group III sympathetic "hypo-responders," in homage to the relative strength of the sympathetic nerves specifically. Overall, in his testing of normal volunteers, the greatest number, between 80 and 90 percent, of subjects fell into Group II, with a balanced autonomic system, with smaller numbers in groups I and III.

Dr. Funkenstein, creative scientist that he always was, observed the responses of his normal volunteers under a variety of circumstances, some relaxed, some stressful—such as before exam time at Harvard, or during a deliberately stressful interview with one of the supervising scientists. He began to realize that the subjects in each group tended to have very distinctive personalities and unique ways of dealing with stress. Subjects in Group I, with the strong sympathetic system, were very aggressive, often hostile, and "angry at other people," particularly when under stress, blaming others always for their discomfort.

Those in Group III, even under relaxed testing conditions, tended to be melancholic, anxious, and very passive and, when under stress, lapsed into depression, while always blaming themselves, not others, for their discomfort. Those in Group II, the balanced reactors, tended to take things in stride, dealing with stress well, becoming neither angry nor self-hating, but simply attempting to deal with the situation as best as they could. They dealt with the stress and moved on to the next task at hand. So consistent were these reactions that Funkenstein labeled those in Group I as displaying "anger out," and those in Group III as feeling "anger in," directed toward themselves.

Of course, what Funkenstein had done, in his Harvard clinic, was to describe differing levels of sympathetic and parasympathetic dominance, and different personalities to go along with it! He had done so clearly, objectively, scientifically, and reproducibly. And he began to believe that the autonomic nervous system—not the brain, its cortex, or Freud's unconscious—perhaps to a very large degree, determined our personalities, how we behave, and how we respond to life and its stresses.

Funkenstein then turned his attention to psychiatric patients—again with normal blood pressure—whom he put through the same routine of testing mecholyl, under both relaxed and stressful circumstances. He used a population diagnosed with a variety of illnesses, including depression and schizophrenia, and invariably he found that the patients, like the normal volunteers, fell into three general groups: the sympathetic hyper-responders (with a weak parasympathetic system), the balanced autonomic group, and the sympathetic hypo-responders (with a strong parasympathetic system).

However, the distribution of the patients was quite different from that of the student subjects. In the normals, remember, 80 to 90 percent of subjects fell into the "balanced" category, but in the patients, the number of Group II was considerably less, ranging, depending on the study, from about 30 to 50 percent, but no higher. Far more patients fell into the Group I and Group III categories, with an imbalanced autonomic system. Funkenstein's studies indicated that autonomic imbalance routinely accompanied mental illness and, he began to believe, might be a cause!

Funkenstein observed that his depressed patients routinely and invariably fell into Group III, the sympathetic hypo-responders. Schizophrenics seemed to be evenly divided between groups I and III, but long-term, chronic schizophrenics tended to be Group III responders. Funkenstein also noticed that when these mentally ill patients improved, whatever their underlying illness, their response to mecholyl and, in turn, their autonomic grouping changed, inevitably toward Group II, that of the balanced responders. Mental illness, Funkenstein seemed to be witnessing, occurred when the autonomic system was out of balance, and mental health returned when the two systems came into balance.

As early as the late 1940s, Dr. Funkenstein performed a series of studies on patients before and after they received electroshock therapy. Though widely controversial today, and in some circles portrayed as barbaric, for many years, before the advent of the antidepressant class of medications, electroshock was a commonly used and at times effective treatment for certain forms of mental illness, particularly depression—though until Funkenstein, no one seemed sure how it might work. Funkenstein would, in his test subjects, administer the mecholyl test before treatment, and then afterward, and assess the change in response.

He made several observations. First, he noted that the treatment worked only for those patients who initially were sympathetic hypo-responders, placing them in Group III. These would include the vast majority of patients with depression and the Group III schizophrenics. After treatment, he noted that if there was an improvement, the patients then responded to mecholyl as if they now had a balanced autonomic system, with neither system hyper- or hypo-reactive. Group I patients receiving electroshock, usually schizophrenics or other psychotics, invariably had a worsening of symptoms!

Funkenstein realized that electroshock treatment stimulated the sympathetic nervous system, a boon particularly to depressed Group III patients with a weak sympathetic response but a disaster to those in Group I with an overly strong sympathetic system. Similarly, he found that tranquilizers helped sympathetic hyper-reactors of Group I but made the Group III hypo-reactors worse. Tranquilizers, he realized, suppressed the sympathetic nerves, useful for those in Group I but a nightmare for those in Group III whose sympathetic system was already too weak. Such drugs turned Group I patients into Group II balanced responders in the mecholyl test.

Interestingly, Funkenstein appears to have discovered that the Group I patients, those with the strong sympathetic system, tended to respond best to psychotherapy—which, if effective, seemed to calm down their overly active sympathetic nerves. Psychotherapy, like tranquilizing drugs, tended to turn these patients into Group II mecholyl reactors. Thus, Funkenstein had not only isolated and identified different autonomic groups but also carefully documented their unique responses to different treatments. He could, in essence, predict which patients, based on their response to mecholyl, would respond to what treatment. This, to me, was an extraordinary accomplishment that, had it been taken more seriously, would have changed the course of psychiatry forever.

Despite his position at Harvard and his groundbreaking publications, Funkenstein's autonomic approach to mental illness was never widely accepted. Instead, psychiatry went off to chase neurotransmitters, believing that the answer to all mental illness would be found in these molecules and how they worked. The physiological approach never became dominant, I believe, tragically.

There was however, at least one fellow scientist working at the same time, during the 1940s, '50s, and '60s, who did take Funkenstein very seriously. That would be the pioneering neurophysiologist Ernst Gellhorn, MD, PhD, who for years toiled to untangle the complexities of autonomic function and autonomic balance. In a strange twist, one of those coincidences that seem to govern my life, I am brought again back to Robert A. Good, my former mentor. It was at the University of Minnesota during the

1940s, '50s, and '60s, where and when Dr. Good studied and worked until moving to Sloan Kettering, that Ernst Gellhorn did much of his most outstanding research.

In Memory of Robert A. Good

I have always been amazed by the ironies and coincidences that follow my life. While I was writing this essay, shortly after I had finished my autobiographical section, my mentor and guide, Robert Good, MD, PhD, died of esophageal cancer on June 19, 2003, at his home in St. Petersburg, Florida. He was thereafter honored in lengthy obituaries, including one in the *New York Times* that referred to this great scientist as the Father of Immunology, a title he without doubt deserved.

Dr. Good's accomplishments were indeed astounding. He received his combined MD-PhD degrees at age twenty-five at the University of Minnesota (the PhD in physiology). He subsequently trained as a pediatrician but from the beginning of his career concentrated his efforts on research. From early on, he excelled not only in physiology but also in microbiology and pathology as well as the infant science of immunology. For years, he was chairman of the department of pathology at the University of Minnesota, though he had never pursued a formal residency in pathology. He once told me over dinner that he was so intrigued by pathology that he had done more than one hundred autopsies with the pathologists at Minnesota so that he might truly understand this discipline.

Though his accomplishments crossed many boundaries, during the 1950s he began to make his name for his research in immunology, which at that time was still in its infancy as a scientific discipline. It was Dr. Good and his colleagues who discovered that the thymus was not a useless vestigial organ, as previously thought, but the center for the body's immune control. He proved as well that the tonsils were an important immune organ and was one of the first to argue against their routine removal—a warning ignored by my own doctor, who arranged that my sister, my brother, and I should all have this "trivial" gland cut out. Subsequent studies in Europe confirmed Good's advice, showing that populations without their tonsils have much higher levels of many diseases, including cancer, than those who still have the glands intact. Importantly, Dr. Good, with his colleagues, performed the first bone marrow transplant at Minnesota in 1969, essentially opening up an entire new branch of medicine.

Dr. Good came to Sloan Kettering in 1973 to great acclaim, with great promise and with unprecedented media attention. Besides his *Time* magazine cover, in those days he could be seen routinely on TV, earnestly discussing his latest findings and hopes for the future. He was indeed always earnest. Dr. Good was charismatic and affected everyone who came into contact with him—students, colleagues, friends.

There are indeed many very bright and very brilliant men and women in medical research, individuals of great accomplishment and great dedication. Of course, Dr. Good had all those qualities, but he had far more, a hunger for knowledge, for new ideas, for new intellectual experiences. That's why, I know, he supported my own somewhat unconventional research for so long.

He also was the most prolific author in the history of the biomedical sciences. Dr. Good published more than two thousand papers in the scientific journals, authoring or coauthoring fifty books, a record I doubt anyone will ever beat. He was a good writer, publishing in fields ranging from organ transplantation to zinc metabolism. I went to Cornell because of Dr. Good's enthusiasm for nutrition, an interest that developed long before the subject became acceptable in academic circles.

Dr. Good was an unusual man for other reasons. He loved to travel, and by the time I worked under him during the 1980s, I don't think there was a place on earth he hadn't been. He traveled constantly, to attend international conferences, to lecture abroad, to meet with fellow scientists and world leaders. After every return, he would talk with great animation about what he had learned and what he had seen, and the fascinating and brilliant people he had met, even the new food he had tasted. During the 1970s, he was one of the first American scientists to travel extensively through China as a guest of the Chinese government.

He also loved good food and wine and was himself a superb cook whose greatest pleasure was, it seemed to me at least, to cook up a meal for a group of some of his many cherished friends. When I was in Oklahoma with Dr. Good, he hosted a party at his home for the late Lewis Thomas, who was still president of the Memorial Sloan Kettering Cancer Center, as well as an award-winning author. Dr. Good did all the cooking and loved every minute of it. The meal was perfect, with a number of courses, including baked salmon as the main event. Dr. Thomas may have been the honored guest, but Dr. Good made the party. He loved to be surrounded by people: his family, his students, and particularly his colleagues.

Dr. Good had many extraordinary qualities—his intelligence, of course, but also his drive, his ambition, his ability to inspire others, and his charisma—but there is one quality I found always most unusual. Dr. Good, despite his achievements, despite his position, despite the adulation poured on him, approached life always as a student, as if each day was a chance to learn something new and exciting. In any medical center, there are, in any given week, many lectures to attend, given by staff scientists and physicians or visiting academic dignitaries. Particularly, when Dr. Good ran Sloan Kettering, and later, at the University of Oklahoma and then at All Children's Hospital in Florida, Dr. Good attracted many fine lecturers doing all types of work in many areas of medicine. The lecture schedule, when Dr. Good was around, was always full and usually interesting.

At these lectures, Dr. Good always sat in the front row, in the middle. He invariably carried with him a legal yellow pad, and no matter what the topic, Dr. Good would listen intently as if the subject were without doubt the most interesting topic ever presented. He always wrote copious notes, whatever the topic. He once told me, a daydreamer who usually sat in the back, that there is no point in going to a lecture if you're not going to sit up front "where the action is."

After he said that, I would sit with him, with my own yellow pad, taking notes. I could never generate the honest enthusiasm he had no matter how dry the presentation or esoteric the topic. I once asked him what he did with his legal pads, and he laughed. "I read them," he said, not really answering the question.

I figured he had over the years attended thousands of lectures all over the world, and I wanted to know whether those yellow pads with his handwritten notes ended up in the garbage, or were stored away in some extraordinary site somewhere. Those yellow pads, I knew, would make a very personal history of medicine in the twentieth century as seen through the eyes of one of its great leaders. Unfortunately, I never did learn the fate of the yellow pads.

Certainly, Dr. Good deserved to win the Nobel Prize many times over, for any number of his discoveries. Though nominated three times, he never did get the ultimate medical honor. I know this bothered him, particularly because the reason had more to do with politics than his achievements. It was only shortly after Dr. Good arrived at Sloan Kettering that he became the center of a well-known scandal, perhaps the most sensational scandal in medicine of the twentieth century, which tarnished his reputation to the day he died.

He had supported a young physician researcher by the name of Dr. Summerlin, an apparently bright young man who appeared to be on the verge of greatness. In his preliminary research at Sloan Kettering, supported by Dr. Good, Dr. Summerlin seemed to have uncovered a method to allow transplantation of tissues and organs between genetically unrelated animals. Remember, normally, a transplant of tissue between such animals will be rejected as a foreign invader. Immune rejection placed, and still places, formidable limits on transplantation medicine. Summerlin seemed to have solved the problem.

In a dramatic gesture, in 1974—after Dr. Good had been at Sloan Kettering only a year—Summerlin presented the proof that he had solved the transplantation riddle. Right in Dr. Good's office in the Sloan Kettering building, he showed a white mouse with a black patch of skin, which Summerlin proudly announced had been transplanted from a mouse with black skin, without rejection! The buzz at Memorial, and in the scientific community, I understand—because this is long before I worked under Dr. Good—was electric. The only problem was that a technician became suspicious and was able to wipe the black color off the white mouse's skin with an alcohol swab. It was a hoax: Summerlin had colored the skin with a black felt pen, and Dr. Good had not seen the fraud.

News of the deception hit the scientific community, and the media, with an explosion. I was a journalist at the time and remember the story well. Part of the problem, as I have heard, is that Dr. Good was already talking up Summerlin's supposedly extraordinary discovery among his colleagues, so when the truth came out, Dr. Good tragically looked foolish, though he himself had had nothing to do with the actual fraud. His mistake was that he believed Summerlin.

A subsequent inquiry at Sloan Kettering absolved Dr. Good of any direct involvement with the deception but did reprimand him for not supervising his students and underlings more closely. He was allowed to continue at Sloan Kettering as president, but the damage was done. The media continued having a field day with the scandal, as always, I suspect, enjoying the prospect of making a great man look foolish. A book came out sometime later, *The Patchwork Mouse*, chronicling the whole sorry affair.

I know the Summerlin fiasco haunted Dr. Good, in many ways. During the summer after my third year of medical school, I had with great enthusiasm told my advisor that Dr. Good, the president of Sloan Kettering, had agreed to support and supervise an independent study of Dr. Kelley. I felt honored. My advisor laughed at me, dismissing Good as "a has been" who was "finished in medicine." He used other derogatory terms I would rather not mention, and all this from a middle-level associate professor who never had done anything memorable in his career. I chose to ignore my advisor and follow my instincts—a course of action that caused me enormous trouble, but that I have never, not for one second, regretted.

Years later, this scandal continued to affect Dr. Good's career. I think it was likely one of the reasons he was finally told to leave Sloan Kettering. I think the way he was fired was terrible. He had trouble finding a job worthy of his talents and background after he was terminated at Sloan; he took the job at the University of Oklahoma, where he was asked to set up a cancer research section, because he felt he could build something from the beginning. I know he was hurt, deeply, and I know he missed New York. His wife told me that, when they first arrived in Oklahoma, he cried daily because he felt so rejected by his profession.

It was this awful scandal that I and others believe ultimately cost Dr. Good the Nobel Prize. After the Summerlin affair, he simply wasn't going to get it, ever, despite three nominations. I think, knowing him as I did, that there was enormous jealousy from colleagues for any number of reasons. First and foremost, Dr. Good had the gall to be so good in so many different fields—something rare, of course, in medical research. But perhaps even more, he had a quality of greatness that always evokes contempt in lesser souls.

I know also that the Summerlin affair, fifteen years later, ultimately affected the way Dr. Good responded to me and my determined efforts to have Kelley's work properly evaluated, tested, and, if it was found to be of value, mainstreamed. Dr. Good had been far more than a teacher to me. He was a mentor, but a mentor who did far more than any mentor—particularly one of his stature—would ever be expected to do. During my internship year, he invited me to spend Christmas with him, his family, and his kids. That was a kind gesture, a gesture I will never forget. He knew at the time how difficult I found my internship and the routine of medicine, and how I longed to be in research, resuming my Kelley project. He knew I needed a few days away, and he was right.

When I joined his group in Oklahoma, I lived in his house for weeks, until I found a place to live. He didn't have to do that. He accepted me as part of his family, I would not be so pretentious to say like a son, but at least like an intellectual son, someone he cared about and cared for. We would sit at breakfast and at dinner and talk science, and medicine, and Kelley, and pancreatic enzymes. He wanted to hear the whole history of Dr. Beard, and his theory, and how Kelley had learned about Beard, and how Kelley had treated his own presumed pancreatic cancer.

He wanted to hear, over and over again, about the cases I had uncovered in Kelley's office files. During this time, I was in Oklahoma City, as far away from New York as I could imagine being, but it didn't matter because I would have gone anywhere to work under Dr. Good. When he asked me to follow him to Florida, I agreed happily, immediately. Just as his group was moving to Florida, I got married, in Virginia, with Dr. Good serving as best man. He didn't have to do that, either, but that was the kind of man he was.

I knew, however, that his attitude began to change when I tried to publish my Kelley monograph that I had completed under his supervision. I initially approached editors of medical journals and medical texts whom Dr. Good knew well. In each case, the editors chose not to write to me, but directly to Dr. Good. He read some of the letters to me; his "friends" warned him that this had to be fraudulent, that I was conning him, and that he was about to find himself involved in another terrible scandal. Dr. Good just didn't have the stomach to fight my battles, and I accepted it wasn't his job. That's one reason I returned to New York.

Then, when my work began generating interest, and inevitably controversy, Dr. Good backed off even more. I know that Victor Herbert had contacted him repeatedly, trying to poison Dr. Good's opinion of my work. I heard that Dr. Good had "renounced" my efforts, an odd turn of events because never during my five years working with him did he ever express anything but support for my investigation of Kelley.

I then witnessed Good's dismissive comments on national television, when he, to my embarrassment, tried to minimize his relationship with me as well as any value in my five-year study. It was a shame, and it left me feeling saddened that Dr. Good, instead of defending me, chose instead to protect himself by going on the attack. His statements, which he knew weren't true, had, I remember, a sad quality—not the words I would have expected from the great scientist he was.

At one point, he sent out a document to selected colleagues, announcing that my work had no scientific basis by any standard he knew, a statement that I again found sad, because he had always told me that great, new ideas that change medicine are always going to be revolutionary and at odds with the science that went before. He was the one who taught me that the fact that a new idea doesn't fit what we believed doesn't matter. He knew that, so well.

It's ironic that Dr. Good should have felt the way he did, because so much of what I do in my office today, and what Kelley did in the past, had been proposed fifty years ago by his colleague at Minnesota—irony of ironies—Dr. Ernst Gellhorn. Dr. Gellhorn, like Dr. Good, had both an MD and a PhD and was a professor of physiology at the University of Minnesota Medical School during the period when Dr. Good was first a medical student, then a doctoral student in Dr. Gellhorn's very own department, and eventually a professor at the same medical school! There is no question that they knew each other, because so much of Dr. Good's early work was in physiology, and because both were so prominent at the same medical center.

I suspect, as erudite a man as Dr. Good was, and as wide ranging as his interests were, that he probably never paid much attention to what Dr. Gellhorn was doing. I know that when I would discuss Pottenger's and Kelley's concepts of autonomic balancing, the thoughts seemed very foreign to Dr. Good. I suspect that if Dr. Good had paid any attention at all to Gellhorn's work, it must have seemed peculiar, far out of the mainstream of most academic research.

Who was Dr. Gellhorn, and why is he important to this story? Dr. Gellhorn was one of the preeminent experts in autonomic physiology, a man who spent the better part of his professional life investigating the mysteries of the way this system works. But more importantly, he laid out, in study after study, in paper after paper, and in book after book, the concept that this collection of nerves might be the foundation for much if not most human behavior—and that imbalance in this system might be at the root of much human illness.

I am repeatedly astounded at the coincidences in my life. I have purchased most of Dr. Gellhorn's books, which are long out of print, from secondhand book services. One has the name of a previous owner on the frontispiece, and that owner was none other than Dr. Good's brother, also a physician trained at Minnesota.

Dr. Ernst Gellhorn and Autonomic Tuning

Ernst Gellhorn was born in 1893 in Breslau, Germany. He received his MD degree from the eminent German institute, Heidelberg University, and his PhD from the University of Muenster. He taught in medical schools in Germany until 1929, when he immigrated to the United States to become professor of physiology at the University of Oregon. He moved to the University of Illinois in 1932, then to Minnesota in 1943—while Dr. Good was still a medical student. At Minnesota, he was appointed professor of neurophysiology. He stayed at Minnesota until retiring in 1960, with professor emeritus status.

His initial research efforts, both in Europe and in the United States, were in the traditional physiology of the day—in subjects such as muscle contraction and the physiology of cell membranes. In Illinois, and subsequently during his tenure at Minnesota, he switched gears, thereafter focusing entirely on autonomic function, an area of interest he pursued until his death in 1973. He was a prolific writer, if not as prolific as Dr. Good, authoring more than four hundred scientific papers and nine books that I know of. His monographs include *Autonomic Regulations* (1943), *Physiological Foundations of Neurology and Psychiatry* (1953), *Autonomic Imbalance and the Hypothalamus* (1957), and *Emotions and Emotional Disorders: A Neurophysiological Study* (1963). (For more biographical information, see the University of Minnesota Senate Minutes, May 24, 1973, announcing Dr. Gellhorn's passing.)

Dr. Gellhorn's earlier work in autonomic physiology centered on the role of the brainstem and hypothalamus in regulating both the sympathetic and the parasympathetic systems. He first documented that autonomic activity can occur as a reflex, such as the baroreceptor reflex, at the level of the medulla. Here, reactions are very fast, to respond to changes in metabolism—such as lowered blood pressure from blood loss—without any information from the thinking areas of the cerebral cortex. Much of this has been confirmed, and today we know that brainstem autonomic centers such as the nucleus tractus solitarius can regulate, without the need for input from any higher brain centers, such activities as blood pressure, heart rate, breathing, secretion and contraction in the GI tract, and bladder function (Guyton 1956, 106).

If you were to transect the brain at the top of the brainstem—in effect putting an end to any input from the higher centers—we could still maintain normal blood pressure, digest food (though we couldn't feed ourselves), and urinate. Brainstem nuclei, remember, connect directly to the sympathetic and parasympathetic preganglionic nerve cell bodies, which are the starting point for the entire autonomic system.

But Gellhorn, more than any other investigator at the time, carefully documented that though the brainstem could do a lot on its own, the hypothalamus in a normal brain had ultimate control over brainstem autonomic centers. In the hypothalamus, just as in the brainstem, there are centers for cardiovascular function, for digestion, for glandular secretion, and for the bladder. The hypothalamic centers aren't simply redundant duplicates of the brainstem areas, spare tires so to speak.

Remember, the hypothalamus sits literally at the crossroads between the lower brainstem areas, which are involved in basic unconscious physiological responses, and the higher levels of the cerebral cortex, our sophisticated "thinking" brain. It receives sensory input from both the brainstem, lower down, and from the cerebral centers, higher up. This information originates, as we have seen, in all corners of the body—in the pain, temperature, and touch receptors of the skin; in the proprioceptors of the muscles; and in the mechanoreceptors, pressure, and chemoreceptors of the internal organs.

Information coming in from higher up in the cortex can begin in the nerves for the special senses of the head, which carry impulses related to smell, vision, taste, and sound. All this funnels into the hypothalamus, from both above and below. In addition, our own thoughts and perusings, which are the province of the frontal and temporal areas of the cortex, can set off action potentials that also make their way downward to the hypothalamus. It is in a pivotal position, anatomically, and in a critical position functionally.

Gellhorn realized that, in the hypothalamus, the mass of incoming information from the brainstem and the cortex—and it is a huge amount of information every minute—is beautifully and quickly sorted out. An appropriate response is then determined. However, neurons in the hypothalamic centers do not connect directly—as do those of the brainstem—to autonomic nerves. Instead, they travel downward and end in the various brainstem nuclei, which in turn synapse onto the preganglionic autonomic neurons. In this way, the hypothalamus exerts control over the brainstem and the autonomic system at large.

In essence, Gellhorn carefully, over the years of his research, documented that there were at least two levels of control of autonomic activities: at the brainstem level and in the hypothalamus, with the hypothalamus in charge. I like to think of the brainstem as the captain of an infantry company who is given responsibility to react in the field as needed, in a very limited, local way, and to give orders to subordinates in response to immediate crises. The hypothalamus is more like a colonel who has a greater picture of the entire field and the flow of troops and can override the captain or change the orders as needed. They are both officers and both have authority over troops, but one has a greater authority.

Gellhorn learned that the hypothalamus does not only regulate the autonomic centers in the brainstem and ultimately the autonomic nerves themselves. In a series of very elegant experiments, he uncovered that different parts of the hypothalamus affect autonomic function differently. In laboratory animals such as rats and cats, he surgically inserted tiny cannulas, or tubes, directly into different parts of the hypothalamus. This allowed him to inject different drugs directly into specific areas of the hypothalamus, while at the same time monitoring the effect. When he injected Pentothal, a powerful tranquilizing drug related to phenobarbital, into the anterior, or front half, of the hypothalamus, the parasympathetic system would turn off and sympathetic activity would increase. The pulse and blood pressure of the animals would rise, and the animals would become more alert, more hostile, more aggressive.

However, if he injected phenobarbital into the posterior hypothalamus, the exact opposite response followed. In this case, the sympathetic tone would diminish and that of the parasympathetic system would increase. Pulse and blood pressure would fall and the animals would become nonaggressive and docile; they might even fall asleep. He also performed experiments in which he inserted a small electrode into either the anterior or the posterior hypothalamus. These probes would allow him to stimulate a particular area repeatedly.

When the anterior hypothalamus was electrically stimulated, the parasympathetic system would become strongly active, and the sympathetic system weak. When he sent currents into the posterior hypothalamus, he observed the opposite response. Dr. Gellhorn designed a variety of experiments, injecting stimulants as well as tranquilizers into the anterior and posterior hypothalamus. He also was able, using certain high electrical currents, to actually destroy specific regions. He repeatedly came to the same conclusion in many experiments and with different species of laboratory animals.

All this difficult laboratory work led Dr. Gellhorn to formulate what now is taken as law among neurophysiologists, that the anterior hypothalamus controls the parasympathetic system, and when it is active, parasympathetic nerves become active. On the other hand, the posterior hypothalamus regulates the sympathetic system, and when it is active, the sympathetic nerves fire.

From these experiments, Dr. Gellhorn also formulated his "law of reciprocity." Scientists long before Gellhorn, such as Langley, had already reported the opposing actions of the sympathetic and parasympathetic system: when one system fires, the other is inhibited. No one really understood how this might happen in the nervous system. Gellhorn's experiments taught him, first, that the anterior and posterior hypothalamus controlled the parasympathetic and sympathetic systems, respectively, but also that when one half of the hypothalamus was active, the other half was inhibited by nerves that connected the two areas.

When for example, the anterior hypothalamus and, in turn, the parasympathetic system are firing, through such reciprocal innervation, the posterior is inhibited, and vice versa. I have already mentioned this relationship, when I earlier discussed the hypothalamus. This law, this phenomenon, was another one of Dr. Gellhorn's firsts, and a very important one in our understanding of autonomic function. Now scientists knew why, when one branch of the autonomic system was busily firing, the other turned off. It happened in the hypothalamus.

I would like to quote Dr. Gellhorn's own pronouncement of the reciprocity principle, appearing in *Principles of Autonomic-Somatic Integrations* (Gellhorn 1967, 24–25):

> Lesions in the posterior hypothalamus . . . lead to an increased parasympathetic reactivity of the anterior hypothalamus. Conversely, lesions in the anterior hypothalamus cause a release of the sympathetic division of the hypothalamus. Moreover, states of increased reactivity of the posterior hypothalamus are associated with a lessened responsiveness of the anterior hypothalamus and vice versa.

In this way, Gellhorn carefully demonstrated that the hypothalamus orchestrates, like a conductor, much of what goes in the brainstem autonomic centers and, globally, in the autonomic system itself. This, in a sense, means that the hypothalamus intricately regulates what is going on "lower down" in the brain and in the autonomic nerves that travel outward to the organs, tissues, and glands of the body. This was certainly an important lesson to have learned, more than most of us could hope to achieve if we lived a scientist's lifetime. For Gellhorn, this was still only the beginning.

In his experiments, Dr. Gellhorn was, in the case of tranquilizing drugs or electrical ablation, directly inhibiting one of the two halves of the hypothalamus.

With stimulating drugs such as Metrazol or mild electrical currents, he was directly stimulating a target area in the hypothalamus. Of course, such laboratory models were—and are—extraordinarily useful, determining what happens when the hypothalamus is either inhibited or stimulated. Again, directly, they did not prove, as Gellhorn knew, that the hypothalamus indeed responds from impulses coming from above and below. It was already known that there were neuron connections from both the cortex and the brainstem to the hypothalamus, but nobody before Gellhorn was quite sure what these nerves did.

In a number of laboratory investigations, Gellhorn devised a method to stimulate the cerebral cortex itself, while measuring what was going on specifically in the hypothalamus with an electroencephalogram (EEG), an instrument that measures naturally occurring electrical activity in the brain. He could adjust the EEG so that it specifically measured only hypothalamus responses. In one series of experiments, he applied the poison strychnine directly to areas of the cerebral cortex. Strychnine was already known in Gellhorn's day to be a very potent stimulant of nerve activity that, when applied directly even to a small area of the cortex, would cause the entire cortex to become diffusely, to use Gellhorn's word, active.

Every time he performed this experiment, the posterior hypothalamus, and the sympathetic system under its control, would start firing, and the anterior hypothalamus, along with the parasympathetic system, would become quiet. On the other hand, if he applied a tranquilizing drug such as Pentothal directly to the cortex, cortical impulses diffusely diminished, the animal would become somnolent, and the anterior hypothalamic and parasympathetic impulses increased, while the posterior pituitary and sympathetic system turned off.

Though these results did indicate the hypothalamus responded to cortical influence, he knew his laboratory model represented a very artificial situation. We, and most animals, don't walk around with strychnine or tranquilizing drugs inserted directly onto the brain surface. But creative scientist that he was, he developed another approach, which told him how the cortex influenced the hypothalamus and, in turn, the autonomic system under far less artificial conditions. It had been known for decades that information on sound travels to the auditory cortex via cranial nerve VIII, the auditory nerve. EEG recordings had shown that any loud noise, such as the ringing of a bell, caused increased nerve firing not only in the auditory cortex, but also throughout the cortex. The sympathetic nerves would also become active. Laboratory animals exposed to irritating noise invariably became very alert and aggressive.

Gellhorn then exposed a variety of laboratory animals to loud disruptive noises while monitoring hypothalamic EEG recordings. Invariably, he found that first the cortex became activated, then the posterior hypothalamus, and then the sympathetic nerves. If he tranquilized the posterior hypothalamus specifically with Pentothal, however, the posterior hypothalamus stopped firing, and the sympathetic nerves became quiet. The cortex, as sophisticated as it is, could not influence the autonomic system, except through the hypothalamus. In such experiments, repeated over a number of years, Dr. Gellhorn demonstrated that indeed the hypothalamus responded to impulses coming in from virtually all areas of the cerebral cortex. That was an important fact to have documented.

He then sought to prove that the hypothalamus did indeed react to sensory information coming in from lower down, from the brainstem, and in turn directly determined how the autonomic system would respond. By the early 1950s, Dr. Gellhorn was very much aware of the pioneering work of Dr. Funkenstein at Harvard, who had used the mecholyl test to measure sympathetic reactivity in his test subjects. Mecholyl, remember, was a drug used to lower blood pressure.

It was Gellhorn who proposed that Dr. Funkenstein, in his various experiments, was observing the effect of reduced blood pressure on the baroreceptors, which in turn controlled sympathetic responses. When the pressure fell, the baroreceptors turned off and their inhibiting effect on sympathetic centers in the brainstem lessened. In turn, the sympathetic nerves fired, attempting to bring pressure back to "normal."

Gellhorn clearly saw the importance of Funkenstein's finding that both patients and normals fell into three distinct groups based on sympathetic activity: Group I, the sympathetic hyper-responders; Group II, the balanced responders; and Group III, the sympathetic hypo-responders. Gellhorn himself, in investigations with both patients suffering mental illness and normals, repeated Funkenstein's experiments at the University of Minnesota, using a far larger number of patients. He too, found what Funkenstein had first reported—that both normals and mentally ill patients could be divided into three groups, based on sympathetic responsiveness. He too found that far more normal subjects tended to fall into Group II, with a balanced autonomic nervous system, than the patients, who far more frequently were either sympathetic hyper- or sympathetic hypo-responders. Gellhorn was convinced that autonomic imbalance was the cause of the patient's illness.

As I read through his writings, covering several decades of this thinking, I can see how deeply affected Gellhorn was by these findings. He thought that Funkenstein was on to something very important, not just to psychiatry, but also to medicine in general. He repeated the test over and over again, in far more patients than Funkenstein himself had studied, and also took Funkenstein's testing approach to another level. He knew that Funkenstein was measuring sympathetic reactivity, but not that of the parasympathetic system.

Indirectly, Gellhorn knew one could assume that the parasympathetic would be behaving in a contrary, or opposite way. If the sympathetic system was hyperactive, the parasympathetic system would be hypoactive, and so on. The contrary behavior of the two systems had been known for fifty years at that point. The mecholyl test still really measured only sympathetic reactions; parasympathetic responsiveness could only be inferred.

Until, that is, Gellhorn devised a method of measuring parasympathetic reactivity. He began injecting norepinephrine, the sympathetic neurotransmitter that had been isolated at the beginning of the twentieth century, into both laboratory animals and then human volunteers. He had postulated that whereas mecholyl would lower blood pressure, hence setting off a sympathetic counterresponse in subjects with normal blood pressure, norepinephrine would raise the blood pressure, through its direct action on the heart and on the vasculature. This pressure increase would stimulate the baroreceptors to fire more aggressively, in turn further inhibiting the sympathetic nerves while directly activating the parasympathetic nerves. This would lower the blood pressure back toward normal. This test, he thought, would be a measure of parasympathetic responsiveness.

Gellhorn found his norepinephrine approach worked well, and again, his normal subjects and patients fell into three neat groups: parasympathetic hyper-responders, balanced autonomic responders, and parasympathetic hypo-responders. Again, most normals fell into the balanced category, while far more patients fell into the hyper- and hypo-responder groups. They correlated precisely with the reactions of the patients to mecholyl.

Having now established the validity of the mecholyl and norepinephrine tests to measure sympathetic and parasympathetic responsiveness, respectively, he turned to the laboratory, his animals, and the hypothalamus. Using a variety of animal species, he tested the effect of mecholyl and norepinephrine on the hypothalamus, measuring its activity, or lack thereof, with the EEG. He found invariably that when he gave animals mecholyl, which lowered blood pressure, posterior hypothalamus activity increased significantly. At the same time, anterior hypothalamus firing slowed. When he gave animals norepinephrine, raising blood pressure, he observed the opposite. The anterior hypothalamus, and in turn the parasympathetic system, became active; the posterior hypothalamus and the sympathetic nerves became quiet. Very quiet.

Interestingly, if he gave mecholyl, while at that same time tranquilizing the posterior hypothalamus, the sympathetic nerves would not fire and the blood pressure would stay low. There would be some counterresponse, in the brainstem, but not a significant one. If, on the other hand, he gave norepinephrine but tranquilized the anterior hypothalamus, there would be only a minimal parasympathetic response and the blood pressure would stay high. These elaborate experiments documented carefully, and to me rather definitively, that the hypothalamus ultimately controlled the autonomic system. It didn't matter whether information was coming in from the sophisticated cortex or from reflexes lower down; the autonomic system wasn't going to do much unless the hypothalamus was involved.

There is something else Gellhorn observed through all these experiments that is really critical for our story. Just a few paragraphs ago, I mentioned that Gellhorn tested the influence of the cerebral cortex on the hypothalamus by either applying strychnine directly to the cortex or ringing a loud bell and then measuring, with the EEG, anterior and posterior hypothalamic nerve activity.

Normally if he rang an irritating bell, the cortex began to diffusely fire, meaning that all areas of the cerebral cortex became active. In turn, the posterior hypothalamus began to fire along with the sympathetic nerves. However, if he tranquilized the posterior hypothalamus, no sympathetic firing followed. He also noticed something else. In order to measure the state of cortical firing, he had EEG electrodes inserted into the cortex of his animals. He found that when he applied strychnine, or rang a loud bell, and at the same time applied Pentothal to the posterior hypothalamus, activity there would diminish as expected and the sympathetic nerves would not fire—again, as he had expected.

What he didn't expect is that when he tranquilized the posterior hypothalamus, the cortical discharges were also significantly lessened. This to him didn't initially make any sense, because with either strychnine or the loud bell he was directly stimulating the cortex. He didn't initially understand why the state of the hypothalamus should make any difference. He discounted a tranquilizing effect of the drug itself spreading from the hypothalamus to the cortex, because when he directly ablated the posterior hypothalamus with a minute amount of electricity—which would affect no other area—he got the same result, diminished cortical discharge. The hypothalamus seemed to be regulating not only the brainstem, but also the cortex itself! This to him explained the behavior in the animals he had observed: when he blocked the posterior hypothalamus, invariably the animals became quiet, somnolent, even sleepy.

On the other hand, if he applied strychnine in small amounts to the posterior hypothalamus or stimulated the posterior hypothalamus directly with a microscopic electrical probe, in addition to heightened sympathetic activity, the cortical discharges would increase dramatically. The animals would become alert, aggressive, and restless. As Gellhorn said, they became more conscious. The hypothalamus received input from all cortical centers—Gellhorn knew that and had confirmed it repeatedly—but now he had shown that the hypothalamus was sending directions upward to the cortex as well as downward to the brainstem.

The cerebral cortex, in effect, seemed to be dependent on the state of the hypothalamus. This wasn't an esoteric finding; Gellhorn was uncovering that the cerebral cortex, the center for our highest intellectual functioning, the part of the brain that makes us distinctly human, really couldn't do very much without the input of a lower, supposedly unconscious area, the hypothalamus. It was an interesting phenomenon to have seen, to say the least.

Gellhorn then repeated his mecholyl and norepinephrine experiments with various laboratory animals, but this time, he monitored cortical discharges with the EEG. In these experiments, he was essentially measuring the effect on the cortex of sensory information coming into the hypothalamus from lower down, from the baroreceptors. When he injected mecholyl into the animals, lowering blood pressure and stimulating the posterior hypothalamus, the entire cortex, from front to back, itself became active. The animals again were more alert, more aggressive, and more active.

When Dr. Gellhorn injected norepinephrine, thus raising blood pressure and stimulating the anterior hypothalamus, the cortex became electrically very quiet. The animals appeared subdued and quiet, and they would even fall asleep. These findings confirmed what he had seen when he had directly applied strychnine, or electrical currents, to the hypothalamus. Whether he stimulated the posterior hypothalamus directly—by strychnine or a mild electrical current—or reflexively, by mecholyl, the cortex diffusely discharged. It was clear from the EEG readings. However, when he inhibited the posterior hypothalamus directly with Pentothal or electrical ablation, or reflexively by norepinephrine, cortical discharge diminished.

One more point needs to be made about Gellhorn's wonderful series of experiments. In certain of his investigations, as I have mentioned, he would study the response of the brain to the ringing of a loud bell. Under normal circumstances, such a noise would increase cortical and posterior hypothalamic discharges diffusely, and the sympathetic system would fire. If he tranquilized the posterior hypothalamus, the sympathetic system, as expected, would remain quiet. But Gellhorn found, in addition, that the auditory sensory areas in the cortex would be less active and less receptive. He found this repeatedly, not only with sound, but also with other sensory information such as pain, for which there are specific cortical sensory areas.

In other words, the brain's ability to perceive special sensory information also depended on the state of the hypothalamus. The cortex couldn't hear sound or feel pain effectively, unless the posterior hypothalamus was active. In a state of anterior hypothalamic-parasympathetic firing, our awareness of such sensations is significantly lessened. Our ability to be aware of, our ability to perceive the world, seemed to Gellhorn to depend largely on the hypothalamus.

Dr. Gellhorn, in his book *Autonomic Imbalance and the Hypothalamus* (1957, 195–97), summed up his twenty years' worth of detailed investigations in several succinct paragraphs:

> 1. Direct and reflex excitation of the posterior hypothalamus is associated with a diffuse excitation of the cerebral cortex. The intensity of this hypothalamic-cortical discharge is directly related to the excitability of the posterior hypothalamus. . . .
>
> 2. The hypothalamic-cortical discharge is associated with the state of wakefulness. Conditions which interfere with this discharge cause somnolence and coma. . . . These observations indicate that perceptions are . . . altered by changes in the intensity of the hypothalamic-cortical discharge.

In these simple principles, Dr. Gellhorn presented his belief that consciousness, perception, our ability to see the world, and behavior itself were in large part determined by the state of hypothalamic "tuning," as he called it, meaning the state of hypothalamic balance. For a hundred years, psychologists and psychiatrists had definitively stated that behavior, either animal or human, was primarily if not entirely the province of the cerebral cortex. Dr. Freud particularly, with his elaborate theories of the unconscious and its conflicts with the conscious, could see behavior primarily as an issue and a problem at the level of the cerebral cortex. Dr. Gellhorn, in his quiet but masterful way, was saying something quite different. Behavior, he claimed, might very well be primarily an autonomic function.

Dr. Gellhorn, Muscles, and Dr. Pavlov

It was Dr. Gellhorn who also ultimately solved another neurophysiological riddle. Scientists long before him had divided the motor nervous system into the somatic, or voluntary, collection of nerves that control the striated skeletal muscles, and the autonomic nervous system, which regulates physiological functions not requiring conscious input. Scientists stressed how different the two were, in their anatomy and in their physiology. The control centers for the voluntary muscles were in the higher areas of the brain, in the motor strip of the cortex, in the basal ganglia and cerebellum. Impulses for action traveled from the spinal cord in motor neurons that connected directly to the target muscles.

Autonomic centers, on the other hand, were known to be in the brainstem and, as Gellhorn had now shown, in the hypothalamus. Information from these areas traveled from the spinal cord along a series of two nerves, arranged in complex arrays of ganglia. When I was in medical school twenty years ago, the distinctions were made clearly: there was the somatic nervous system and the autonomic nervous system, and they did very different things.

There were perplexing questions, raised during the 1940s and 1950s, indicating the separation might be more artificial than real. From my reading of the scientific literature, it seems that researchers before Dr. Gellhorn had reported that when the sympathetic system fires, all the skeletal muscles of the body become tense, technically more contracted. When the parasympathetic nerves are active, the somatic striated muscles, and all of them, will relax—invariably. This was an interesting finding, because it indicated that there was some sort of communication going on between the somatic (voluntary) and autonomic nervous systems.

But, though these phenomena had been observed for some fifty years, no one seemed sure what to do with these observations, or what they meant, or how such a connection might work—because everyone in neuroscience stressed the differences in the two sets of nerves. Clearly, there had to be a link-up somewhere, because when the sympathetic or parasympathetic nerves were active, predictable changes happened in the muscles.

It was Dr. Gellhorn who finally put the pieces together. In his laboratory and clinical investigations during the 1940s and '50s, he had carefully unraveled the role of the hypothalamus in both autonomic and cortical function. He had carefully documented what followed in the autonomic nerves, and in the cortex, after he stimulated or inhibited the anterior or the posterior hypothalamus. But he also carefully observed—and noted—in each of his painstaking experiments what was going on in the somatic nervous system. He began to understand just how closely linked the two systems really were.

Early on in his work, Dr. Gellhorn began to suspect that the connection between the two sets of nerves happened, not surprisingly, in the hypothalamus. To confirm his hypothesis, he first evaluated the effect of the mecholyl test on the voluntary striated muscles. Remember that mecholyl caused the blood pressure to drop, a situation that slowed baroreceptor firing, relieved the inhibition on the posterior hypothalamus, and ultimately stimulated the sympathetic system into action. Blood pressure would return to normal.

As the sympathetic system became more active, he observed always the same changes in behavior: the animals became more alert, more restless, and more aggressive. They became more active; they would move more, pacing around their cages restlessly. There was an obvious increase in tone in all the striated muscles. The "knee jerk reflexes," for example, a simple measure of striated muscle tension, showed a definite heightened response: the limbs would kick out with far greater strength after the animals had received mecholyl, and the sympathetic system was firing. (Yes, knee jerk reflexes can be measured in laboratory animals, though I wouldn't try it on a grizzly bear.)

Dr. Gellhorn then decided, in one group of experiments, to see whether increased posterior hypothalamus activity would have any effect on convulsions, which are the ultimate state of severe muscle contraction. Convulsions occur because the muscles contract without restraint.

In one group of animals, he injected mecholyl and a drug known to produce convulsions. A control group received the convulsive drug, without mecholyl. Gellhorn found that the animals receiving both drugs had far more intensive seizures than the control group, indicating again that, when the posterior hypothalamus, and in turn the sympathetic nerves, fire, muscle contraction is stronger. Far stronger.

The mecholyl experiments showed Dr. Gellhorn what happened when he reflexively stimulated the posterior hypothalamus, by dropping the blood pressure. He wasn't doing anything directly to the hypothalamus; it was all happening through the baroreceptor reflex. He then decided to see what happened to the muscles when he stimulated the posterior hypothalamus directly with a mild electrical current. He got the same result as he had with mecholyl:

> Stimulation of the posterior part of the hypothalamus (and some adjacent areas) resulted in sympathetic effects which were associated with a state of increased reactivity of the motor system. . . . The direct excitation of the hypothalamus or the reflex excitation of sympathetic centers through their release from the antagonistic action of the baroreceptors . . . is associated with an increased excitability of the motor system. (Gellhorn 1957, 140)

He then repeated his norepinephrine studies, this time observing specifically the response of the muscles. Norepinephrine, as I discussed earlier, when injected raised the blood pressure, and this caused the baroreceptors to fire more strongly, thus inhibiting the posterior hypothalamus and the sympathetic nerves. The anterior hypothalamus instead becomes active, as do, in turn, the parasympathetic nerves. Blood pressure then drops back again toward normal.

The effects on the animals were always the opposite of that seen with mecholyl. According to Gellhorn (1957, 140), "When the pressure was raised, the unanesthetized animals became quiet, reacted less to environmental stimuli, and had a tendency to fall asleep." They moved less, their muscles became flaccid, and he could not elicit a knee-jerk type of stretch reflex. He could move the animals' limbs into odd positions easily, because the muscles offered no resistance. In his descriptions, it seems as if the limbs were like soft clay.

Furthermore, he noted that if in these "parasympathetic" animals he injected a convulsion-causing drug, nothing happened. They simply would not convulse. In essence, their parasympathetic state had in effect protected them against the drug.

Then, in the next investigations, he directly stimulated the anterior hypothalamus with an electrical current, and he found again a significant reduction in muscle tone in the animals: "the stimulation of the anterior hypothalamus leading predominantly to parasympathetic symptoms was accompanied by a lessened reactivity of the neuromuscular system. . . . The direct or the reflex activation of the parasympathetic system is accompanied by a marked loss of tone in the skeletal muscles" (Gellhorn 1957, 140–41).

Because the results were consistent in both his reflex and his direct stimulation studies, Dr. Gellhorn assumed that the point of connection between the somatic and autonomic nervous systems was indeed in the hypothalamus. Though he had shown, convincingly, that the hypothalamus, and the autonomic system, profoundly affected somatic nerves and muscles, he wondered if the corollary held true. Did the muscles influence the hypothalamus? Did the influence work both ways?

This question led him to curare, the famed drug of legend and lore that in the more mundane research laboratory was known to block transmission of action potentials at the neuromuscular junction, hence preventing muscular contraction. When injected, curare caused muscles to relax, very profoundly. The drug, even in Gellhorn's day, was widely used by anesthesiologists to put patients into a state of muscular relaxation before major surgery. Curare, as it turned out, was an ideal drug for Gellhorn's use, because it had no effect directly on the central nervous system and worked only at the point where the motor nerve met the muscle, blocking the attachment of neurotransmitters. There would be no influence on the brain itself, to confuse the issue.

Gellhorn decided to evaluate what happened when he injected curare into laboratory animals and then sent an electrical current directly into the posterior hypothalamus. Normally, this would quickly activate the sympathetic system, sending the pulse and blood pressure up, etc. In the curarized animals, when he stimulated the posterior hypothalamus, nothing happened—no change in pulse, no change in blood pressure, no dilation of pupils, no sympathetic response whatsoever anywhere. The sympathetic system stayed quiet. In similar experiments, the results were the same.

These were extraordinary findings, because they indicated that if the muscles were relaxed, the posterior hypothalamus and the sympathetic nervous system could not fire! Yes, previously he had shown that when either the anterior or the posterior hypothalamus was stimulated—either reflexively or directly—predictable muscle responses followed, relaxation or contraction, respectively. Now he had shown the reverse, that the tone of the muscles remarkably influenced the hypothalamus.

Gellhorn then went a step further. He knew, from his previous work, as we have seen, that the hypothalamus not only regulated the autonomic downward discharges, but also seemed to control activity in the cerebral cortex, higher up. If muscle tone could influence the hypothalamus, he wondered, what occurred in the cortex, when the state of muscle contraction changed? Could the tone of the striated muscles have any effect on the cortex, our highest centers for thinking and action? This was yet another important question to ask.

In another set of experiments, Gellhorn measured electrical activity in the posterior hypothalamus and cerebral cortex while subjecting animals to various stimuli, such as pain. Invariably, firing in both areas increased dramatically, as did overall sympathetic tone. He then injected curare into the animals, relaxing their muscles, and repeated the experiments. This time, with curare on board, there was no stimulation in either the posterior hypothalamus or the cortex—the enforced muscle relaxation blocked the expected response. The cortex, the posterior hypothalamus, and the sympathetic nerves all became quiet and calm, and the animals behaved accordingly, becoming quieter and calmer.

Gellhorn's (1957, 144) own words expressed the observed changes better than any I could use:

> Moreover, cats which before the injection of the drug [curare] were quite alert appeared sleepy and returned to this state almost immediately after an arousal reaction had been produced by hypothalamic stimulation. In some instances aggressive tendencies, indicated by growling, hissing and spitting, and forward movements suggesting that the cat was ready to jump at the experimenter, disappeared, and there was a tendency for the cat to crawl into a corner (escape reaction?). A cat that after hypothalamic stimulation had previously bitten one of the observers reacted to the same or an even stronger stimulus mainly by walking forward a little and then turning to the back corner away from the experimenter. . . . The tendency of previously aggressive cats to retire to the farthest corner even if pulled forward by the experimenter is noteworthy.

When the muscles relaxed, the behavior of the cats changed, dramatically. Aggressive cats became docile, alert animals, sleepy. These were not subtle changes but quick, profound, and obvious. They did not involve years of cat psychotherapy, or training, just relaxation of the muscles. The system did work both ways: the hypothalamus influenced the muscles, and the muscles influenced the hypothalamus—and in turn, the cerebral cortex. As Gellhorn (1957, 144) wrote in *Autonomic Imbalance*, summing up his findings with great understatement, "it may be suggested that emotional reactivity is related to the tone of the striated muscles, which in turn determines the intensity of the proprioceptive discharge." The muscles, he now believed, helped determine behavior.

These findings from forty-six years ago succinctly and convincingly help us understand, perhaps as much as anything published since, why relaxation therapies such as biofeedback and the various meditation techniques that reduce muscle tone influence sympathetic activity, and even the way we think, the way we respond to the world, and the way we behave. Pioneering researchers such as Elmer Green, at the Menninger Foundation during the 1970s and '80s, and, more recently, Dr. Herbert Benson at Harvard Medical School have proposed that methods that diminish muscular contraction also calm an overstressed brain. In most of these approaches, patients are taught how to relax their muscles at will, an effort scientists suggest in turn relaxes both our thinking brain and our sympathetic function.

Many popular books, including several by Dr. Benson such as *The Relaxation Response*, describe the power of simple muscle relaxation and the benefit it provides for a host of stress-related illnesses such as heart disease, headaches, and anxiety. The proponents of such approaches usually suggest everyone would benefit by incorporating relaxation therapies into their lives, something that in our model would be a big mistake. Relaxation techniques are valuable for those with a heightened posterior hypothalamus–sympathetic system, but counterproductive—at least in our, and Gellhorn's, model—for those with strong anterior hypothalamus–parasympathetic activity. Such patients are already too relaxed. Dr. Gellhorn showed all this fifty years ago.

Dr. Gellhorn, Dr. Pavlov, and Dr. Funkenstein

Through his years of careful experimentation, Dr. Gellhorn had indeed accomplished much. He had shown that the anterior and posterior hypothalamic areas were the real centers for autonomic control, through their downward discharges into the brainstem, but that the hypothalamus also enormously influenced behavior, through its upward connections with the cerebral cortex. He had established the "law of reciprocity," finally demonstrating why, when one branch of the autonomic system fires, the other becomes still. He had documented that the anterior and posterior hypothalamus affected muscle tone directly and in opposite ways, but also that muscle tone affected the hypothalamus, and in turn both autonomic and cerebral responses. He had rather forcefully proven that the actual connections between the autonomic and somatic nervous systems allowing for such interactions were right in the hypothalamus.

While he was working so hard in the laboratory, he was at the same time refining the mecholyl test of Dr. Funkenstein, which tested sympathetic tone, and developing the norepinephrine test, which revealed the state of parasympathetic activity. He had expanded Dr. Funkenstein's work with both "normal" humans and those suffering psychiatric illness, confirming importantly that human populations generally fall into three groups: sympathetic hyper-responders, balanced autonomic reactors, and sympathetic hypo-responders. Or, in Kelley terminology, sympathetic dominants, balanced metabolizers, and parasympathetic dominants.

It was this last finding, this idea that humans could be divided into three populations according to their state of autonomic balance, that seemed to dominate Gellhorn's thinking in his later books. He believed—as Dr. Kelley, in his own pioneering way, was to believe years later—that this concept might help explain much of human behavior and human illness.

In his 1963 book *Emotions and Emotional Disorders*, Dr. Gellhorn included a chapter entitled "Vagotonia and Sympathotonia," terms to describe states of "parasympathetic and sympathetic" dominance, respectively. The terms literally mean "strong vagus tone," the vagus being the main parasympathetic nerve, and "strong sympathetic tone." Here, in this chapter, he summed up decades of animal and human studies, both his own and those of others, documenting his thesis that individuals can differ in their state of autonomic dominance.

In the opening paragraph of this particular chapter, he nicely outlined what had brought him to think as he did. Note in the following that he maintained that most humans fell into the balanced category—something Kelley in his practice a decade later, and ourselves, in our practice today, did not and do not find. Nonetheless, his words in so many ways do confirm how we approach patients:

> Should it be assumed that the activity of the autonomic centers varies considerably between different persons, the majority being characterized by an intermediate activity of the sympathetic system, while the minority at either end of the scale comprises persons with either a greatly increased or a markedly reduced sympathetic activity? And should not this normal "distribution curve" be expected in like fashion for variations in parasympathetic activity?
>
> The close relation existing between emotional processes and central autonomic activity and the great variability in emotional responsiveness of individuals certainly points in this direction. The investigations reported in Chapter 6 on the Mecholyl and noradrenaline tests support this assumption. . . . Consequently on the basis of these tests one could distinguish between different degrees of sympathotonia and vagotonia. (Gellhorn 1963, 244)

Here, in this chapter, Dr. Gellhorn emphasized that differing degrees of sympathetic or parasympathetic dominance are found among normal populations, that this is a normal state of affairs among humans. Furthermore, using the results of his own studies, and those of other scientists who seem to have been intrigued by Gellhorn's ideas, he convincingly showed just how different these human classes are, in a basic biologic sense. He had, in many different ways, already done this in much of his published work, of course, but now he selected two areas—cardiovascular physiology and brain wave studies—to make the point.

In the heart studies, Gellhorn and colleagues evaluated several parameters in normal volunteers identified as vagotonics, balanced metabolizers, and sympathetics. One factor considered was minute volume, the amount of blood pumped out of the heart each minute. This measures essentially the combined effect of pulse and the strength of cardiac contractility. Another was total body oxygen consumption, a marker for the rate of overall total body metabolism—a fancy way of saying how quickly the body uses energy. Gellhorn reported that there were indeed significant differences in both minute volume and oxygen consumption among the three groups:

> Normal persons could be divided into three groups. The vagotonic group is characterized by a low minute volume of the heart and a low oxygen consumption . . . and low values for pulse rate, work of the heart . . . . In the sympathotonic group these values are high. . . . The mixed group shows partially sympathotonic, and partially parasympathotonic symptoms. (Gellhorn 1963, 245)

These results confirmed what Gellhorn had already suspected from his years of research. He suspected that individuals with a high parasympathetic tone would have a reduced minute volume, and a sluggish overall metabolism, compared with sympathetic dominants, with their high pulses, strong cardiac contractility, and high metabolic rate.

Gellhorn then described a series of studies in which researchers, using the EEG instrument, recorded the actual alpha brain wave patterns of normal volunteers, while determining their cardiac minute volume and rate of oxygen consumption. Alpha waves are one of a number of clearly identifiable brain waves that can be measured on the EEG, each reflecting a different state of brain activity. Gellhorn reported that studies

> led to the conclusion that the alpha frequency is low in vagotonics, intermediate in mixed types, and high in sympathotonic individuals. It is not unlikely that these findings are based on a shift in hypothalamic autonomic balance in vagotonia and sympathotonia and corresponding changes in the degree of the tonic discharges of the sympathetic division of the hypothalamus which manifest themselves in the alpha frequency of the EEG on the one hand and the level of oxygen consumption and the minute volume of the heart at rest on the other. (Gellhorn 1963, 248)

Dr. Gellhorn also discovered that even the standard blood chemistry profile differs very distinctly among the three autonomic classes—a claim Dr. Kelley would make some twenty years later. For example, calcium tended to be high and potassium low in sympathetics, whereas in vagotonics calcium tended to be low and potassium high. Dr. Gellhorn suggested that the potassium/calcium ratio might prove to be a useful screening test to determine the state of autonomic balance.

These various studies showed that though they were all human, of course, the vagotonics, mixed types, and sympathetics had entirely distinctive patterns of cardiac function, basal metabolism, brain nerve firing, and even blood chemistry, patterns as unique, in a sense, as a fingerprint, and all the result of different states of hypothalamic-autonomic dominance.

Like Dr. Kelley, Gellhorn believed that genetic factors largely determined autonomic balance, whether one was vagotonic, mixed (Dr. Gellhorn's word for the balanced types), or sympathetic. Our state of autonomic dominance was, to Gellhorn, a part of our basic biological inheritance. In *Emotions and Emotional Disorders*, he discussed data from twins to support his contention. Keep in mind that identical twins have the same genetic makeup, but fraternal twins do not:

> The role of genetic factors is apparent from the examinations of these parameters [meaning minute volume, etc.] in identical and fraternal twins. Although the number studied thus far is small, it is worthy of emphasis that identical twins were found to belong to the same autonomic type and show only slight quantitative variations, whereas fraternal twins show marked differences and may belong to different autonomic types. Earlier work involving various pharmacological tests showed already that autonomic reactions may be quite similar in identical twins. (Gellhorn 1963, 247)

Such data, I believe, should have attracted the attention of the entire medical research community. Unfortunately, they did not. Undeterred, Gellhorn kept following leads. Somewhere in his intellectual wanderings, he had discovered Dr. Pavlov and his extensive writings.

I can't tell from Dr. Gellhorn's writings when he first began to study Pavlov's work. I do know that in his earlier books from the 1940s and 1950s, references to the Russian scientist are notably absent. But in *Emotions and Emotional Disorders*, published in 1963, Gellhorn devoted entire sections to Pavlov and his concepts of conditioned reflexes. By that point, he had not only discovered Pavlov but had repeated many of his animal experiments. It is this work, based so much on Pavlov's earlier investigations, that finally led Gellhorn to believe that autonomic imbalance was the basis of much, if not most, mental illness.

Pavlov's demonstrations of the "conditioned reflex" pointed Gellhorn in this new direction. Though in my historical discussion I previously described the meaning of terms such as "unconditioned" and "conditioned" reflexes, before we move on a brief review is in order. I thought the section "The Exploration of the Mind through the Conditioned Reflex" in *Emotions and Emotional Disorders* summed up decades of Pavlov's work as well as anything anyone could write, so I repeat his words at some length:

> An unconditioned reflex is inborn, a conditioned reflex is acquired and therefore the result of the individual's experience. The stimuli eliciting the unconditioned reflex and conditioned reflex are called unconditioned and

conditioned stimuli respectively. In most experiments the salivary reflex in response to food or the withdrawal reflex of the leg to a painful stimulus is used as the unconditioned reflex. Any other sensory stimulus (light, sound, touch, etc.) may be used as a conditioned stimulus. It is a stimulus which does not evoke the response (salivation, for example) until it has been presented sufficiently often in combination with the unconditioned stimulus. If the unconditioned stimulus routinely follows the conditioned stimulus at the proper time interval, the latter will become an effective stimulus. Thus, if a sound is presented a few seconds before food is placed in the mouth of a dog, and if this procedure is repeated a number of times, the sound will become an adequate stimulus and elicit a salivary secretion although it is no longer followed by feeding. In a similar way, the sound stimulus can be combined with the withdrawal reflex and will elicit it even when the painful stimulus is omitted. The sound may become the signal for food and pain respectively and evoke therefore a conditioned reflex, either salivation or withdrawal. (Gellhorn 1963, 175–76)

In the classic example, Pavlov would provide food to a dog, and the dog would salivate. This is an unconditioned reflex, something that happens instinctively, that doesn't have to be taught. The food is the unconditioned stimulus. He then would ring a bell, before providing food, and repeat this sequence of events over and over. Eventually, of course, the dog began to salivate just at the sound of the bell, even if no food appeared. This was now a conditioned reflex, with the animal responding to a stimulus—the bell—not usually associated with salivation. This is a trained, not an innate, response, hence the word "conditioned."

In the case of the painful unconditioned stimulus, if Pavlov administered a mildly painful electrical shock to a dog's leg, the dog would immediately withdraw the limb. This too is an unconditioned reflex, though unpleasant, something the dog doesn't have to learn how to do. The shock is the unconditioned stimulus. However, if Pavlov rang a bell and then shocked the dog, and did this repeatedly, eventually the dog would withdraw its leg at the sound of a bell, even if no shock followed. This is a conditioned reflex, with the bell the conditioned stimulus. Importantly, in the salivation and withdrawal experiments, the dog responded to the same stimulus, the bell, with salivation in one case and withdrawal in the other. The dog could be trained to respond to a neutral stimulus, the sound of a bell, completely differently depending on the unconditioned stimulus presented.

Interestingly, conditioned reflexes could involve either the autonomic nervous system, as in the case of salivation, which is a vagal response, or the somatic nervous system, as in the case of the withdrawal response, which requires contraction of the striated, voluntary muscles.

In later experiments, Pavlov took his conditioning experiments a step further and learned how to provoke "experimental neurosis" in his laboratory animals.

By experimental neurosis, Pavlov meant distressed, confused, abnormal, even self-destructive behavior. In the simpler form of experimental neurosis, Pavlov learned, he could evoke such responses by using a particularly strong, as opposed to a mild, electrical shock as the conditioned stimulus during the leg withdrawal training. As mentioned in the earlier discussion of his work, Pavlov also found that if he used the bell as the conditioned stimulus upon presenting food but used, instead of a bell with a single pitch, a series of bell ringings confusingly close in pitch, neurosis resulted.

In a more complicated version, Pavlov would develop a pleasant conditioned reflex by ringing a bell and then providing food. But once the reflex had been established, he added an unpleasant step: the ringing of a bell followed by the appearance of food, but this time as the animals began eating they would be shocked. Eventually, at the sight of food the animals became so upset they would not eat, but rather starved—even if the electrical current was no longer turned on. They had been very effectively trained to view food as the enemy.

Gellhorn, as he studied Pavlov's reports, realized that experimental neurosis developed in two general sets of circumstances. In the first case, when the animals were strongly shocked, it appeared that an excessive painful or uncomfortable stimulus, if repeatedly administered, was enough itself to provoke neurotic behavior. Gellhorn referred to such a stimulus as a negative conditioned stimulus. On the other hand, the situation was a little more complicated in the case where animals had been trained that a certain pitch of a bell meant food was coming, but were then presented with a series of bell sounds very close together, only one of which indicated food was coming. The series of sounds seemed only to confuse the animals initially and eventually provoke neurosis.

The situation was also complicated when Pavlov, and later Gellhorn, first trained the animals to expect food at the sound of a bell and then, after this positive conditioned reflex had been established, complicated the situation by shocking the animals when food appeared. Here again, the animals responded initially with signs of great confusion, which over time deteriorated into erratic and neurotic behavior. It seemed that a strongly uncomfortable or painful stimulus repeatedly administered, or confused signals, led to abnormal behavior. Interestingly, Gellhorn found that the training with conflicting signals, that is, food and pain, for example, were far more effective in producing abnormal behavior than simply shocking the animals.

Gellhorn was also very much aware that Pavlov in his initial experiments repeatedly found that some dogs were difficult to work with in a laboratory setting. Some would be very aggressive, at times attacking the handlers. Other dogs were difficult because they were so timid, very cowed, and would urinate and defecate at the sight of a handler. Other dogs were easy to handle, sociable, and friendly. Pavlov found that the happy dogs could easily be trained to form nonneurotic conditioned reflexes, but they rarely developed experimental neurosis, even when stressed to the extreme with unpleasant stimuli. The aggressive or timid dogs did not easily develop standard conditioned responses but were the most vulnerable to forming experimental neurosis.

Eventually, Pavlov subdivided his laboratory dogs, and even his cats, into the four groups previously mentioned, based on their personalities before undergoing any experimental testing. Type I were "aggressive and unrestrained" (see Gellhorn 1963, 199). These animals responded to neurosis-evoking training with fierceness, fighting the handlers all the way to the laboratory. Gellhorn clearly identified such dogs in his own experiments decades after Pavlov:

> Increased activity and struggling prevail and it may be difficult to take the animal to the experimental room. On the bench the formerly quiet animal is constantly moving and howling. Cats appear restless and trembling and respond to minimal stimuli with startle reactions. On presenting the conditioned stimulus, the signal for food, the neurotic cats show signs of increased anxiety and attempt to escape from the vicinity of the food box. Even with the food openly displayed in the food box used in the conditioning experiment, the hungry neurotic animal starves itself. Dogs presented with food turn away from it and this abnormal behavior persists outside the experimental laboratory. It may last indefinitely and the social as well as the individual behavior of the animals is altered. . . . The neurotic dog kept in the same kennel with a normal dog is unable to get at the food placed on a single pan. (Gellhorn 1963, 192)

Type IV dogs were timid, anxious dogs that only with great difficulty formed nonneurotic responses but very easily developed their own peculiar form of mental illness with neurosis training. These animals could become at times nearly catatonic, as Gellhorn (1963, 192) reported: "In such animals (dogs and sheep) the activity is subnormal, and the movements are performed slowly. Hypnotic and sleeplike conditions, and a cataleptic state in which the neurotic animals become rigid and tend to retain a fixed posture, have been observed by Pavlov and others."

Pavlov's types II and III were the happy, well-adjusted dogs, which did not develop, except rarely and under extreme conditions, an experimental neurosis.

What I find still so amazing about Pavlov's findings, and those of Gellhorn a generation later, is that a simple neutral stimulus such as the bell, or something desirable such as food, could in one set of experiments evoke pleasant anticipatory reactions such as salivation, while with different training, the same stimuli became a sign of terror, capable of producing overt mental illness that could last the duration of the poor animal's life. Even food, something necessary for life, could become so frightening that the animals would rather starve than face the pain they had come to associate with it.

Pavlov assumed that conditioned reflexes, and experimental neurosis in particular, formed in the brain at the level of the cerebral cortex. Neurosis, he believed, resulted because of conflicts between what he proposed as activating versus inhibitory centers in these higher brain centers. As Gellhorn studied Pavlov's intricate experiments, and as he confirmed Pavlov's findings in his own extensive laboratory studies, he became aware of something Pavlov never grasped. That had to do with the role of the autonomic nervous system in the development of nonneurotic conditioned reflexes and "experimental neurosis."

Though, ironically, Pavlov in the early days of his remarkable career had mapped out the nervous input to the heart, pancreas, and GI tract in general, once he began studying conditioned reflexes, he never thought much about autonomic function—even after Langley's pioneering papers at the turn of the last century helped put the system on the neurological map. He just never seemed to have made any connection. He, like so many neuroscientists of his time, and during Gellhorn's time, and even today, tended to look higher up, into the cortex, for answers—not lower down, to the less esteemed realm of the hypothalamus, the brainstem, and the autonomic nerves.

Gellhorn, on the other hand, having spent most of his professional life immersed in autonomic physiology, had no such prejudices. And when he looked at Pavlov's four groups of dogs and repeatedly identified such groups among his own laboratory animals, he saw immediately what Pavlov had missed. The Type I dogs, which were aggressive and angry and so easily became neurotic, were "sympathetic" dogs, dogs with an overly active sympathetic nervous system and weak parasympathetic nerves. Type IV dogs, the anxious, timid, frightened dogs that couldn't form normal conditioned reflexes but quickly became catatonic when faced with painful stimuli or conflicting messages, were "vagotonic," with an overly developed parasympathetic but weak sympathetic nervous system. The happy types II and III were "mixed," or balanced autonomic types, with equally developed sympathetic and parasympathetic nerves. In them, mental illness just didn't happen.

Gellhorn made several observations. He noted that the sympathetic-dominant Type I dogs, when given extreme or conflicted training signals, developed a neurosis that correlated with a wildly firing sympathetic system. The animals became aggressive and violent, their heart rate and pulse increased, their pupils dilated, and their muscles tensed. He also noticed that these animals at the same time showed signs of parasympathetic hyperactivity, such as vomiting, uncontrolled urination, and defecation. If the neurosis-inducing testing persisted, eventually these animals would even pass out—a sign of strong parasympathetic action.

In these Type I dogs, the sympathetic symptoms were predominant, but unquestionably the parasympathetic nerves were firing at the same time. It appeared to Gellhorn that in these sympathetic-dominant dogs subjected to high-stress stimuli, the reciprocity principle that seemed to universally hold true under more normal conditions broke down. Both branches of the autonomic system, contrary to what he had previously thought possible, were active at the same time, though not equally so.

Type IV dogs, when exposed to strongly painful or ambivalent signals, showed signs of excessive parasympathetic activity, such as extreme fear, timidity, and eventually catatonic states of immobility. They also showed signs of sympathetic activity, though erratically. At times their pulses would slow, a sign of parasympathetic activity, but then their pulses would race wildly, an indication of sympathetic firing. There would even be variability in their catatonic states. At times, the muscles would be very flaccid; at other times, the muscles would be very tense and contracted, associated with strong norepinephrine release from sympathetic nerves. The parasympathetic symptoms in these Type IV animals were dominant, but there were, Gellhorn was sure, signs of sympathetic activity as well. Just as in the Type I group, there seemed to be a loss of reciprocity, of inhibition between the strong and weak autonomic branches.

Gellhorn carefully and slowly began to sort out what he was witnessing. He first considered what was happening when the animals were confronted repeatedly with a painful stimulus, such as a strong electrical shock. With Type I animals, measurements of brain activity indicated that, in this situation, there was a massive discharge of electrical energy in the posterior hypothalamus, the sympathetic center, and the cerebral cortex. In addition, there was strong activation of the anterior hypothalamus, the parasympathetic center, which normally shuts down when the posterior hypothalamus fires.

In Type IV animals, the reverse held true. There was a massive activation of the anterior hypothalamus and reduced cortical activity diffusely, associated with a lessened firing in the posterior hypothalamus. There was in each case indeed a loss of reciprocity, the usual inhibition that runs between the two halves of the hypothalamus and between the two branches of the autonomic system. Instead of inhibiting each other, the two halves were firing rather strongly at the same time.

Gellhorn surmised that when animals with an imbalanced autonomic system, with either overly strong sympathetic or parasympathetic tone, were confronted with a painful, threatening stimulus, the dominant system would fire so powerfully that neuronal circuits misfired and the entire hypothalamus, both the anterior and posterior halves, became active, with the dominant half always more so.

In the case of ambivalent training—animals being shocked when eating, for example—the signals were contradictory and confusing. Feeding behavior classically elicits strong parasympathetic reactions, such as salivation, pancreatic enzyme secretion, and peristalsis. Pain activates the sympathetic fight or flight reactions, so you have the case where contrary signals stimulate both branches of the autonomic system at the same time. Apparently, if the stimuli are uncomfortable enough, both halves of the hypothalamus will fire together, with the dominant half leading the way.

In either situation, the cortex received completely contradictory signals from the hypothalamus, both excitatory input from the posterior half and inhibitory discharges from the anterior. Inevitably, the cortex ends up in a state of complete neurological and electrical chaos, with excitatory and inhibitory action potentials telling it to behave in contradictory ways. It wasn't surprising, thought Gellhorn, that the result of all this would be very abnormal behavior.

In the balanced animals, the law of reciprocity did not break down, no matter how painful or confused the stimuli the animals faced. The two hypothalamic halves and the two branches of the autonomic system remained in balance, neither system firing out of control. Neurosis simply would not develop. The animals might be appropriately unhappy in the testing rooms, but once back in the kennel they resumed their normal dog or cat behavior. Gellhorn concluded that hypothalamic and, in turn, autonomic imbalance was the key to neurosis, and hypothalamic and, in turn, autonomic balance was the key to mental health!

Gellhorn summarized his thoughts about experimental neurosis nicely in *Emotions and Emotional Disorders*. He used the word "tuning" to mean a state of autonomic dominance:

> Sympathetic tuning normally leads to an increased sympathetic and decreased parasympathetic reactivity, while parasympathetic tuning causes opposite effects. Under normal circumstances (autonomic balance or "mild" tuning) an ambivalent stimulus would increase the reactivity of both by further facilitating the "tuned" system and partially canceling the reciprocal inhibition of the antagonistic system. However, in a situation in which the reactivity of one system is already quite high due to a strong tuning influence, an ambivalent stimulus may further facilitate it to the point of massive discharge. In this circumstance, the antagonistic system, instead of remaining suppressed, may also discharge. Thus in the so-called "excitatory neurotic state" although there is general sympathetic dominance and increased psychomotor activity, an ambivalent stimulus may cause simultaneous parasympathetic phenomena such as vomiting, defecation, etc. In the "inhibitory neurotic state" [parasympathetic dominance] an ambivalent, neurosis producing stimulus would lead to both an augmentation of the inhibitory (parasympathetic) discharge and a simultaneous excitatory (sympathetic) discharge, in similar fashion. For example, in human catatonia, the prevalent parasympathetic inhibitory state is combined with an increased excretion of noradrenaline, indicating a concurrent sympathetic discharge. (Gellhorn 1963, 200–201)

All of this experimental data confirmed rather forcefully what Dr. Funkenstein had observed up at Harvard and what Dr. Gellhorn had himself with his clinic patients and normal volunteers subjected to the mecholyl and norepinephrine tests. Both Dr. Funkenstein and Dr. Gellhorn had repeatedly found that mentally ill patients fall into extreme categories of autonomic dominance far more regularly than do non-mentally ill volunteers. Gellhorn could now explain why these states of autonomic imbalance, either sympathetic or parasympathetic dominance, could make these patients far more susceptible to developing overt mental illness. The problem didn't happen in the higher thinking brain, in the unconscious, wherever that may be. It happened in the hypothalamus, in the autonomic centers. It happened because of autonomic imbalance.

Of course, with any form of mental illness we will find disordered and confused thinking patterns, and thinking is a function of the cerebral cortex. Remember, the hypothalamus, through its upward discharges, to use once again Gellhorn's terms, in a sense controls what is going on in the cortex, and this abnormal cortical activity in mental illness, Gellhorn believed, is the result of chaotic hypothalamic firing. As he wrote in *Emotions and Emotional Disorders*, "The physiological and pathological states of altered hypothalamic balance are characterized by changes in autonomic reactivity and also by an alteration in the whole personality. It is believed that the changed hypothalamic-cortical discharges are, at least in part, responsible for these effects" (Gellhorn 1963, 273).

I always find it instructive to view how a genius works. Like the geniuses I have been fortunate to see in action, Dr. Gellhorn, like Dr. Beard, was a masterful interpreter of other colleagues' work. He was able to take the investigations of Pavlov from decades earlier and weave them together with the findings of his contemporary Dr. Funkenstein into a very profound theory of mental illness.

And to wax philosophic for a moment, Gellhorn's thesis also helps answer, hopefully definitively, the often asked question "Is it nature or nurture?" Is our behavior, both normal and abnormal, genetically determined or environmental in origin? In reality, if Gellhorn was right, and I believe he was, it's most often clearly both. Excessive or strongly ambivalent stimuli in our environment may be a precipitating factor for mental illness, but it is our neurological makeup that often, if not always, allows it to happen. And from his twin studies, Gellhorn knew that our state of autonomic dominance—or balance—is largely genetically determined.

Gellhorn was amazed at how difficult it was to produce neurosis in his balanced dogs and cats, no matter how hard he tried—and how easy it was in the sympathetic and parasympathetic dominants. Left alone to do what dogs normally do, the Type I and Type IV would survive just fine, even if they had their own particular personality quirks, such as heightened aggression (sympathetic dominants) or timidity (parasympathetics). But once confronted with difficult or conflicting stimuli, they rapidly decompensated into very disturbed behavior. Of course, no one would disagree that there are syndromes of abnormal human behavior, such as autism, that seem largely if not entirely biological in origin. For many forms of mental illness, the problem might well be one of an imbalanced autonomic system responding to abnormal environmental stimuli.

Gellhorn also came to appreciate Funkenstein's reports on the different responses of sympathetic and parasympathetic dominants to therapeutic interventions such as electroshock and insulin shock. Funkenstein learned, and Gellhorn confirmed this to be true, that these seemingly drastic treatments stimulate the sympathetic nervous system and would be of benefit only in his Group III patients, those with a strong parasympathetic and weak sympathetic set of nerves. The treatment essentially brought an out-of-balance autonomic system back into balance, and with balance, the underlying problem would resolve. For Group I patients, the sympathetic dominants, electro- and insulin shock were a disaster, invariably making their symptoms worse. Of course, this now makes sense, in Gellhorn's encompassing model. In such patients, these treatments would further stimulate an already too strong sympathetic system, in effect making these patients even more neurologically unbalanced, more vulnerable to strong or conflicting environmental cues and influences, and more susceptible to worsening illness.

In this, we have both a warning and a guide. Because autonomic imbalance might very well be the basis of much mental illness, both neurosis and psychosis, Gellhorn advised that the therapist always consider the patient's state of autonomic balance. Any effective therapy must, Gellhorn further claimed, aim to bring an out-of-balance autonomic system back into balance. Otherwise, the treatment might very well be doomed to fail, often times, as Funkenstein had learned the hard way, with disastrous results. As Gellhorn (1957, 273) wrote in his usual humble fashion, "It is suggested that psychiatric therapy be directed toward restitution of the normal sympathetic hypothalamic reactivity."

In his book *Emotions and Emotional Disorders* from 1963, Gellhorn included long sections on electro- and insulin shock, how they work, which patients might benefit from their use—and which patients might be harmed by the treatments, all based on his autonomic hypothesis of mental illness. He also had a very unusual chapter titled "Some Contributions of Psychopharmacological Research." During the 1950s, when Gellhorn was bringing so much to fruition in his own thinking, other researchers in other laboratories around the world were beginning the first organized investigations into the biochemical basis of mental illness.

Drug companies had patented and promoted the first generation of antipsychotic and antidepressant medications, such as thorazine, chlorpromazine, and imipramine, during the 1950s and 1960s. Most often, the early antipsychotic drugs were developed for some other intended purpose, and then during clinical trials, an effect on behavior was noted. No one was really quite sure how they worked, though many theories were proposed with great emphasis placed on synaptic neurotransmitters in the brain. No one working in the field of psychopharmacology seems to have paid much attention to Gellhorn and his autonomic thesis.

Gellhorn saw clearly how well his concepts could explain how and why these early drugs might work. For example, chlorpromazine was one of the first of the modern tranquilizing drugs to hit the market, initially intended to calm uncontrolled psychotic patients. Though it had severe side effects, such as sedation, it worked fairly well in some cases and is still used today. Like so many drugs developed at that time, no one was sure, that is, no one outside of Gellhorn's group seemed to know how it worked.

Yet Gellhorn meticulously documented with EEG recordings and other tests that chlorpromazine reduced posterior hypothalamic and sympathetic firing, and in turn upward discharges to the cortex, while at the same time establishing a tranquil state of parasympathetic dominance. It sedated because it blocked the sympathetic system.

As such, it was predictably useful for sympathetic hyperactivity but was potentially disastrous for parasympathetic-dominant patients, who could be pushed into a severe cataclysmic depression by the drug.

Gellhorn described the action of amphetamine as having the opposite effect of tranquilizers such as chlorpromazine on autonomic nerves. Amphetamines, he reported, increased sympathetic activity intensely:

> In contrast to the action of tranquilizers which reduce the responsiveness of the sympathetic system, amphetamine and its derivatives induced increased sympathetic discharges. They lead to a rise in blood pressure and heart rate, vasoconstriction, dilatation of the pupils, dryness of the mouth, etc. The fact that the action of the drug increases activity of the somatic nervous system . . . is apparent from the enhanced motor activity in man and animals and the facilitation of spinal reflexes. The psychological changes observed in normal individuals include a feeling of increased mental alertness, restlessness, and euphoria. . . .
>
> From this description it is obvious that the action of tranquilizers and that of the analeptic [stimulant] drugs exemplified by amphetamine is diametrically opposed. Chlorpromazine lessens the hypothalamic sympathetic responsiveness and relatively large doses elicit catatonic-like effects. In contrast, amphetamine enhances the reactivity of the ergotropic [another word for sympathetic] system at the hypothalamic level. (Gellhorn 1963, 335–36)

The point of all this is that Gellhorn proposed that the observed actions of the tranquilizers, stimulants, antidepressants, and even psychoactive drugs such as LSD result from their direct influence on the hypothalamus and autonomic system. Summing up his thesis, he wrote the following:

> It is suggested that this mechanism is likewise involved in the emotional and mental changes induced by tranquilizers, analeptic and some psychoactive drugs. . . .
>
> The core of this hypothesis lies in the fact that changes in the intensity of the hypothalamic-cortical discharges which are reflected in mood and emotional behavior are determined by the state of the hypothalamus. It is rather immaterial whether the sympathetic division of the hypothalamus is depressed by appropriate changes in the visceral brain, by a diminution of afferent impulses as in our curare experiments, by a lesion in the posterior hypothalamus, by a tranquilizer such as chlorpromazine . . . . In each case the emotional reactivity is diminished. This principle applies also to the relation between increased sympathetic hypothalamic activity and emotional hyper-reactivity. The range of the excitability of the hypothalamus determines that of emotional states. (Gellhorn 1963, 342)

Had the psychiatric profession heeded Dr. Gellhorn's suggestions from 1963—all backed by meticulous data—I believe that so much confusion that persists even today in the field, so many wrong turns, and so much patient suffering might have been prevented. We currently live in what has been billed as the "revolution" in psychopharmacology, particularly with the advent over the past ten years of the selective serotonin reuptake inhibitors (SSRIs) such as Prozac and Paxil. When introduced not too long ago, these drugs were hailed as the answer to many behavioral and psychiatric problems such as depression, anxiety, insomnia, attention deficit disorder, obsessive compulsive behavior, and childhood behavior problems; the list of proposed targets goes on.

I have heard psychiatrists propose, only half-jokingly, that such drugs be put in the water supply because they seem to help with people's basic level of psychological functioning. Unfortunately, though these medications have been extraordinarily useful for millions of patients, and indeed have saved lives as their developers point out, their initial promise has paled considerably. Many patients do not respond well to these drugs, some get significantly worse, and the effect often wears off. We all have read stories of patients who claimed they became psychotic, even violent, while on these drugs. Lawsuits have been filed. Books have been published attacking the enthusiasm with which these drugs have been promoted.

In my own practice, though I treat mainly cancer, I have had patients consult me who have been on half a dozen antidepressants, all of which worked for a time before failing. Patients can become disillusioned and desperate. At times, it seems that doctors are guessing at what drug to use, trying one after another, hoping that one finally sticks.

If nothing else, Gellhorn's research, his model of autonomic physiology, could very precisely guide the use of these drugs and avoid many of the pitfalls that are becoming increasingly evident in their use. Gellhorn forty years ago reported that there really are two types of depression. One is the classic lethargic depression, the deep-seated melancholy associated with exhaustion, hopelessness, a sedated mentation, problems with memory and cognition, feelings of spaciness, grogginess, and slowed thinking. There is also an agitated depression, associated with anger, aggression, and severe insomnia. Patients often feel "dysphoric," meaning not themselves, unable to concentrate, prone to obsessive thinking and rumination.

These two types of depression are not the same. The deep melancholic depression occurs in Funkenstein's Group III parasympathetic dominants. The agitated depressions develop in sympathetic hyper-reactors, Funkenstein's Group I patients. Not only are they different autonomically, physiologically, and biochemically, but they also need to be treated, as you might predict, completely differently.

Serotonin reuptake inhibitors do, at least it seems, exactly that: they block uptake of serotonin into cells, keeping the molecule in the synapse, where it is active. The net result is an increase in serotonin concentration at the nerve endings. This has been perceived to be of great benefit, because in the serotonin hypothesis, behavior problems such as depression, anxiety, and insomnia result from too little serotonin in the brain synapses. It is believed that many severe behavior problems result from such a serotonin deficiency.

Unfortunately, this is an oversimplification. Serotonin, as Gellhorn knew and as researchers today now report, is the ultimate stimulant of parasympathetic activity in areas such as the anterior hypothalamus. It tones down sympathetic activity strongly. Sympathetic-dominant patients, with their correspondingly weak parasympathetic axis, tend to be deficient in serotonin, at times very deficient. For these patients, a serotonin uptake inhibitor can be indeed of great benefit, increasing serotonin levels and in turn parasympathetic activity. Usually, these patients feel very calm and at peace on these drugs, as their autonomic systems come into balance.

For a parasympathetic-dominant patient who already has too much serotonin floating around in the central nervous system, however, such drugs can be a potential disaster, pushing the patient deeper into the hole of parasympathetic activity and depression and disordered thinking. Such patients I believe can become paranoid, psychotic, even violent. These are predictable results, based on their autonomic state.

I have one patient, a very bright individual, who has suffered depression since her twenties. Her well-meaning psychiatrists—and there were a number of them—had diligently tried many different serotonin reuptake inhibitors, each of which had no effect, some of which made her chronic depression worse. Her doctors tried different doses, different combinations, all to no avail. As far as I was concerned when I first met her, she had the classic parasympathetic depression, deeply so, associated with a feeling of spaciness, bone-wrenching fatigue, feeling always as if she were chronically sedated. She said the drugs that had been tried, all of which raise serotonin levels, had made all these symptoms worse.

When we tested her, she did appear to be strongly parasympathetic dominant. Her newest psychiatrist then coincidentally tried her on Imipramine, an old-line antidepressant that raises norepinephrine, not serotonin levels, and stimulates the sympathetic system into action. On this old-fashioned drug, which has fallen out of favor in the psychiatric profession, she enjoyed significant improvement within only several weeks, having spent years failing on the other drugs. She continues doing great.

Over the decades, Gellhorn concentrated much of his energies on uncovering the role of the autonomic system and autonomic imbalance in behavior and mental illness. However, like Dr. Kelley in subsequent years, he begin probing the role of autonomic imbalance and dominance in visceral problems, particularly hypertension and peptic ulcer, two common and often debilitating problems today as well as in Gellhorn's day. In *Emotions and Emotional Disorders* (1963), he had separate chapters devoted specifically to these two problems. Both, he came to believe, must be interpreted as problems in autonomic activity.

In terms of hypertension, Gellhorn suspected that the problem was in the baroreceptors of the carotid sinus and the aortic arch. These two sensory receptors, remember, respond to changes in blood pressure, with high blood pressure activating the receptors and low blood pressure turning them off. When their activity increases, the baroreceptors ultimately, through connections in the brainstem, inhibit the sympathetic system, and when inactivated by low pressure, the sympathetic nerves become uninhibited.

Gellhorn knew that researchers before him had observed that if they surgically removed the baroreceptors in a laboratory animal, the blood pressure would go very high due to the loss of the inhibitory effect. Based on his own laboratory and clinical observations, Gellhorn began to suspect that, in patients suffering hypertension, the baroreceptor set point was too high, meaning they didn't begin their inhibitory round of firing even though the blood pressure might be abnormally elevated. In such patients, the sympathetic tone was chronically too strong, hence explaining chronic hypertension. These were, of course, his sympathetic-dominant patients, who appeared to be very susceptible to hypertension because of their innately strong sympathetic system. Though of course not all sympathetic dominants develop hypertension, it did appear to Gellhorn that in this group the set point for the baroreceptors could easily be pushed higher by environmental stressors, particularly, he claimed, emotional stress.

He reported on a study done by a fellow researcher, in which cats were exposed to barking dogs for a period of several months. Half—though not all, interestingly enough—of the animals developed chronic high blood pressure (Gellhorn 1963, 229). These must have been the sympathetic-dominant cats. Not only did these animals develop hypertension, but microscopic examination of heart tissue showed considerable damage. "These findings," wrote Gellhorn, referring specifically to the barking dog studies, "support the assumption that increased hypothalamic sympathetic discharges may play an important role in the genesis of hypertension."

In another set of studies, some monkeys exposed to neurotic conditioning experiments, specifically involving a shock administered while they ate, developed chronic hypertension:

> From these and other experiments it is inferred that: (1) emotional strains of many kinds produce temporary or permanent increases in blood pressure which may be accompanied by severe cardiovascular changes; (2) not only the intensity and frequency of the emotional excitation but also the individual susceptibility of the animal plays an important part. Genetic differences probably play a major role in this respect. (Gellhorn 1963, 229–30)

Gellhorn described a series of studies with human volunteers that showed importantly how conditioned reflexes could lead to high blood pressure in susceptible patients, that is, sympathetic dominants. Subjects would dip one hand in cold water, an action that immediately caused vasoconstriction along with systemic sympathetic activity and higher blood pressure. This was essentially an unconditioned reflex, a normal response to cold water, that didn't require training. However, if researchers coupled an unconditioned stimulus such as a light or a bell with the water dipping, eventually the light or the bell by itself—without any dipping—would cause sympathetic discharge and elevated blood pressure.

After a period of training, blood pressure would go up in some patients—but again, not all—if they just thought about the light, or the bell! Here we have an illustration of just how influential conditioning can be in our lives. "This suggests," wrote Gellhorn (1963, 231), "that any factor associated with an emotional situation may evoke sympathetic discharges long after the crucial event!"

Clearly, in Gellhorn's model—and later in Kelley's—it was, and is, the sympathetic dominants who are prone to hypertension. Of course, it is a question of both genetics and environmental stressors. A sympathetic-dominant patient living a reasonably quiet life might never have to worry about hypertension. But stress, particularly if prolonged, or conflicting stressful signals put such patients at risk. According to Gellhorn (1963, 235),

> It is believed that emotional excitation leads to increasing sympathetic discharges and a rise in blood pressure. Severity, frequency, and duration of these discharges seem to be related to certain personality traits and to depend on both external circumstances and genetic factors. Both are reflected in sympathetic hypothalamic reactivity and possibly also in the level of tonic sympathetic discharges.

Now, a few words about ulcer disease before we bring our journey through autonomic physiology to a close. Even in my professional lifetime, I have seen remarkable changes in the way physicians and the lay public think about ulcers. When I was in medical school during the early 1980s, we students were taught that ulcer disease was a fairly simple problem of too much acid, or in some cases, a weakened mucosal lining in the stomach or duodenum, where ulcers occur. At the time, there was great enthusiasm among my professors for the then-new generation of anti-ulcer drugs, such as cimetidine, and ranitidine, both of which block stomach acid secretion. Carafate, fairly new on the market in those days, worked in a different way, by coating the stomach with a protective barrier against the deleterious actions of hydrochloric acid.

The problem was, as we learned in the clinics and in practice, that though the drugs worked initially, often the effect lessened with time and the ulcers recurred repeatedly. Drug companies kept researching the problem and kept developing newer and allegedly better types of medications, particularly the proton pump inhibitors such as the currently available Nexium and Prevacid, which specifically block the gastric enzyme used to manufacture hydrochloric acid in the parietal cells of the stomach.

While all this was going on, however, Dr. Barry Marshall, a family practitioner from a small town in Australia, had the audacity during the 1980s to suggest that the great majority of gastric and duodenal ulcers had little to do with acid secretion and everything to do with the presence of the bacteria *Helicobacter pylori*, an organism Dr. Marshall consistently found in the mucosal lining of his ulcer patients. *H. pylori* was well known at the time as a cause of severe gastroenteritis, but no one before Dr. Marshall had linked the bug to ulcers. Dr. Marshall then proposed that the proper treatment for ulcers was not any of the antacid medications, but antibiotics that could knock out *H. pylori*.

In a dramatic demonstration worthy of at least a TV movie, Dr. Marshall drank a hefty dose of the bacteria, allowing himself to develop an ulcer—all documented by endoscopy—and then cured himself with antibiotics. He began administering antibiotics regularly to his ulcer patients, with apparent success, a result that only brought on the venom and hostility of the gastroenterologists of the world. Marshall was initially branded as falling somewhere between a quack and a pure psychopath, but he refused to give up this theory.

JP Jones, PhD, a chemist by training and, before his retirement at the young age of fifty-seven, vice president in charge of health care research at Proctor and Gamble, somehow heard of Dr. Marshall and subsequently got P&G to finance Marshall's controversial research. P&G even brought Dr. Marshall to the United States, to a safe professorship in Virginia where he could continue his research in some degree of peace. JP, who has long been a strong supporter of my own research and a close friend, has over the years related some harrowing adventures that occurred during his association with Dr. Marshall. At one medical gastroenterology conference in the early 1990s, when, through the prestige of P&G, Dr. Marshall was allowed to present his work, JP feared for Marshall's safety, so great was the hostility to the *H. pylori* hypothesis. Dr. Marshall, with the help of P&G, did ultimately prevail, so much so that antibiotic treatment has become a standard approach to ulcer disease. Dr. Marshall has since returned to Australia, now respected as a medical pioneer and medical-cultural hero.

Unfortunately, again, the situation doesn't appear to be that simple. While many ulcer patients do respond to the antibiotic regimen, many don't, and even if they do, often the ulcers recur. Furthermore, it turns out, as we now have learned, *H. pylori* is not necessarily an insidious demon-germ, but instead a member in most of us of the normal bacterial flora of the gut, where it might have a useful purpose. It seems that H. p*ylori* may protect against esophageal cancer, because we are starting to see higher rates of this aggressive cancer in patients in whom this type of bacteria has been eradicated. Currently, while antibiotics are still commonly used to treat ulcers, often acid-blocking medications are given at the same time. Though in no way do I wish to diminish Dr. Marshall's truly heroic struggles, nor in any way minimize his achievements, so much for simple answers.

Which brings me back to Pavlov and Dr. Gellhorn. It was Pavlov who at the turn of the nineteenth century had shown that the vagus nerve was largely responsible for acid secretion in the stomach. This had been confirmed repeatedly, and by Gellhorn's day it was known that acid production was indeed a parasympathetic function. If hypertension was to him a problem of an overactive sympathetic system, then ulcers in the Gellhorn universe were clearly a problem of vagotonia, heightened parasympathetic tone, and chronically increased acid production.

In support of this, by the 1950s, researchers had carefully demonstrated that ulcer patients tended to produce considerably more hydrochloric acid than "normals" did. In his chapter on the disease, Dr. Gellhorn (1963, 236–37) described a large-scale study showing that nighttime secretion of acid was four to twenty times greater in ulcer patients. When in one group of patients surgeons simply cut the vagus nerves to the stomach, hence reducing stomach acid production, "90% of more than 1000 cases of duodenal ulcers" enjoyed what appeared to be a cure, with documented healing of the lesions.

As with mental illness, and as with hypertension, Gellhorn proposed that ulcer disease resulted from a combination of hereditary and environmental stresses. The hereditary component would be a dominant parasympathetic system and with it a tendency to hypersecretion of stomach acid. The environmental part included any number of environmental influences, particularly those producing emotional stress. Such stimuli might lead to negative unconditioned reflexes in these vagotonic individuals, reflexes that further increased acid production.

Gellhorn cited a number of studies that demonstrated how negative conditioning with conflicting stimuli could lead to ulcer disease:

> Moreover, experiments on rats in situations arousing fear and conflicts led to the formation of ulcers. In these experiments the animals were kept in a box provided with a grid adjacent to the food and water supply. The grid was electrically charged for 47 out of 48 hours. Consequently, attempts to secure food or water were punished with pain. The experimental animals developed ulcers and some died from gastrointestinal hemorrhages but control animals kept without food and water for 47 out of 48 hours remained normal. "In experimental human subjects and patients emotional stresses increased acid secretion. This was found in students during the examination period, and in patients in whom anxiety, anger, or resentment were elicited by an interview. . . .
>
> The experiments imply that numerous factors associated with an emotion arousing situation may through conditioning increase acid secretion for prolonged periods of time and thereby contribute to the development of peptic ulcers. . . . These data suggest that the anterior hypothalamus, which largely controls parasympathetic reactions that occur on an emotional basis, may be in a state of heightened excitability in the ulcer patient, and recent investigations seem, indeed, to show that such patients are "vagotonic." (Gellhorn 1963, 238)

Forty years later, I suspect that Gellhorn was right. Parasympathetic-dominant patients, already prone to acid hypersecretion, under prolonged environmental stress of any type, could easily produce too much acid. Ulcers then follow. Perhaps these stressed-out parasympathetic-dominant patients are also susceptible to *H. pylori* infection in the stomach. I don't know if this is true, but it warrants some thought. Regardless, though theories about ulcer causation come and go, and treatment regimens come and go as quickly, perhaps it is time to reconsider Gellhorn's hypothesis.

Dr. Gellhorn clearly considered mental illness, hypertension, and ulcer disease as problems, fundamentally, in autonomic function. Throughout his writings, he makes his case strongly and thoroughly, his arguments always backed by careful experimental and clinical documentation. Though he never discussed the relationship of autonomic imbalance to other diseases, such as cancer for example, he suggests in his writings that many illnesses might have as their cause imbalance in autonomic physiology. He proposes this scenario in *Emotions and Emotional Disorders* at the conclusion of the chapter on ulcers. He just didn't, I suppose, have the time to look further.

One final point: At some point in their autonomic education, all students of physiology learn, as I have myself learned, that the sympathetic system is the classic "stress system," or the "fight or flight system," the system we supposedly rely on when confronted with any type of physical, emotional, or psychological stress. The parasympathetic system, on the other hand is, as I have myself stated and implied, more the workhorse of the body, involved in maintaining the basic metabolic functions of digestion, assimilation of nutrients, excretion of wastes, etc.

Well, as you've probably surmised, these traditional caveats are only half right. Gellhorn, in his long career, really showed us that our response to stress depends largely if not entirely on our state of autonomic balance—or imbalance. If you are a sympathetic-dominant individual facing some sort of difficult situation, indeed, your sympathetic system will turn on more strongly, and—due to the law of reciprocity—the parasympathetic nerves will turn off. However, if you are genetically or functionally in a state of parasympathetic dominance, under stress your parasympathetic nerves rev up and the sympathetic system will become not more but less active. In this case, the "stress fight or flight" sympathetic system does very little.

That's why, if life is chronically tough, sympathetic "hyper-reactors," to use Dr. Funkenstein's words, become angry and develop high blood pressure, while parasympathetic hyper-reactors dealing with the same pressures fall into depression and form ulcers. Their reactions to an identical stressful situation, just like the reactions of Pavlov's Type I and Type IV dogs, will be completely different.

Of course, I haven't yet mentioned those balanced people among us, with equally strong sympathetic and parasympathetic nerves. In these people, under stress, both systems turn on, but mildly, neither to excess. The responses are in turn mild, controlled, and usually appropriate for the difficulty, whatever it might be.

We've come a long way, through what I see as wonderful neurophysiology that explains so much about our lives, who we are, and why we behave the way we do. So when I hear my critics proclaim, sometimes very loudly, that "there is no scientific basis" for what we do in our office, I would laugh if their ignorance weren't so sad. It's sad not for any egocentric reason, or because I am thin skinned. It's sad to me because today

Gellhorn seems to have been completely forgotten. In my contemporary textbooks of autonomic physiology, I find no mention of his name, no reference to his work.

It's not that he was ever discredited; that never happened, and in his own time he seems to have been highly regarded among those working in his field. His scientific accomplishments stand the test of time. His experimentation appears to have been impeccable, his references accurately quoted. Like Dr. Beard before him, he was in his lifetime largely ignored by the medical and psychiatric community and is now unknown.

When I called the department of physiology at Minnesota to try to get some background information on Gellhorn, no one there, not even the head of the department, knew who he was. A very helpful librarian in the university archives finally found a biography of him in the records, actually an obituary in the university files written in his honor at the time of his death. However, no one today was familiar with him or with his great contributions.

Even Dr. Kelley, always open as he was to new ideas and certainly open to support for what he claimed, never once in the years that I worked with him mentioned Gellhorn, nor did I ever see copies of Gellhorn's books in Kelley's extensive library. Dr. Kelley did frequently refer to Beard and to Pottenger, and I did see the books of both men in his home, well marked and clearly well read. He just didn't seem to be aware that only a decade earlier, the superb academician Dr. Gellhorn had carefully laid out the details of autonomic dominance and autonomic imbalance and, in essence, had already explained what Kelley was to observe in his humble Texas dental office.

Postscript

As you may have noticed, this book comes to a rather abrupt end, just as Dr. Gonzalez's life came to an abrupt and unexpected end on July 21, 2015. It is fitting, in a way, that the book and the life follow a parallel process. Dr. Gonzalez had much work yet to do, with his patients, his writing, and his teaching, and with developing and teaching his model. Because that life's work was so suddenly brought to an end, others are now striving to ensure that his legacy survives and is transmitted to others who can carry the work forward.

The present volume is an essential part of the foundation for that future-oriented project, along with volumes 1 and 2 of *Conquering Cancer* (volume 2 to be published in 2017). Combined with books and papers published during his lifetime, these three volumes place the work solidly in the mainstream of scientific medicine. Of course, this doesn't mean that mainstream medicine will accept The Gonzalez Protocol any time soon. As with any new model or theory in any field of science or medicine, there is resistance and delay before the new way of looking at things is accepted and, eventually, becomes part of regular, normal science.

Before reading and lightly editing the manuscript, I was aware of the nutritional types derived from the work of William Donald Kelley, and the vitamins and minerals required as supplements for each of them. I was also aware of the theory of sympathetic-dominant, parasympathetic-dominant, and balanced metabolizers. But I didn't really understand where all of this came from. Now I do.

Similarly, with the technical aspects of pancreatic enzyme preparation, I knew that Dr. Gonzalez did quite a lot of work getting this ironed out, but I didn't grasp how technical and detailed his efforts were. I did nine months of immunology research in medical school and published two papers in immunology journals, one as first author. During that time, I acquired a pretty good grasp of how technical basic lab research can be and how much time, effort, and creativity go into solving technical problems. I listened to lectures by visiting professors describing their ingenious solutions to technical problems in biochemistry, virology, immunology, and related fields.

In my opinion, Dr. Gonzalez was a scientific student of the technical processes involved in enzyme preparation at the intellectual level of a university professor. This fact is one more piece of evidence that Dr. Gonzalez was not a quack or a fringe practitioner. He was a scholar, a scientist, and a clinician.

Clearly, not all of the details of The Gonzalez Protocol are scientifically proven to be valid. However, to be scientific, a theory does not have to be proven or even correct. Once proven correct, the theory becomes a fact and is no longer a theory. In the present day, no one says that bacteria causing pneumonia is a theory; it is a fact. But not that long ago, even the concept of a bacterium was a disputed theory. The Gonzalez Protocol is grounded in science and is formulated in a manner that makes it a scientifically testable theory.

The two volumes of *Conquering Cancer* provide conclusive evidence that The Gonzalez Protocol can be amazingly effective for biopsy and MRI-confirmed advanced and otherwise lethal cancers. This doesn't mean that every detail of the protocol is necessarily correct, indispensable, or immutable. But it does mean that the protocol should be taken seriously by mainstream medicine. More evidence is required, including prospective clinical trials, animal studies, and in vitro studies. However, there is now sufficient evidence of the effectiveness of the protocol, and of its scientific foundations, for it to be taken seriously by academia, organized medicine, and grant agencies. The treatment of cancer with pancreatic enzymes, combined with nutritional support, should be an option for patients to consider within mainstream medicine.

Colin A. Ross, MD

About the Author

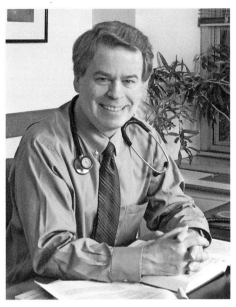

Nicholas James Gonzalez, MD, age sixty-seven, passed away suddenly at his home in New York City with his wife, Mary Beth, at his side. Born in Flushing, New York, he graduated from Brown University, Phi Beta Kappa, magna cum laude, with a degree in English literature. He subsequently worked as a journalist, first at Time, Inc., before pursuing premedical studies at Columbia. He then received his medical degree from Cornell University Medical College in 1983. During a postgraduate immunology fellowship under Dr. Robert A. Good, considered the father of immunology, he completed a research study evaluating an aggressive nutritional therapy in the treatment of advanced cancer.

Dr. Gonzalez had been in private practice in New York City since 1987, treating patients diagnosed with cancer and other serious degenerative illnesses. His nutritional research received substantial financial support from Proctor and Gamble and Nestlé. Results from a pilot study published in 1999 described the most positive data in the medical literature for pancreatic cancer.

Dr. Gonzalez is the author of several books published by New Spring Press:
- *The Trophoblast and the Origins of Cancer*
- *One Man Alone: An Investigation of Nutrition, Cancer and Dr. William Donald Kelley*
- *The Enzyme Treatment of Cancer and Its Scientific Basis* by Dr. John Beard, foreword by Dr. Gonzalez
- *What Went Wrong: The Truth behind the Clinical Trial of the Enzyme Treatment of Cancer* (Independent Book Publishers Association 2013 Silver Award Winner)
- *Conquering Cancer: Volume One—50 Pancreatic and Breast Cancer Patients on The Gonzalez Nutritional Protocol*

Dr. Nicholas Gonzalez leaves a legacy of faith, healing, and genuine love for the truth, people, and the pursuit of medicine. For more information about Dr. Gonzalez and The Gonzalez Protocol, visit The Nicholas Gonzalez Foundation website at www.thegonzalezprotocol.com.

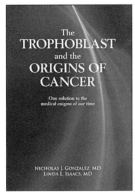 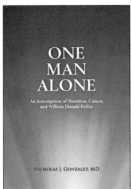 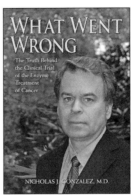 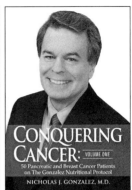

Dr. Gonzalez's books have provided both a theory about cancer and the scientific evidence. In *The Trophoblast and the Origins of Cancer*, Dr. Gonzalez reveals Dr. John Beard's theory for the likely origin of cancer and his pioneering use of pancreatic enzymes for cancer treatment. In *One Man Alone*, Dr. Gonzalez summarizes his assessment of Dr. William Donald Kelley's fifty patients and their remarkable recoveries. Then, in *Conquering Cancer: Volume One—50 Pancreatic and Breast Cancer Patients on the Gonzalez Nutritional Protocol*, Dr. Gonzalez details the evidence through his own cancer patient case reports. *Conquering Cancer: Volume Two* will be released in 2017.

Together, these revolutionary books answer the question of which alternative therapy is most effective in treating and reversing cancer. Cancer patients and their families throughout the world owe it to themselves to demand increased access to the appropriate pancreatic enzymes and The Gonzalez Protocol to reduce the severity and incidence of cancer. The solution to cancer is here, and you can recommend these books to those who do not believe it.

For more information, visit
The Nicholas Gonzalez Foundation website at www.dr-gonzalez.com.